"I predict **Health Basics** will be the standard medical reference for most Americans."

—Harry A. Nurkin, Ph.D.,
Past President and Chief Executive, Carolinas Health Care System

"A carefully comprehensive, well written and understandably practical guide to help explain bodily ills, function and how to stay healthy, and how modern medicine might contribute toward this end."

—James A. Bryan II, M.D., M.P.H.,
Professor Medicine, University of North Carolina School of Medicine

"It is refreshing to read such a clear and focused book that can be a great guide for those interested in learning more about how to keep their bodies healthy."

—Bradley Evanoff, M.D., M.P.H.,
Associate Professor of Medicine, Chief Division of General Medical Sciences,
Washington University in St. Louis, School of Medicine

"Dr. Richardson's new book not only covers the human body from head to heel, but does so in a way most non-clinicians can grasp and apply in their personal quests for healthy living. My hat is off to Dr. Richardson for an excellent and timely book."

—Peter S. Anderson, President,
Carolinas Physicians Network, Inc., Carolinas Health Care System

"He had produced an easy-to-read guide that breaks through medical-ese to speak to the average reader. Anyone with half an interest in his or her own well being should have a well-thumbed copy at home.

—Merry Tipton, Vice President,
Corporate Communications, Sea Island Company

"Dr. Richardson has succeeded where many others have failed in providing up to date medical information on topics of interest to everyone, in a manner that conveys depth but is easy to read. His answers to commonly asked questions are right on target."

—Marschall Runge, M.D., Ph.D.,
Marion Covington Distinguished Professor of Medicine,
Chairman, Department of Medicine, The University of North Carolina School of Medicine

"Dr. Richardson has provided a terrific service to the intelligent public interested in their own health."

—Carolyn E. Hart, President,
Mecklenburg Medical Society

i

HEALTH BASICS

*A Doctor's Plainspoken Advice
About How Your Body Works
and What to Do When it Doesn't*

By

Michael S. Richardson, M.D.

*Physician, Charlotte Medical Clinic,
Carolinas Physicians Network*

*Clinical Associate Professor of Medicine
The University of North Carolina School of Medicine
at Chapel Hill*

Published by

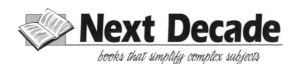

Next Decade
books that simplify complex subjects

Health Basics
A Doctor's Plainspoken Advice About How Your Body Works
and What to Do When it Doesn't

Published by:
Next Decade, Inc.
39 Old Farmstead Road
Chester, New Jersey 07930-2732 USA
www.nextdecade.com
email: info@nextdecade.com

Book cover and interior design:
Sherry Stinson, The Printed Image, Bartlesville, OK.

Library of Congress Cataloging-in-Publication Data

Richardson, Michael S., 1960-
  Health basics : a doctor's plainspoken advice about how your body
works and what to do when it doesn't / by Michael S. Richardson.
      p. cm.
Includes index.
   ISBN 0-9700908-5-4
  1. Medicine, Popular. 2. Health. I. Title.
   RC81 .R55 2003
   616—dc21
                                        2002015194

$22.95 Softcover

Dedication

This book is dedicated to four individuals as representatives of hundreds of educators who have influenced the development of my thoughts and helped to reasonably direct my actions and ambitions over the years:

Mrs. Lynn H. Roberts, my 5th grade science teacher in Hendersonville, North Carolina, who first instilled in me a passion for the Life Sciences and awakened a consciousness of my self and the world around me.

Mr. Peter Iver Kaufman, a professor of religious studies at the University of North Carolina, Chapel Hill, who taught me to be aware of how I know what I think I know, and to question whether my hidden assumptions are correct.

Dr. Phillip A. Sellers, an internist in Hendersonville, North Carolina, who showed me how to successfully balance the practice of medicine with life and family.

Dr. Clay W. Richardson, a family doctor in rural North Carolina, a role model and hero, my friend and brother.

A heartfelt thanks.

Foreword

My grandfather was a country doctor. Dr. Flave Hart Corpening was born the seventh of seven children in the mountains of western North Carolina in 1902. He was raised in the Brevard area, graduated from N.C. State University in Raleigh, and then returned to Brevard to teach mathematics. He eventually made his way to Jefferson Medical School in Pennsylvania and, upon completing his studies, originally practiced in New Jersey. When the health of his brother-in-law, a physician, failed, Dr. Corpening moved back to North Carolina to take over the family practice. At the age of 37, he settled with his family in rural Mills River, North Carolina where he practiced medicine for 14 years until his death at age 51 of Amyotrophic Lateral Sclerosis. I never met my grandfather, but through the stories about him I feel a family and professional kinship with him.

Dr. Corpening built his office next to his home. My mother recalls the small and always crowded waiting room, with two examination rooms and an office in the back. A single assistant helped patients, bartered doctor's fees for canned goods and poultry, and assisted with surgeries and autopsies. The dispensing pharmacy was essentially a closet lined with large brown glass bottles, each filled with pills that were ceremoniously doled out in white paper sacks at the end of each consultation. Smaller versions of these bottles were lined up in his black bag, accompanying him on frequent trips into the hills and backcountry surrounding Mills River. Mom remembers the pungent chemical air of the dispensary to this day.

When my mother returned to visit the area in the late 1990s, she was approached by a woman in a diner who recognized her as Dr. Corpening's daughter. "Your father delivered me and then saved my life!" she exclaimed. She then told the story of when she was rushed to Dr. Corpening's office as a very sick infant at three weeks of age. After examining her, Dr. Corpening immediately closed the office and drove mother and infant across the mountains to the nearest hospital in Asheville, where against rather formidable odds she survived.

It is through this and similar stories, as well as through eulogies recorded at his funeral, that my grandfather taught me about being a physician. The best physicians are both scientists and humanitarians—passionate in their craft and compassionate with their patients. They understand the foundations of their knowledge and the limits to which it can be extended. They integrate the physical, psychological, social, and spiritual aspects of health and disease. As their level of knowledge and experience grows, so does their humility in their lack of understanding and influence over life and health.

The science of medicine has seen tremendous advances since my grandfather's practice 50 years ago. The understanding of how the body functions and what goes wrong in disease continues to grow exponentially. Many strong mentors, as well as excellent training, helped me develop my medical skills; computer programs and Internet resources help keep them sharp. Laboratory tests and imaging studies are readily available to help me probe every recess of the body, as is immediate access to specialists when my own knowledge is insufficient.

Other changes have also occurred. Patients' expectations are different. In my grandfather's day, a farmer sought enough relief of his knee pain to allow him to continue to work and support his family. My patients expect their knee injuries to heal immediately and completely so that they can get back to their 10K races and step aerobics. My grandfather was pretty much a solo act; I work in a group of 30 physicians owned by a "Health System." My grandfather traded services for ham; our group includes several individuals whose only responsibility is to help us negotiate through the maze of managed care reimbursement.

My challenge in trying to live up to my grandfather's standards and expectations is to strive to use the knowledge and tools that I am blessed with to provide compassionate medical care. To orchestrate these resources, I command not to simply seek out and cure disease but to address the human needs of my patients. I have come to realize that I can have the greatest impact by educating my patients. The more people know about how their body functions, and how things go wrong, the better they are able to assist their doctor in helping them. My goal in writing this book is to provide a reasonable understanding—in everyday language—of how the body functions, what happens in sickness, and how to optimize your chances for good health.

My apologies in advance for writing a book that will start becoming out of date the moment I put down my pen. Other than certain basic guidelines (eat right, drink lots of water, get plenty of exercise and sleep, love someone and be loved), most of modern Medicine is subject to constant fluctuation and is based on theories and reasoning that may be brought into question with the next published journal article.

In Medicine, there is little truly absolute knowledge about anything. Our understanding of how the body works and what goes wrong in disease are fluid and continually refined. Our knowledge is constantly expanding; as the biochemical basis and molecular genetics of health and disease unfold for us, fundamental changes in Medicine have and will continue to occur.

Let's look at a couple of examples of how we view conditions differently as we learn more about them:

- **Peptic Ulcer Disease:** Ten years ago, most physicians were taught to believe that ulcers of the stomach and duodenum were caused by excessive acid. It was felt that acid ate away at the lining of the stomach—forming a crater—and treatment of the resulting ulcer required correction of the "acid problem" with diet and medications. Most patients with ulcers developed more ulcers over time and were either treated again or placed on long-term medication to "control the acid."

  Researchers identified the real culprit, a 3-millimeter bacterium called Helicobacter pylori, in 1983. A series of articles beginning in 1991 provided evidence that H. pylori was related to ulcers and that treatment helped prevent ulcers from returning, eliminating the need for costly ongoing therapy in most patients. Despite this convincing evidence, the excessive acid theory was so deeply believed that it was years before H. pylori was widely accepted as responsible for most ulcers and the approach to ulcer treatment changed.

- **Atherosclerosis:** We believed that atherosclerosis (hardening of the arteries) was a progressive process where hard cholesterol plaques developed in the wall of an artery, slowly blocking it up like a clogged septic drainage line. When the blockage became severe enough to choke off flow through the vessel, patients developed chest pain or had heart attacks. Because this was felt to be a slowly progressive process, patients without symptoms of heart disease underwent periodic exercise stress tests to try to detect these plumbing problems in time to prevent damage. (A blockage of 70 percent or above is required to affect flow rates through a tube such as a blood vessel, and when the heart can't get enough blood supplied to it through highly blocked coronary arteries, the heart muscle experiences changes that show up on an exercise stress test.)

  However, recent studies show that 90 percent of heart attacks occur in areas of cholesterol plaque blocking only 30 to 55 percent of the vessel—not enough to significantly reduce blood flow. We are now developing an understanding of the dynamic nature of a cholesterol plaque and why soft, smaller plaques rupture, causing blood clots to form on them, which blocks the vessel completely and results in a heart attack. This has led to major advances in new therapies for heart disease and prompts us to question the whole premise of screening stress tests, since they typically do not detect these subcritical blockages. How do we detect heart disease early, then? Doctors are not sure.

Medicine has evolved over time. We will continue to learn new information and develop better ways to understand health and disease. However, my challenge lies in the fact that my patients can't wait to see what the next insights into health and disease will show us; they are having problems and seeking assistance now. I also realize that the information I have about each patient is incomplete. I might not ask that one crucial question about a subject that they didn't feel was related to their current problem. The tests and procedures I ask my patients to submit to give me likelihoods and probabilities, often not yes or no answers. Yet hourly I, as any physician, must make tough decisions amid incomplete, changing, and at times contradictory information. It is a daunting task.

The purpose of this book is to educate you, the patient, about how your body works and what goes wrong in disease. The greater your own understanding of the concepts reviewed in this book, the better you will be able to assist your physician in understanding your symptoms and optimizing your personal health.

This book provides a basic understanding of the functioning of an adult body and how diseases—as we understand them today—interfere with these functions. It covers common medical issues I have experienced in a primary care office; more unusual or exotic illnesses are beyond the scope of the book. In addition, the medical issues I discuss pertain only to adults. I have no experience in doctoring children other than my own, and I would not advise readers to attempt to apply the concepts in this book to children.

The initial sections of this book discuss general but crucial topics in health, including sound nutrition and exercise. I then present a medical view of the benefits and risks of Alternative Medicine, including a review of common supplements. This is followed by a basic look into how I practice preventative care. I close the first section with suggestions on how to get the most out of your medical providers; that is, how to help your doctor best help you.

The second part of this book discusses specific body systems and the problems that occur with them. These chapters are not meant to be comprehensive, but they do cover most of the common problems that my patients and I have encountered over the past decade of our practice together.

Good health.
Mike Richardson, M.D.

Disclaimer

The purpose of this book is to provide interested individuals with a general understanding of how your body works. It is presented with the understanding that the publisher and author are not engaged in rendering medical advice or other professional services in this book, and that without personal consultation the author cannot and does not render advice or judgment about a specific patient or medical condition. When medical or other expert assistance is required, the services of a competent professional should be sought.

Health Basics was not written to provide all the information that is available to the author/and or publisher, but to complement, amplify and supplement other texts and available information. While every effort has been made to ensure that this book is as complete and accurate as possible, there may be mistakes, either typographical or in content. Therefore, this text should be used as a general guide only, and not as an ultimate source of health information. Furthermore, this book contains current information only up to the printing date.

Information herein was obtained from various sources whose accuracy is not guaranteed. Opinions expressed and information are subject to change without notice.

The author, editor, and Next Decade, Inc. shall not be held liable, nor be responsible to any person or entity with respect to any loss or damage caused, or alleged to be caused, directly or indirectly by the information contained in this book.

If you do not wish to be bound by the above, you may return this book to the publisher for a full refund.

Table of Contents

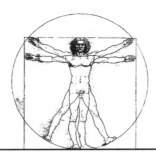

PART I

Staying Healthy

In Part I, we talk about general but crucial topics in health, including exercise, a healthy diet, and how the body reacts to allergens, antibiotics, pain, tobacco, and alcohol.

Part I also discusses screening techniques for common types of cancer, how vaccines work, how to stay healthy while traveling, the benefits and risks of dietary and nutritional supplements, and how to get the most from your office visits.

CHAPTER 1

Physical Fitness

Exercise—if I had to choose one thing I would like to be more successful at, it would be in motivating my patients to exercise. Everyone has heard that being active is the right thing to do. Exercise helps keep your body healthy, it releases stress and tension, and it helps develop and maintain a positive self-image. Active people live longer and remain more independent as they get older. Exercise enhances the quality of life. Yet, only one-fourth of the adult population in the United States exercises regularly.

From the doctor's stool, it is usually obvious when a patient exercises regularly and when they do not. Most men can get away without a good health program until about 35 before I start to see the differences. In women, the changes don't often seem as obvious to me until about 40. Patients who exercise regularly simply look and feel better. I see them much less often for nuisance complaints such as minor upper respiratory infections, generalized aches and pains, chronic fatigue, or sleep disturbance. Contrary to what you may expect, patients who exercise seem to come in less often with joint pain and other musculoskeletal complaints. Stronger muscles function as shock absorbers, cushioning the day-to-day stresses on joints. Those who exercise regularly develop better balance, strength, and coordination and are able to protect themselves from injury when life throws a curve. My patients have no difficulty understanding the need for a financial plan for their retirement years and they invest and save most of their adult lives. A regular exercise program is an investment in your body for the future, and should be pursued with the same commitment as financial investment. Just as those individuals who do not save for retirement will experience financial difficulties, a 60-year-old man who has been sitting in his recliner for 30 years cannot expect the same vigor in health as his counterpart who has been going to the gym regularly.

What medical evidence proves that exercise is a healthy thing to do? Several well-controlled medical studies bear this notion out.

- **Exercise and the immune system.** Studies at Appalachian State University in North Carolina show that specialized white blood cells called Natural Killer Cells, a first line in the body's immune defense, are 54 percent more active in fit older women than in their sedentary peers. Surveys consistently show that people who exercise vigorously, but not to the point of exhaustion, get sick less often. In one study of 91 women, half of the women were randomly assigned to walk briskly for 45 minutes a day, five days a week. This study showed that the exercise group had half as many sick days in the follow-up period as the sedentary group.

- **Exercise and cancer.** More than ten large observational studies show a reduction in cancer death rates in those who exercise regularly. The immune system is responsible for identifying and eliminating cells that have mutated before they can turn cancerous. In theory, exercise benefits to the immune system should help in cancer prevention. In a study of 25,000 people followed by the Cooper Clinic in Dallas, total cancer mortality was 80 percent lower in the most physically fit individuals. Why? Colon cancer may diminish because exercise speeds up the passage of waste and toxins through the colon, reducing the exposure of the lining of the colon to possible cancer-inducing substances. Exercise inhibits the release of pituitary hormones that trigger estrogen release, possibly reducing the risk of estrogen-related breast cancer. Exercise reduces total body fat, which is a second source of estrogen. Exercise also reduces levels of testosterone, which is known to fuel the growth of prostate cancer.
- **Exercise and diabetes.** In a study reported in *The Journal of the American Medical Association*, 70,000 women were followed over 8 years. Of these women, 1,419 developed Type II diabetes during the study period. Women who exercised at least 30 minutes 5 days each week reduced their risk of developing diabetes by 41 percent. This reduction in risk correlated directly with the intensity of exercise, showing a 30 percent reduction in diabetes in women who routinely walked from two to three miles per hour and a 60 percent reduction in women who walked at a faster pace.
- **Exercise and heart disease.** Patients who have had one heart attack and then begin a regular exercise program are less likely to develop a second heart attack. Many insurance companies pay for cardiac rehabilitation programs because of this data. Exercise improves cholesterol profiles by raising the healthy HDL cholesterol subcomponent and lowering total cholesterol and triglycerides. Exercise beneficially affects the level of Interleukin-1, which makes arteries narrow, and Interleukin-2, which helps keep arteries open and clog free. 40-year-old males placed on a regular exercise program experienced a 60 percent reduction in Interleukin-1 levels and a 35 percent rise in Interleukin-2 levels. In another study reported in *Circulation* in 1999, walking more than 1.5 miles a day cut the risk of developing heart disease by 50 percent. In the Nurses Health Study, briskly walking three hours per week cut cardiac events in women by 35 percent.
- **Exercise and gallbladder.** The Nurses Health Study, which involved 60,000 women, showed that the more a woman exercised, the lower her risk was for gallbladder surgery. A 20 percent reduction in gallbladder surgery was noted in women who exercise at least 30 minutes, 5 days each week. A Harvard study of 45,000 males showed that physically active men were 25 percent less likely to have gallbladder symptoms.
- **Exercise and osteoporosis.** Regular, weight-bearing exercise builds healthy bone. In a study of 10,000 women over age 65 at the University of California in San Francisco, the risk of hip fracture was much lower in active versus sedentary women.

Exercise was found to build bone density and enhance balance and coordination. Being physically fit reduced the risk of falling and improved the ability of women to protect themselves from injury in a fall.

- **Exercise and the brain.** In a study reported in *Nature*, 120 sedentary older adults gradually worked up to a brisk 45 to 60 minute walk, 3 days each week. A similar number of individuals in the control group spent an equal amount of time toning and stretching, but not aerobically exercising. After six months, the exercise group achieved a 20 percent improvement in tests that measured mental abilities including the ability to switch rapidly from one task to another. These physically fit, older adults were found to be as mentally agile as unfit younger adults in their 30s.

- **Exercise and death.** In 1998, a study of 25,000 men examined what lifestyle factors could most closely predict the risk of premature death from any cause in subsequent years. Low physical fitness scores were more highly correlated with premature death than any other factor, including cigarette smoking, hypertension, elevated cholesterol, and obesity.

Are you convinced? I am.

Goals for an Exercise Program

You should start your exercise program with the following goals in mind:

- **Improving cardiovascular endurance and aerobic fitness.** This type of exercise seeks to boost the ability of the heart and lungs to supply muscles with oxygen. It requires a minimum of 30 minutes of sustained activity at your target heart rate, either continuously or in three 10-minute chunks.

You calculate your target heart rate using a combination of your age and fitness level, as follows:

1. Calculate your *predicted maximum heart rate* by subtracting your age from 220.
2. Use the following chart to determine your *target heart rate* (that is, based on your fitness level, the heart rate you should aim to maintain throughout your exercise session).

If you are...	Start with a heart rate goal of...
Just beginning an exercise program	55% of your predicted maximum heart rate
In fairly good shape and striving to improve physical conditioning and burn fat (that is, you have been exercising 3 to 5 days a week for the past 4 weeks)	65% of your predicted maximum heart rate
In good shape and striving to boost aerobic capacity (you know all the regulars on a first name basis and consider the exercise equipment in the gym as your personal property)	75% of your predicted maximum heart rate

For example, a 40-year-old person who is just starting an exercise program should try to sustain a maximum heart rate of 99 throughout his or her exercise session (subtracting 40 from 220 equals 180; multiplying 180 by .55 equals 99). After the first month of injury-free exercise, the heart rate target can be increased to 117 (65 percent of predicted maximum heart rate).

Avoid exercise that pushes the sustained heart rate greater than 90 percent of predicted maximum.

Find Your Target Heart Rate
1. Subtract your age from 220.
2. Multiply the result by the fitness percentage indicated in the table on page 5.

- **Building muscular strength.** After age 30, there is a natural and continuous decline in the amount of muscle tissue. Lifting weights can help preserve muscular strength and endurance. Strengthening exercises build bone and fight osteoporosis. Weight-lifting programs have proven to reduce the risk of fall and injury in elderly patients.
- **Building and maintaining flexibility.** Stretching and other flexibility exercises increase the active range of motion of joints and prevent injury.
- **Improving body composition.** Regular aerobic and strengthening exercises increase lean body mass and reduce fat. Muscle requires more energy, both at rest and during exercise, resulting in a body that burns calories faster. A leaner body reduces the risk for diabetes, hypertension, cholesterol disorders, heart disease, and cancer.
- **Improving the mind.** In addition to the proven cognitive benefits of better mental performance in elderly patients who exercise, regular exercise helps with stress reduction, alleviates depression and anxiety, and helps develop self-confidence and a sense of well-being. Those who exercise regularly report a higher general quality of life. Physical exercise is a great temporary diversion from the cares of the day.

Exercising Safely

Following are some tips for staying safe while you exercise:

- **Get your doctor's approval.** If you are over age 45, get a medical checkup before you begin a new exercise program.
- **Warm those muscles.** Warm up five to ten minutes by walking, light jogging, or biking. If you are an early morning exerciser, extend your warm-up time. Muscles are stiffest in the early morning after the prolonged inactivity of bed rest.
- **Stretch.** Flexibility is crucial for a healthy body. Don't confuse stretching with warming up; muscles must already be warm to stretch properly. Stretch each muscle

group to the point of tension, not pain. Do not bounce your stretches; this increases the risk of tendon strain or muscular tear. Hold each stretch for 10 to 30 seconds.

- **Cool down after exercise.** After the strenuous part of your workout, continue exercising lightly until your heart rate returns to near normal. This helps continue to supply your muscles with extra blood and prevents lactic acid build-up from exercise, reducing muscular soreness. Stretch again after cooling down.

- **Stay adequately hydrated.** Most individuals do not drink enough fluid during exercise. A good rule of thumb is to drink 8 ounces of water immediately before exercise, 4 ounces of water every 20 minutes during exercise, and 8 ounces of water afterwards.

- **Listen to your body.** Tenderness and pain are warning signals of greater problems and should prompt you to adjust your exercise program. Muscle pain and soreness may signal excessive stress from a workout, indicating that you should be cautious with the intensity of your efforts. Pain at a joint surface is more serious; you should immediately reevaluate your exercise efforts and—for persistent pain—seek medical evaluation.

- **Wear appropriate footwear.** In addition to the exercise surface that you choose, your footwear is a primary means of absorbing shock and protecting your joints. In those who exercise regularly, the shock absorbing features of their shoes wear out long before the tread does. Most regular exercisers need to change their footwear three or four times a year.

- **Lift weights safely.** If you are not a regular weight lifter, seek a professional trainer before you begin your weight-lifting program to ensure that your form is correct and to reduce the potential for injuries. To give your muscles time to respond to training and heal—thereby reducing the chances of muscular injury and injury to tendons and ligaments—restrict your strength-training exercises for a particular muscle group to two or three times a week. During weight lifting, you should exhale with exertion to avoid strain and be aware of working opposing muscular groups for balance. Vary your workout to maintain your interest and to provide balanced strength. Change your resistance program completely every three months. Move weights slowly and smoothly—jerking the weights increases the chance of injury. Don't bend a joint beyond 90 degrees when lifting weights.

- **Don't overdo it.** Pushing exercise to the point of exhaustion is not beneficial. In this state, the body produces adrenaline and cortisol, which help to cope with the physical stress of exercise-related injuries but have other adverse health consequences. Excessive exercise suppresses the function of the immune system. In studies at Indiana University, riding a stationary bike vigorously to the point of exhaustion created a decrease in the function of Natural Killer Cells that took 20 hours to recover. In surveys of those participating in the Los Angeles Marathon, those who trained more than 60 miles a week were twice as likely to report colds or flu-like illnesses than those who trained less than 20 miles per week.

There are plenty of reasons to exercise; what becomes difficult is staying motivated enough to continue. Often, three months of regular exercise will produce such profound physical and mental benefits that exercise becomes its own motivation to continue. Here are some hints for reaching this magic three-month mark:

- Develop a buddy system; find an exercise partner to encourage you.
- View exercise as a stress reliever or pick-me-up.
- Be realistic about the time of day you wish to exercise and the amount of exercise you can routinely do. Once you have decided this, vigorously protect this time for yourself.
- Vary your workout so that it stays interesting.
- Set goals for your exercise and celebrate them.
- Above all, choose as your exercise something that you enjoy doing.

Good luck!

Common Sense Nutrition

As far as nutrition is concerned, it is time to get back to basics. Good nutrition is a lifelong habit; don't be tempted by the latest fad diet. It is important to understand and follow a reasonable nutritional plan, one that can be maintained indefinitely. Fad diets do not teach good nutritional habits that can be maintained over time and are not effective in reaching the goal of sustained good health.

A sound nutritional diet should consist of 50 percent carbohydrates, 20 percent protein, and 30 percent fat. Most American diets have much too much saturated fat, processed sugar, and salt and not enough fiber and water. Total calories should be calculated to reach or maintain proper weight. If your weight is stable, keep a careful dietary record for a few weeks and calculate your average daily caloric intake. If you wish to lose weight, reducing your intake by 500 calories a day will cause you to lose about a pound a week. One gram of carbohydrates has 4 calories; one gram of protein has 4 calories; one gram of fat has 9 calories.

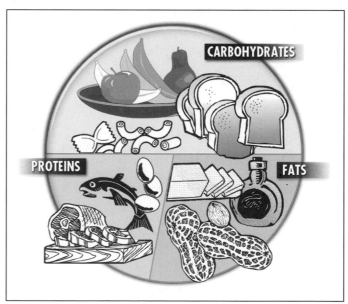

Illustration: Sherry L. Stinson

If you wanted to take in 1,800 calories a day, for example, how many grams of fat can you eat? Calculate your allowable fat grams as follows:

1. Multiply 1,800 calories by 30 percent (remember we said that a sound nutritional diet should consist of 30 percent fat). The result is 540 calories allowed from fat.
2. Divide the 540 fat calorie allotment by 9 calories per gram of fat. The result is 60 fat grams a day.

See How Many Fat Grams You Can Eat

1. Figure out how many calories you want to consume in one day.
2. Multiply that number by .30 to get the number of calories allowed from fat.
3. Divide that number by 9 to get the number of grams allowed from fat.

Almost all food labels denote fat grams, making it easy to monitor and limit fat intake.

The traditional food pyramid still has much merit. Daily intake should include:

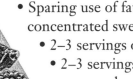

- Sparing use of fats, oils, sugars, and concentrated sweets
  - 2–3 servings of milk, yogurt, and cheese
    - 2–3 servings of meat, poultry, fish, dry beans, eggs, and nuts
      - 3–5 servings of vegetables
        - 2–4 servings of fruit
          - 6–11 servings of bread, cereal, rice, and pasta

Illustration: Sherry L. Stinson

What's a Serving Size?

Most patients greatly overestimate serving sizes, particularly when it comes to commercially prepared foods and restaurant portions. (Serving sizes at an all-you-can-eat bar? Good luck maintaining that degree of discipline!) Here are some tips for estimating serving sizes:

- For commercially prepared foods, read labels! Weigh or measure foods if you aren't sure.
- Use "handy measurements." A clenched fist = 1 cup; an average thumb = 1 ounce of meat or cheese; the tip of the thumb to the first joint = 1 tablespoon; the tip of a finger to the first joint = 1 teaspoon; a cupped hand holds 2 ounces of grain or nuts.
- Use exchange lists. A committee from the American Diabetes Association and the American Dietetic Association publishes large lists of serving sizes for various foods. This information is available from their web sites.

General rules for 1 serving size: 1/2 cup of cereal, grain, or pasta; 1 ounce of bread; 1/2 cup of cooked vegetables of juice; 1 cup of raw vegetables; 1/2 cup of fresh fruit or juice; 1/4 cup of dried fruit; 1 cup of milk; 3 ounces of meat (about the size of a deck of cards).

Here is the skinny on fat:
- Increase your use of meatless main dishes. Balanced, low-fat meals are easily prepared using combinations of brown rice, vegetables, beans, soy products, and fruit.
- Plan fish, chicken, turkey, and veal for your menus.
- Remove skin and all visible fat prior to cooking.
- Broil, roast, bake, boil, steam, and microwave. Avoid frying.
- Use low-fat dairy products, skim milk, and skim milk products rather than whole milk, cream, and cheeses. Substitute low-fat yogurt or cottage cheese whipped in a blender for sour cream or mayonnaise.
- Limit egg yolks to two a week. Substitute two eggs without yolks for every whole egg needed in baking.
- Avoid organ meats such as liver and kidney.
- Instead of animal fats, use corn, olive, or safflower oil. Use cooking spray when technique allows. Use soft tub margarine rather than stick margarine. Reduce the use of fat in sauces; season with herbs and spices instead.
- Avoid processed foods with "partially hydrogenated oils," which contain trans-fatty acids that have an adverse effect on the cholesterol profile.
- Replace store-bought baking goods with homemade goods containing egg whites, recommended fats, and skim milk.

Sugar

Sugar provides only empty calories with no other nutritional value. The average American diet includes 20 teaspoons of sugar a day, largely from commercially prepared food, which is twice the recommended amount. Research at Harvard shows that a high-sugar diet increases the risk of diabetes by 40 percent. Commercially prepared low-fat foods are often high in sugar, so be sure to read labels before buying.

Water

The average person exists in a state of mild chronic dehydration. How can you tell you're not drinking enough water? Symptoms of dehydration include muscle cramps, headache, fatigue, and lightheadedness. These symptoms usually worsen towards the end of the day. Most people begin to feel thirsty when they have lost about 2 percent of their body weight. If they don't drink fluids when they feel thirsty, they will continue to lose water through the breath, skin, urine, and bowel movements. When they have lost 4 percent of their body weight, they are considered severely dehydrated and their blood volume and blood pressure drops, resulting in sensations of weakness, dizziness or light-headedness when upright, headache, and muscle fatigue. Elderly adults, along with those on certain medications and with certain diseases, have a weakened sense of thirst and often do not stay well hydrated. In addition, they are more prone to both minor and serious effects of dehydration.

To calculate the number of eight-ounce glasses of water recommended daily, divide your weight in pounds by 100 and then multiply the result by 8. Thus, a 150-pound woman should drink 12 eight-ounce glasses of water daily. Drinks containing caffeine or alcohol act as diuretics and therefore do not count toward the fluid intake.

> ## How Much Water Should You Drink?
> 1. Divide your weight, in pounds, by 100.
> 2. Multiply the result by 8.

There are other benefits of drinking water. A Harvard study of 50,000 men reported in 1998 that those who consumed the most fluid daily had one-half the incidence of bladder cancer as those who consumed the least. Water intake lessens the chance of kidney stones, leads to fewer asthma attacks in asthmatics, provides better dental health, and helps to curb appetite.

High-protein Diets

Don't go on a high-protein diet. Studies that look at the health of large groups of people over time show that people who eat the least fruit, vegetables, and whole grains (all relatively high-carbohydrate foods) have the highest risk of a variety of deadly diseases, including heart diseases and cancer.

High-protein diets have been around since the 1970s. Their virtues are extolled in best-selling books, not peer reviewed medical journals. Weight is gained or lost based on the total amount of calories consumed, not the source of the calories. Analysis of prescribed meals in high-protein diets shows that these diets consist simply of less food and fewer total calories. There is nothing magical about a high-protein diet that boosts metabolism. High-protein diets are relatively high in fat; the early stages of the Atkins diet derive two-thirds of their calories from fat.

To function normally, the body needs frequent doses of carbohydrates. These provide the main fuel for muscles and the only fuel for brain cells. If the body is deprived of carbohydrates, it acts like it is starving. When the diet lacks carbohydrates, the body first uses its limited stores of carbohydrates. Unlike fat and protein, which are packaged quite tightly in the body, carbohydrates are loose chemicals that are packed in water. Therefore, when the carbohydrate stores are lost, several pounds of water-related weight are also lost. While this may be cosmetically beneficial for an upcoming high school reunion, it has no long-term health benefits. Once the carbohydrate stores are exhausted, the body then goes after stored protein (muscle) and fat. On extremely low-carbohydrate diets, the body switches metabolism to a process called ketosis. As protein and fat are digested, ketones are produced. These create side effects of queasiness and lightheadedness that decrease appetite. Excessive ketones also increase urine output, resulting in thirst and high water consumption, which in turn decreases appetite. Unfortunately, ketones that pass into the urine take important salts with them such as sodium, potassium, and magnesium, which can ultimately lead to dehydration and problems with the heart rhythm.

Passing up fruits and vegetables misses out on a whole range of nutrients that protect the heart, strengthen bones, fight cancer, and boost immunity. We are just starting to understand the complex interactions of nutrients and foods, and do not understand these well enough to safely rely on vitamins and supplements to replace these missed nutrients.

What happened to the millions of Americans on high-protein diets in the 1970s? They became tired of the side effects and the limitations of the diets and stopped them. Those who continued a high-protein diet learned that eventually their bodies adjusted to the process of ketosis, hunger returned, and the weight loss achieved was regained.

Omega-3 Fatty Acids

A study reported in the *New England Journal of Medicine* in 1997 showed that two servings of fish a week reduced the risk of fatal heart attack by 50 percent. Fish oil was found to reduce triglycerides and inhibit blood clotting. It also serves as an anti-inflammatory agent; the types of chemicals (prostaglandins and leukotrienes) made with these fatty acids are less inflammatory than those produced with common fats. Inflammation is now understood to play a key role in the development of atherosclerosis (thickening of the artery walls) and its complications. It is recommended that fish be included in the diet two to three times a week. Mackerel, salmon, halibut, herring and less so tuna, cod, and flounder are good sources of omega-3 fatty acids. Oils such as olive, safflower, and corn are also good sources of healthier oils.

Soy

Since October of 1999, the FDA has allowed manufacturers of soy products to label them with claims of reducing heart disease. Soy products, such as soybeans, tofu, and prepared meat substitutes are full of isoflavones—a group of estrogen-like chemicals. In studies of those already on a low-fat, low-cholesterol diet, replacing 100 calories of animal protein with soy protein caused an additional 5 to 10 percent drop in cholesterol levels.

Other benefits of soy relate to its estrogen-like effects. One study showed improvement in bone density in postmenopausal women eating soy. Observational studies of women whose cultures prompt them to consume more soy in their diet show a reduction in hot flashes in menopause and a reduced incidence of breast cancer. It is hypothesized, but not yet proved, that the soy proteins may partially interact with estrogen receptors in women, activating them enough to help with hot flashes but blocking the ability of true estrogen to reach the receptor and thus reducing the incidence of estrogen-sensitive breast cancer.

It is uncertain what part of the soy product provides the health benefits; therefore, it is best to stick with soy products, not processed pills.

Fiber

A large percentage of fiber is not absorbed through digestion; rather, it is passed through to the colon where its bulk and water retaining properties prevent the hard, dry stools of constipation. You should consume between 20 and 35 grams of fiber a day by eating produce, whole grains, beans, and high-fiber cereals. Some evidence suggests that fiber reduces cholesterol and blood pressure, and may have a role in preventing colon cancer.

Calcium

Calcium is essential for proper bone development and maintenance. Adequate calcium is needed in childhood to reach peak bone densities. Calcium is obtained from the diet in dairy products and, when necessary to make up the difference, by taking calcium supplements. See *Calcium* on page 78 for more information about how much calcium you need, when to take calcium supplements, and how to help your body best absorb this important element.

B Vitamins

B vitamins such as B_6, B_{12}, and folic acid are crucial to maintaining normal heart and neurological function. Folic acid helps reduce the rate of defects in the central nervous system in pregnancy; supplements should begin several months before attempting to become pregnant. B vitamins reduce homocysteine levels, which are linked to heart disease. Too little B vitamin intake may contribute to heart disease and stroke, dementia, mental decline, and depression. As adults age, the ability to absorb B vitamins from the diet declines; therefore, adults should add a B vitamin supplement to their diet by age 50.

Antioxidants

Oxidation is a chemical process that produces free radicals in the body. These free radicals are thought to be responsible for creating chemical damage in a variety of tissues. Oxidation has been linked to heart disease, cancers, cataracts, the aging process, and macular degeneration. Antioxidants are other chemicals that mop up the damaging free radicals that cause oxidation. Antioxidants include vitamins E and C, beta-carotene, lutein, and others. The recommended 5 to 9 servings of fruits and vegetables a day provide most of the needed amounts of antioxidants. It is not yet known whether taking antioxidants in pill form has any benefit; in fact, recent studies have suggested a detrimental effect from supplemental forms of beta-carotene, vitamin C, and vitamin E; see *Chapter 12: Herbals, Vitamins, and Other Nutritional Supplements* for more information about using nutritional supplements.

The Mediterranean Diet

The Mediterranean diet is so named because it follows the traditional diets of some cultures based in Greece, southern France, and parts of Italy. It emphasizes eating whole, natural foods, olive oil, fish, nuts, and wine. Current cardiovascular research provides significant evidence that the Mediterranean diet is more effective than traditional low-fat diets in preventing heart disease. Instead of concentrating on fat reduction, the diet emphasizes the importance of the type of fat consumed.

Diet Guidelines

The guidelines for this diet are fairly simple—lean more toward the good fats and avoid the bad:

Consume...	Avoid...
Foods high in omega-3 fatty acids such as fatty fish (salmon, trout, sardines, tuna), tree nuts (walnuts, almonds, pecans, hazel nuts, Brazil nuts)	Saturated fats (red meat, butter, cheese, milk)
Monounsaturated fats found in olive oil, canola oil, flax seed oil, nuts, and avocados	Trans-fatty acids (margarine, shortening, and other processed foods with partially hydrogenated oils such as baked goods, chips, and fried fast foods)
Seven to ten servings each day of natural, whole plant foods (fruits, vegetables, salads)	Foods with concentrated sugar (candy, cookies, cakes)
Whole-grain, high-fiber breads and pastas	Oils with omega-6 fatty acids (corn, sunflower, safflower, soybean, and peanut oils)

Consider the regular consumption of a small amount of wine, up to 4 ounces a day for women and up to 8 ounces a day for men, for those with no history of, or no risk for, alcohol abuse.

The Evidence

Let's look at some evidence to support the benefits of this diet:

- The Lyon Diet Heart Study, published in 1999, enrolled 605 heart attack survivors in a four-year dietary study. Those consuming a Mediterranean-type diet had a 55 percent reduction in death rate and a similar reduction in the number of additional cardiac events in comparison to those on a regular diet.
- The GISSI-Prevenzion Trial, also published in 1999, followed 11,000 patients over $3\frac{1}{2}$ years. Patients with high omega-3 fatty acid intake reduced their death rate from heart disease by 45 percent.
- The Diet and Reinfarction Trial, published in 1989, assigned 2,033 men with previous heart attacks to different diets. Those on a Mediterranean-type diet had a 29 percent reduction in mortality.
- Olive oil diets reduce total cholesterol, LDL cholesterol, and triglycerides without lowering the healthy HDL cholesterol levels. Experimentally, this creates a more favorable effect on the whole lipid profile than what can be achieved by simply limiting fats in the diet.

- Olive oil, berries, apples, onions, tea, and red wine are all high in flavonoids, which are antioxidants that inhibit the oxidation of LDL cholesterol (a step necessary in cholesterol related blood vessel damage).
- Trans-fatty acids, avoided in the Mediterranean diet, increase LDL cholesterol levels while reducing HDL cholesterol, resulting in an unfavorable effect on the cholesterol profile that is twice as bad as that from the consumption of a similar amount of saturated fat.

The Mediterranean diet has shown promising results, makes medical sense, is less restrictive than many other dietary approaches to the prevention of heart disease, and is certainly worth considering.

The Ornish Diet

The program promoted by Dr. Dean Ornish includes a rigorous diet, exercise, stress management, and support groups. This diet reduces fat to less than 10 percent and contains no cholesterol. It is a natural food, plant-based diet that concentrates on fruits, vegetables, grains, beans, non-fat dairy products, egg whites, and soy products. Studies of this program have shown a measurable reversal in coronary artery disease, a two-and-a-half time reduction in heart attacks, 91 percent fewer incidences of chest pain, and drops in LDL cholesterol by as much as 40 percent. I have no direct experience with this program, but it appears to be a rigorous program that requires training and support to follow.

Obesity and Weight Loss

You may have noticed that my chapters on exercise and nutrition do not mention weight loss as either motivation for a better exercise and nutritional program or as a goal of such programs. This is intentional. Exercise, nutrition, and obesity are related but nevertheless independent issues.

The National Institutes of Health identifies obesity as an independent risk factor for premature death, hypertension, heart disease, stroke, osteoarthritis, and cancers of the uterus, breast, prostate, and colon. Obesity limits mobility and endurance and leads to fatigue, stress, and social discrimination.

However, regular exercise and a sound diet may reduce the risk of these diseases, regardless of their effect on weight. Exercise and good nutrition improve blood pressure, cholesterol, and blood sugars. Patients seeking weight loss through proper nutrition and exercise don't need to reach normal weights to improve their health; the benefits of proper nutrition and exercise are statistically evident with as little as a 5 to 10 percent loss of body weight. I would rather have my patients concentrate on improving their body composition (lean muscle mass) than focus on the bathroom scale.

What is Obesity?

Important concepts in obesity include the *body mass index*, a measure of weight in comparison to height, and the distribution of that weight on the body. The body mass index is calculated by multiplying the weight, in pounds, by 705—a correction factor that allows us to use inches and pounds rather than metric system measurements—then dividing by the height, in inches. This result is again divided by the height, in inches.

Calculate Your Body Mass Index
1. Multiply your weight, in pounds, by 705.
2. Divide the result by height, in inches.
3. Divide the result of #2 by height again, in inches.

What does the Body Mass Index Mean?

The following table will help you understand what the body mass index means, in terms of health.

A body mass index of...	Means...
Less than 22	You are underweight. A body mass index of 21 or less increases the risk for osteoporosis and provides no reserve bodily tissues should you become seriously ill.
22–25	You are within normal range. There is no health advantage to losing weight.
26–27	You are overweight. This is medically significant if you have hypertension, diabetes, or arthritis. You should modify your lifestyle to avoid additional weight gain. Your physician will also consider the distribution of weight on your body to determine whether you might benefit from medical intervention.
28–30	Your risk of weight-related disease increases dramatically, and medical intervention is needed. Drug therapy may be considered if you also have weight-related medical conditions, such as diabetes, hypertension, elevated cholesterol, arthritis, or heart disease.
Greater than 30	You are 20 percent or more above your ideal body weight, posing a high risk of medical complications.

Weight Distribution on the Body

Abdominal fat is different than fat on the hips or thighs. Abdominal fat is deposited and retrieved through carrier proteins in the bloodstream more easily than fat in other locations. This fat is easier for the body to access when energy stores are needed, but as a consequence leads to higher fat levels in the bloodstream. When metabolized, byproducts of belly fat raise cholesterol and reduce the body's sensitivity to insulin, affecting blood pressure and increasing the risk of heart disease and cancer. Abdominal fat also produces more estrogen, which may fuel the growth of breast cancer. Observational studies show that patients with more abdominal fat increased their risk of hypertension, heart disease, diabetes, colon cancer, and postmenopausal breast cancer.

One way to assess abdominal fat is to look at the waist-to-hip ratio; this ratio is determined by measuring the waist at its narrowest point, then measuring the hips at their widest point. Women should have a waist-to-hip ratio of 0.8 or less; men should have a waist-to-hip ratio of 1.0 or less.

Myths of Weight Loss

Myth # 1: Everyone who loses weight will eventually regain it.

This myth comes from very small studies of people who enter university-sponsored weight loss programs. Often these programs are used as a last resort for those with serious weight problems. The incidence of physical and psychological problems in this group of people is much higher than average and long-term health issues complicate their ability to maintain their weight reduction. Community-based weight loss programs, on the other hand, do show long-term successes.

Myth # 2: Dieting and weight loss make the body's metabolic rate slow down, making it difficult to lose additional weight.

While this is initially true, new studies show that once weight loss occurs and the weight stabilizes, the body's metabolic rate will return to normal. This implies that those patients who need significant weight loss should do it in a stair-step fashion, periodically pausing at weights for several weeks to allow their metabolism to normalize.

Myth # 3: "But I don't eat that much."

Study after study shows that overweight people consistently underestimate how much they eat. Retrospective recordings of nutritional intake are worthless; keeping a diary and recording measured food intake as it occurs is the only reliable way to track calories.

Myth # 4: Reducing fat in the diet will make me lose weight.

Numerous medical studies prove that weight is gained or lost based on the total number of calories consumed, not on the source of those calories. If high-calorie, sugary foods are substituted for the fat, no benefit is obtained. Most "fat-free" commercial foods are very high in sugar. Read labels carefully on these commercially prepared foods before you assume that their low-fat content also means low in calories.

Myth # 5: Gimmicky diets which lead to rapid initial weight loss will help me get started.

I am constantly amazed at what nonsense my patients will swallow in order to try to lose weight. Numerous studies show that short-term weight loss through dramatic dietary changes does not lead to long-term success in weight loss efforts. Weight control is a life-long goal that requires consistency in adopting proper nutritional, dietary, and lifestyle habits. The motivation for this change must come from within; relying on gimmicky diets continues to place hope for a magical solution outside of you, and sets you up for failure.

Myth # 6: Switching to foods I don't like will help me lose weight.

Food is one of the pleasures of life. In designing a nutritional plan, you must take into account personal likes and dislikes or else the plan will fail over time.

Myth # 7: Sleeping less will increase my activity and help me lose weight.

I have two responses to this myth. First, the goal of proper nutrition and weight loss is for a healthier mind and body; sleep deprivation does not foster this goal. Second, studies show that sleep-deprived people are more likely to seek out and consume a high-fat, high-sugar diet to provide rapid energy to the brain.

Myth # 8: One bad meal will wreck my diet.

It is the number of calories consumed per week that matters, not the calorie count of any one meal. Planning a special occasion? Make up for it from other meals that week.

Myth # 9: My doctor should give me a pill to help me get started losing weight.

Numerous studies of the short-term use of appetite suppressants prove that this technique is not beneficial in promoting long-term weight loss. The weight is regained—and then some—after the pill's initial effects wear off. If successful drug therapy for obesity exists, it is life-long therapy for those with medically significant obesity who have attended a supervised weight loss program for greater than 6 months and failed. To date, very limited data exists to indicate that drug therapy, even in this high-risk population, is effective in producing beneficial long-term health outcomes.

How to Lose Weight

The best hints for successful weight reduction come from the National Weight Control Registry, a record of those individuals who have successfully lost 30 pounds or more and kept the weight off more than one year. The following hints come from this source:

- **Do it for you.** Motivation for this type of permanent change must come from within. Gimmicky diets and pills provide false hope for a magical solution outside of yourself and avoid the necessary commitment and responsibility for your own actions.
- **Set realistic goals.** Aim to lose 10 percent of your body weight over the first 6 to 12 months. Most of the health benefits of weight loss (lower blood pressure and cholesterol, reduced risk of diabetes and arthritis) occur with this first 10 percent.
- **Curb your impulses and pause before acting.** Once food is swallowed, it takes 15 minutes or longer for feedback from the stretch and chemical receptors in the digestive tract to let the brain know that sufficient food has entered. Eating too quickly overloads the stomach before the "full signal" is triggered. Slow meals down by pausing for three to five minutes a few times during the initial course. Work on delaying your response to cravings at least 15 minutes; try drinking some water or nibbling on raw vegetables during those minutes to see if your craving will subside.
- **Keep a food diary for at least two weeks.** This provides a realistic picture of where you need to cut back and helps identify situations and stresses that may trigger eating.
- **Watch portions at restaurants.** Eating out prevents you, to some degree, from controlling how food is prepared but not how much of it you eat. Reduce restaurant portion sizes by one-third to one-half. Ask for and pack a "to go box" before you eat your meal.
- **Set up psychological support systems.** Use a diary, buddy system, or group.
- **Relax.** Learn and use relaxation techniques other than food.

- **Expect to slip.** Then get over it and get on with your plan.
- **Eat small, frequent meals and snacks.** In supervised studies, most successful dieters ate five times daily or more.
- **Exercise regularly.** Dieters who exercise are more likely to keep weight off over the long term. Try to exercise a minimum of 30 to 60 minutes a day. Add strength training two to three days a week to build muscle (muscle burns more calories than other tissues, even at rest).
- **Don't rely on "will power."** This concept only serves to make overweight people feel weak and bad about themselves. Weight loss is the result of careful planning and sustained effort over time.

Weight Loss Medications

I do not advise over-the-counter (OTC) weight loss medications. All of these chemicals are marketed as "dietary supplements" under the 1994 Dietary Supplement Health and Education Act. This permits the marketing of any product claimed to affect the structure or function of the body without evaluation or approval of any government agency, as long as the labeling includes a disclaimer saying that it has not been evaluated by the FDA and the product is not intended to diagnose, treat, or prevent any disease. No proof is required to market these products. No safety data is required before they are sold. Manufacturers are not required to reveal reports of adverse effects when they are received. If questions about safety arise, the burden of proof is on the FDA, not the manufacturer.

Numerous medical studies show that the types of chemicals used in OTC weight loss products do not promote long-term weight loss; in addition they have significant side effects and potential for adverse reactions. "Drug-free" weight loss products simply use herbal sources for their active chemicals: ephedrine (heartleaf, Ma Huang) and caffeine (green tea, guarana). For the last few decades, the majority of weight loss supplements used to contain phenylpropanolamine. The FDA pulled this drug off the market in 2000 because of the excessive number of strokes experienced by patients using it. In my considered opinion, OTC weight loss medications have no role in long-term, healthy weight loss.

Currently, three types of prescription weight loss medications exist:
- Stimulants affect the appetite center in the hypothalamus, and are associated with short-term weight loss that is usually temporary. Side effects of these drugs include elevated blood pressure, anxiety, and aggression.
- Medications that suppress appetite by blocking uptake of serotonin and norepinephrine in the brain. Side effects of these drugs include headache, dry mouth, constipation, and insomnia.
- Medications that work on the gastrointestinal tract and limits the absorption of dietary fat. Side effects include abdominal gas, diarrhea, lack of control of bowel movements, and a decrease in the absorption of fat-soluble vitamins.

All of these drugs are expensive. The average weight loss in one year from prescription therapy is less than 10 percent of body weight. The safety and long-term (that is, greater than two years) benefits of these drugs on the ill health and mortality associated with obesity-related diseases have not been established.

Prescription medications are considered only in patients with a body mass index greater than 30 or in patients with a body mass index greater than 27 and certain medical conditions. All available evidence suggests that once drug therapy for obesity is started, it is needed lifelong. These drugs should be considered only in those individuals who have tried and failed other supervised efforts of weight loss for greater than six months. In my opinion, these drugs are safe and effective only when used by experienced providers, and the chance of success is greatly increased when resources including nutritionists, exercise physiologists, and counselors are available. Unless your physician is very familiar with the use of these medications and can provide backup support to you, he or she should refer you to a weight loss specialty clinic.

CHAPTER 4

Allergies

Your body's immune system is responsible for monitoring and responding to any threat from the outside world. When a threat is perceived, the immune system launches a counter attack to destroy the invaders and expel them from your body. While this is good for you if the invaders are a foreign virus or bacteria, the effects are not so healthy when the immune system perceives tree pollen or animal dander as a threat. In the non-allergic patient, substances such as pollen and animal dander are ignored. They are caught by the mucus in the respiratory tract and expelled. In an allergic patient, these same substances are recognized as a threat; the immune system launches a counterattack with the release of histamines and other substances, leading to the typical symptoms of allergies—itchy eyes, running nose, sneezing, cough, and malaise.

A substance that the immune system's allergy mechanisms recognize and react to is called an antigen. The way that the reaction is triggered is through proteins made by certain white blood cells called antibodies, of which there are several types. Most allergic reactions involve antibodies of the IgE class.

Allergic Rhinitis

Allergic rhinitis refers to the reaction caused when an antigen floating in the air is inhaled through the nose. The allergic reaction is caused by antibodies of the IgE class, which are specific to each type of antigen. An allergic reaction occurs only when the body has seen an antigen before, has made antibodies to it, and then is exposed to that particular antigen again. Symptoms include nasal congestion and blockage, postnasal drainage, sneezing attacks, a runny nose, fatigue, and headache. Seasonal rhinitis occurs with predictable seasons, such as when certain plants bloom or when cold weather forces individuals indoors to be exposed to more house dust, and is typically triggered by inhaling pollens, molds, and house dust mites. Perennial rhinitis occurs year around and can be triggered by inhaling house dust mites, animal dander, occupational exposures, molds, or other allergens.

In a non-allergic patient, pollen is caught in the mucus in the nose and is eventually swept out of the body. In the patient with allergies, the pollen stimulates an immune reaction when it is recognized by and bound to an IgE antibody. This combination of antigen and IgE antibody then triggers a series of reactions that result in the release of histamines and other chemicals into the nasal lining, which causes sneezing, itching, and nasal moisture. The blood vessels in the nose enlarge and become more leaky, and secretions from glands increase.

A 23-year medical study of patients with allergies showed that more than half of young adults with allergies either lose them or significantly improve with time. Of the remainder, about a third will not notice a change in their allergies as they age. Ten percent of young adults with allergies will notice a worsening of their symptoms as they get older. The final 10 percent will develop other allergy related diseases, such as asthma, as they age.

Several effective types of treatment exist for allergies:

- **Allergen avoidance.** Reducing the potential exposure to allergy-causing antigens takes time, but is one of the most effective and cost-efficient ways of improving allergy symptoms. Reduce dust mite exposure by keeping the indoor humidity less than 45 percent to retard their growth, eliminating carpeting, stuffed furniture, and clutter from the home, and encasing mattresses and pillows in special fabrics. Reduce animal-related allergies by eliminating circumstances that lead to exposure to animal hair, urine, and saliva. Time outdoor activities carefully to minimize seasonal and weather-related allergen exposures. Close windows and air-condition the home to reduce allergen exposure and lower moisture. Consider other allergen culprits including houseplants, fish tanks, old paper products, and poorly ventilated areas in your home.

- **Antihistamines.** Many medications are available to help relieve sneezing, itching, and drainage. Some older antihistamines are more sedating, causing drowsiness and interfering with cognitive and motor performance. Studies of driving ability show that the driving reactions of patients who take a sedating antihistamine are similar to people who are legally intoxicated with alcohol. Using a sedating antihistamine at bedtime can prolong these effects into the next day. Newer antihistamines, currently only available by prescription, are much less sedating and are the drugs of choice for most individuals. "Non-drowsy" allergy formulas currently available aren't antihistamines at all; they are simply decongestants and have no effect on the actual allergic reaction other than drying up secretions. Side effects include drying of nasal secretions, dry mouth, and constipation.

- **Mast cell stabilizers (cromolyn and others).** Mast cells are specialized white blood cells that live in the tissues and participate in the allergic reaction. When they are activated by an antigen-IgE complex, mast cells release a variety of stored chemicals (histamines and others) that promote localized inflammation. Mast cell stabilizers prevent the mast cell from releasing these irritating substances and, when used routinely, help block the release of chemical mediators of allergic reactions. Most mast cell stabilizers are used in spray (the nose) or dropper (the eye) forms. They must be used four to six times daily, take a few days to reach their peak effect, and have only a modest benefit for most patients. Side effects, other than temporary local irritation, are infrequent. I have had few patients over the years that found these drugs worth the trouble of the frequent applications required to use them.

- **Leukotriene modifiers.** Leukotrienes are another potent class of chemicals in the body that are involved in the process of inflammation. A new class of medications has recently become clinically available that blocks the effects of leukotrienes and prevents them from worsening the inflammatory process, such as an allergic or asthma reaction. These medications are taken once or twice daily in pill form. In asthma patients, benefit can often be measured within the first few doses. Side effects, though rare, include allergic reactions to the drug itself, drowsiness, changes in sleep, and gastrointestinal upset. Although currently only approved for use in asthma patients, the use of this class of medications for allergy sufferers looks promising.

- **Nasal steroid sprays.** These potent, topical, anti-inflammatory medications should be used as the main therapy for most patients with allergic rhinitis. These sprays build up in the lining of the nasal passage and block the allergy response before it gets started. They may require one to two weeks to provide relief, and can take a month or longer until maximum benefit is achieved. Used daily during the allergy season, they have proved to reduce complications of allergies such as sinusitis. Side effects can include a temporary burning sensation in the nose, nosebleeds, and thinning or irritation of the nasal lining with prolonged use. In my practice, I rarely have had patients with side effects significant enough to change therapy.

- **Immunotherapy (allergy shots).** These shots are the only potentially curative therapy for allergic rhinitis. This is a reasonable option that can provide safe and cost-effective management of allergy patients who have a long allergy season, year-round symptoms, poor response to or intolerance of usual allergy medications, or recurrent sinus or ear infections. Long-term studies of immune therapy in children with allergies show that it can significantly reduce the chance that the child will go on to develop asthma. This finding has not been studied in adults. Immunotherapy involves giving repeated injections of antigens under the skin. Over time, this decreases the allergy response through several changes in the immune system. Allergy shots result in the creation of IgG antibodies to the antigen injected. These IgG antibodies get in the way of the IgE-antigen reaction, and thus interfere with the allergy response. Allergy shots also activate parts of the immune system called T-suppressor cells that suppress the allergy immune response.

Food Allergies

Food allergies are more common in the first years of life. Allergies to milk, eggs, and soy are usually outgrown. Allergies to peanuts, tree nuts, fish, and shellfish are not; allergies to these foods make up 90 percent of adult food allergies.

Food allergies also involve IgE. Food allergies can produce symptoms in the gastro-intestinal tract, such as lip swelling, mouth irritation, sore throat, nausea or indigestion, bloating, cramping, or diarrhea. The allergic reactions can occur in other parts of the body, such as skin reactions, nasal congestion, asthma-like responses, and whole body reactions (see *Anaphylaxis* on page 27). The more serious reactions account for 100 deaths each year in the United States and are usually triggered when patients with known allergies unknowingly ingest a food allergen. This is most common with peanuts, cow's milk, eggs, fish, shellfish, or wheat.

Patients with very sensitive allergies do not need to ingest food to react. Exposure to airborne allergens (peanut dust) can trigger a response.

Treatment of food allergies consists mainly of identifying and avoiding the allergen. Allergy skin testing is somewhat useful, though difficult with certain fruits and vegetables because their proteins break down too easily and allergy extracts are hard to prepare. Allergy elimination diets, where possible allergens are excluded and reintroduced one by one until the culprit is found, are also useful.

Patients with severe food allergies should carry warning identification and emergency treatment, including supplies of self-injected epinephrine and antihistamines.

Insect Allergies

Allergies to stinging insects occur in 1 to 1.5 percent of the population. The reactions to stinging insects are classified as one of three types:

- *Local reactions* consist of transient pain, swelling, and redness. These reactions begin to subside in less than one hour.
- *Large local reactions* are greater than 10 centimeters in diameter and/or extend across a joint. They peak in 24 to 48 hours and can last from five to seven days. Large local reactions do not predict future systemic reactions.
- *Systemic reactions* are whole-body reactions. Systemic reactions range in severity from whole-body skin reactions to life-threatening reactions involving multiple body systems, including respiratory and cardiovascular collapse (see *Anaphylaxis* on page 27).

Insect allergies are usually discovered as the result of an initial stinging and reaction. They can be confirmed by skin testing, though this requires an experienced allergist to interpret correctly.

If a patient has a severe reaction to an insect sting, the chance of a similar reaction to the next sting is approximately 60 percent. Allergy immunotherapy with the appropriate insect venom can reduce the subsequent risk of reaction to 2 to 3 percent.

Emergency treatment of an insect sting includes icing the sting site to slow the release of venom and using antihistamines and anti-inflammatory medications such as ibuprofen. People with known severe reactions should also carry epinephrine for self-injection. I give my patients several units of epinephrine to keep in a variety of places and on their person to ensure that it is readily available when needed.

Hives (Urticaria)

Hives are very itchy, red, raised spots composed of dilated blood vessels and localized tissue fluid. Individual lesions come and go in less than 24 hours, leaving no sign of their presence when gone. If you draw a circle around a hive with a pen, there should be nothing in that circle 24 hours later. *Acute hives* are outbreaks of hives with successive crops of lesions that can last a few days. They are "self-limited," which means that they will resolve on their own over time, even if no therapy is given They are common with viral illnesses and affect 10 to 20 percent of the population. *Chronic hives* are a series of outbreaks that last at least six weeks. Fifty percent of people with chronic hives will still have symptoms six months later; 20 percent of them will have symptoms more than 10 years. Unfortunately, more than 90 percent of the time, the cause for chronic hives is never identified.

Hive-like reactions that extend deeper into the skin and subcutaneous tissues—typically involving the face, tongue, and genitals—are referred to as *angioedema*. Hives and angioedema involve the action of histamines and other chemical mediators of inflammation.

If individual hive-like lesions last longer than 24 hours, they are not considered to be true hives. These types of lesions are associated with inflammation of blood vessels and often leave a reddish stain on the skin after they have resolved. This type of reaction should prompt your doctor to search further for underlying diseases that may be associated with them.

Hives and angioedema involve the action of histamines and other chemicals that trigger inflammation. These reactions typically occur as a result of an exposure to an antigen. Common causes include medications such as aspirin, anti-inflammatory medication (ibuprofen, naproxen, and others), or ACE inhibitors (medications used to treat high blood pressure and heart disease). In some individuals, the reactions can be triggered by exposure to environmental changes, such as cold or heat. Other less common causes include hives triggered by the cholinergic portion of the nervous system (responsible for sweating), physical exercise, or pressure on the skin.

Hives are treated by avoiding whatever triggers them, if known. Tepid or oatmeal baths can help relieve symptoms. Avoiding excessive heat and sweating limits the itching. Antihistamines help; often the older, more sedating drugs are more effective. Occasionally, newer chemical modifiers of inflammation are used, such as the leukotriene modifiers. Severe cases may require the use of steroids.

Anaphylaxis

Anaphylaxis is another IgE-related reaction to an antigen that causes skin flushing; hives and angioedema; excessive secretions, swelling, and spasm in the respiratory airways; chest pain and palpitations; and effects on the gastrointestinal tract including abdominal cramping, nausea, vomiting, and diarrhea. The reaction can trigger dilation of large numbers of blood vessels, which can lead to a sudden and severe fall in blood pressure, vascular collapse (inadequate pressure left to supply blood to the brain and other vital organs), and death.

Common causes of anaphylaxis include aspirin, penicillin, bee sting venom, and the allergenic extracts used in allergy skin testing and allergy shots. Shrimp and other shell-fish, as well as peanuts, are the most common food causes of reactions.

The time frame between exposure to the antigen and a life-threatening anaphylactic response may be only minutes. Therefore, this condition is best treated by avoidance of substances known to cause it. Patients with severe reactions to bees, for example, shouldn't tend a flower garden. Patients with a history of anaphylactic responses to medication or other substances should carry clear identification of their allergy (a bracelet or necklace) so they are not inadvertently given the drug in treating another condition. Aspirin is the first drug given to patient presumed to be having a heart attack. If you are rushed to the emergency room semi-conscious from your allergic reaction to aspirin, and your symptoms look like a heart attack, you may well be given more aspirin—which could be a lethal mistake.

 If you have severe drug allergies, wear clear identification indicating so!

Epinephrine, given by injection under the skin, is the first line of therapy for patients in the early stages of an anaphylactic reaction. Patients with a history of anaphylactic reactions are taught to carry and use subcutaneous epinephrine to treat early symptoms while they are waiting for emergency medical care.

Infections and Antibiotics

I wish more of my patients trusted my decision to prescribe—or refrain from prescribing—antibiotics. The same patients who accept my advice regarding life-and-death decisions about cancer and heart disease look at me in surprise when I advise against antibiotics for the treatment of a common cold or sore throat.

Infections occur when organisms, such as viruses, fungi, or bacteria, enter the body and cause disease.

Viruses are tiny infectious agents that are responsible for more than 90 percent of all infections of the upper respiratory tract. Viruses are made up of an outer protein core surrounding genetic material and are not capable of living independently—that is, they must use the cellular machinery of their host to reproduce and they do so only within living cells. Think of viruses as packages of information wrapped in an envelope; when a virus enters a human cell, the information it contains is released into the cell and takes over the cell's own chemical processes for the purpose of making new viruses. Since the chemical processes used are the same for the virus as they are for other human cells, there is often no unique target for a drug like an antibiotic to affect.

Fungi, or yeasts, are parasitic plants that typically cause infections of body surfaces, but can also cause invasive disease when the body is not functioning properly.

Bacteria are single-celled organisms that are able to live independently—that is, use their own chemical processes to grow and reproduce—outside of other cells. Most antibiotics work by interrupting specific chemical processes that are necessary for the bacteria to survive or reproduce. Since these chemical processes are specific to the bacteria, and not the human body, often a drug can be targeted to selectively affect the bacteria and not be too harmful to the human.

Antibiotics are medications that kill bacteria or stop them from growing so that your immune system can destroy them. Antibiotics work by chemically interfering with the key steps that a bacterium follows to get energy, grow, or reproduce. Fortunately, bacteria use different chemical pathways than human cells, which means drugs can be designed to harm them while not having a similar effect on us. Each bacterial species may have differences in its chemical pathways; therefore, some drugs will affect one bacterium but not another. Bacteria also have defenses against these chemical poisons, including enzymes that inactivate an antibiotic by chemically cutting it up, proteins that bind the antibiotic's active sites so that it can't function, methods of blocking entry of the antibiotic into the bacterial cell, or mechanisms to actively pump the antibiotic out of the bacterial cell. The ability of a bacterium to do this is called *resistance*. Some bacteria code the secret for their ability to beat antibiotics in tiny chemical messages that they can give to other bacteria, spreading the resistance.

Bacteria and viruses reproduce at an amazing rate. Some of these organisms make frequent mistakes in copying the genetic material for their progeny. Most often, these mistakes either do not affect the offspring or are lethal. Occasionally, the bacteria or virus will get lucky, and one of the "mistakes" will actually change the organisms in a favorable way. The protein that the antibiotic previously attached to may be subtly changed, enabling the protein to continue performing its function for the bacteria but preventing the antibiotic from fitting onto it, rendering those bacteria resistant to a previously effective antibiotic. This is another way that resistance develops.

Bacteria invade your body; antibiotics can chemically kill certain bacteria (hopefully without harming you). Why the caution in using antibiotics too liberally?

First, not all bacteria are bad. Bacteria exist in the upper respiratory tract and are important for proper digestion and nutrition in the lower colon. These bacteria are called normal flora. They take up the available space and nutrients and act as part of the body's line of defense against invaders. The concept is similar to a well-manicured lawn. The normal flora in the upper respiratory tract are like the blades of grass. They cover the soil and use the available fertilizer and water. Their presence keeps large populations of weeds from growing because there simply isn't room. Despite the best attentions of the caretaker, any yard will have a few weeds in it. If an herbicide is sprayed over the lawn, the sensitive grass will die and a few hardy weeds will survive. Since the weeds' competition is gone, they will rapidly take over the lawn. Likewise, the first casualties from antibiotic use are the normal flora. Their elimination creates the opportunity for a nastier population of bacteria to take residence. These bacteria are now in a position to take advantage of subsequent opportunities to cause infections in the sinuses and lungs, infections that are resistant to some antibiotics. Because of this phenomenon, for any individual patient, taking any antibiotic increases the risk of developing a future infection with a resistant strain of bacteria.

Second, many people do not take antibiotics properly. Each infection involves a large population (millions and millions) of bacteria. In this population, some bacteria may be very sensitive to a given antibiotic, some moderately sensitive to it, and some resistant. When antibiotics are begun, the most sensitive bacteria die first. With continued exposure to the antibiotic, even those less sensitive to it begin to die. Once the numbers of bacteria are low enough, your immune system can take over and mop up the remaining stragglers, even if a few were totally resistant to the chosen drug. A course of antibiotics, usually 5 to 14 days, is designed to eliminate the bacteria; if you stop the antibiotics prematurely—as many people do—the drug hasn't yet killed all the bacteria. To make matters worse, those that are left over may be partially or totally resistant to the drug. If your immune system doesn't win, the new populations of bacteria that grow back are now super bugs, the weak ones have been weeded out, and the first antibiotic now won't work at all.

Because of the improper use of antibiotics, some bacteria are rapidly becoming resistant. In the past five years, Streptococcus pneumoniae, a common cause of upper and lower respiratory infections, has increased in its percentage of penicillin-resistant organisms by 300 percent. In addition, many of these bugs have simultaneously become resistant to other antibiotics including cephalosporins, erythromycin, sulfa drugs, and quinolones. I'm very concerned about this; you should be too.

Contributors to bacteria's increasing resistance to antibiotics include the widespread use of antibiotics outside of the United States, with many countries making antibiotics available off the shelf in the pharmacy for patients to take themselves without medical guidance. Antibiotic use is not restricted to humans; researchers are also concerned about their global use in livestock feed to promote growth. Modern medicine must share in the blame; in the United States alone, an estimated 50 million unnecessary prescriptions for antibiotics are written each year. Studies of doctors' offices show that one-half to two-thirds of patients diagnosed with upper respiratory infections receive antibiotics, when viruses cause 90 percent of these infections. Why? Because patients expect a prescription when they feel bad and have taken the time and expense to see the doctor, and because doctors lack the time and inclination to educate patients properly about the use and misuse of antibiotics. The medical profession is currently involved in a major educational effort to correct this.

Some last words about antibiotics:

- **Take all of your pills, as directed.** Take all of your medication according to the quantity, frequency, and duration specified in your prescription.
- **Don't save leftover antibiotics.** (If you have taken your prescribed course, you shouldn't have any leftover drug anyway.) For most people, having antibiotics available is just too great a temptation during the next cold.
- **Never share antibiotics with another person.** Rarely will it do them any good. Serious allergic reactions do occur, and you can be held criminally liable for adverse effects experienced by another from your medication.
- **Make sure your physician is aware of all of your previous adverse reactions to antibiotics and other medication.** Allergic reactions are usually a class effect, and you may not recognize all the members in any given drug class.
- **Don't consume antibiotics with products that affect their absorption.** These include multivitamins, zinc, magnesium, calcium, iron, and antacids.
- **Be familiar with expected side effects.** Report significant side effects to your physician.

CHAPTER 6

Pain

Pain is part of our body's alarm system. When something is wrong, it gets our attention. The signals of pain are carried along special neurological pathways. These pathways can be activated by a variety of stimuli—some are specific to the type of sensory receptor at the end of each nerve, such as sensations of pressure or heat, while others are triggered by more general stimuli. The brain constantly receives messages from these pathways. When the messages are loud enough, when enough nerve impulses are received in a certain window of time, pain is perceived.

It is apparent in my practice that individuals vastly differ in how loud the message must be before pain is perceived. Some of my patients have very sensitive alarm triggers—the slightest nuance of bodily function is perceived as painful. Other patients literally have to be hit by a brick before they complain of pain. Psychological and social factors play a great role in the perception of—and response to—pain. I am convinced that many diseases, including irritable bowel, fibromyalgia, and chronic fatigue syndrome, have their primary defect as an unusual, and unfortunate, tendency for the brain to classify normal sensations as painful.

A key concept in pain management is the concept of neurological memory. When a certain neurological circuit is repeatedly activated, it "hardens." More connections between the involved nerves develop, and a memory is made. Efforts to provide prompt and adequate control of pain hope to eliminate the painful signals before a pain pathway is burned into the neurological memory, a pathway that is more easily activated in the future. In making this effort, the management of pain usually involves medications that either affect the perception of pain in the brain and spinal cord or confuse the nerve fibers and block the transmission of painful signals.

Another key concept in pain management is the importance of staying ahead of the wave of pain. In patients with ongoing pain, medication given regularly to prevent pain often is more effective, and results in less overall medication use, than waiting for the pain to be unbearable and then trying to catch up to it.

Aspirin is effective for most types of pain. It is cheap, works rapidly, and is generally well tolerated. It has anti-inflammatory activity, which in addition to relieving pain may diminish the cause of that pain. Many of my patients with arthritis or cancer rely on aspirin for some component of their pain management plan. Unfortunately, aspirin interferes with the function of platelets in the bloodstream, which carries an increased risk of bleeding. Some patients with asthma are sensitive to aspirin and experience a flare in asthma activity related to aspirin exposure. Aspirin can also irritate the lining of the stomach, leading to ulcers and bleeding.

Studies have shown that acetaminophen is as effective as aspirin for pain relief. It may be used alone or in combination with other pain relievers to boost their effect. I have several older patients who are at high risk to take other pain relievers that get satisfactory relief from regular doses of acetaminophen alone for arthritis pain. Acetaminophen is metabolized in the liver and can injure it. The maximum safe dose is 4 grams a day—less in patients with liver disease, those who drink alcohol daily, or when combined with other drugs that affect liver function. Overdose can cause serious or fatal liver injury.

NSAIDs (Nonsteroidal anti-inflammatory medications), like ibuprofen and naproxen, are discussed in detail in *Chapter 25: The Musculoskeletal System*. In general, these drugs seem slightly more effective than aspirin or acetaminophen in relieving pain. For reasons that are not fully understood, patients can differ widely in their response—or lack of response—to drugs in different classes of NSAIDs. Very few side effects are noted from the short-term use of these drugs over 2 to 4 weeks. Long-term use carries a risk of ulceration and bleeding of the gastrointestinal tract, fluid retention, and kidney or liver damage.

Opioids (narcotics) are the most effective drugs for the treatment of severe acute pain and some types of cancer pain. They are often combined with acetaminophen to augment their effect. Patients develop a tolerance to these drugs over time, resulting in a shorter duration of pain relief and an overall decrease in the effectiveness of the drug. Side effects include sedation, nausea and vomiting, and constipation. Opioids are more effective when used regularly to control pain, rather than waiting for pain to return and then trying to catch up to it.

Other therapies are used in pain management. Tricyclic antidepressants play a crucial role in the management of chronic pain. They seem to confuse the small nerve fibers responsible for certain types of pain, such as neuropathy, and decrease or eliminate painful sensations. Certain seizure medications reduce other neuropathic pains, such as trigeminal neuralgia and the lingering pain of shingles. Caffeine enhances the effects of many headache medications. Steroids may relieve pain related to an inflammatory process by reducing the underlying inflammation.

Patients, family members, and physicians alike are concerned about the potential for abuse and dependence on pain medications. In reality, significant physical dependence on narcotics develops only after weeks of the regular use of higher doses. Those who take these medications for the relief of physical pain rarely develop the euphoria that leads to psychological addiction in addicts.

If I do suspect the abuse of a pain-relieving drug, however, I look for the following warning signs:

- Frequent problems with drug prescriptions, including pill bottles that are lost or stolen. (No one ever seems to lose his or her penicillin.)
- An overwhelming focus on pain management after the third office visit. (I can usually have things pretty well managed by then.)

- After hours phone calls for drug refills. We no longer provide refills of narcotics after hours in my practice because of this problem.
- Repeated requests for early refills.
- A need for continued increases in drug dosing to control pain in an otherwise stable disease.
- Patients who see multiple physicians for pain medications. I insist that my patients only get their pain medications from one source.
- Patients who claim multiple drug allergies to all but one desired pain medication.

CHAPTER 7

Smoking

S moking is not the smartest thing that you can do for your health. This should not be news to anyone. However, recent surveys show that 25 percent of the adult U.S. population continues to smoke, including 20 percent of adolescents. Cigarette smoking is a powerfully addicting habit. My success rates in assisting patients with other chemical addictions (alcohol, cocaine, other illicit drugs) are higher than with my patients who smoke, which concerns me greatly.

Effects of Tobacco Smoke

Immediate effects of tobacco smoke include effects on the circulatory and respiratory systems. Tobacco smoke contains chemicals that act as vasoconstrictors, causing the smooth muscle in arteries to contract. This raises blood pressure 5 to 10 points. Some heart attacks are caused by spasm in the smooth muscle in the wall of an artery feeding the heart. When an artery is already narrowed by cholesterol deposits, spasm of the muscle in the artery can shut down the blood supply to a portion of the heart, resulting in heart damage.

In addition to interfering with blood flow, tobacco smoke contains carbon monoxide. Carbon monoxide binds to hemoglobin in a way that prevents hemoglobin from carrying oxygen to the tissues of the body. This carbon monoxide takes several hours to "let go" of the hemoglobin so that normal oxygen carrying capacity can return. Thus, we see a tobacco smoke's dual immediate effect: less blood flows to the tissues because the arteries are narrower than normal, and the blood that does get through has less oxygen to deliver.

Tiny hairs called cilia line the upper respiratory tract. Glands beneath these hairs secrete a thin layer of sticky mucus that is suspended over the ends of the cilia. When this system is functioning normally, the cilia beat in unison like the oars of a boat, sweeping the mucus back from the sinuses and up from the lungs to the throat to be swallowed. Dust, bacteria, viruses, and other particles are caught in the flypaper-like mucus, swept to the gastrointestinal tract, and destroyed by acid in the stomach. Tobacco smoke has three detrimental effects on this system. Chemicals in the smoke paralyze the cilia and cause the mucus to stagnate. The mucus produced becomes thicker, gooier, and harder to expel. Finally, the smoke itself contains lots of particulate debris that sticks to and clogs up the mucus. These effects combine to shut down the body's primary mechanism of sweeping the respiratory tract clean. Because invading organisms are no longer cleared rapidly, more infections occur, smokers' cough develops in an attempt to blast out this gunk, and cancer-causing chemicals that are inhaled (in smoke and other substances) stay in contact with the respiratory lining longer.

Tobacco smoke has other effects. We are learning that many disease processes, as well as aging itself, are promoted through a process called oxidation. In this process, free radicals (molecules that need an extra electron), attack proteins and other chemicals in the body, resulting in damage. The chemicals in tobacco smoke produce many free radicals and adversely affect a variety of organs. Tobacco smoke also contains known cancer-causing substances. Exposure to these carcinogens increases the risk of cancers.

Diseases and Conditions Associated with Tobacco Smoking

Many diseases and conditions—affecting every body system and extending into financial and psychiatric implications—are associated with smoking tobacco, including:

- Cancers of the mouth, upper respiratory tract, larynx, lung, breast, colon, kidney, bladder, pancreas, esophagus
- Skin: wrinkling and premature photoaging
- Eyes: cataracts and macular degeneration
- Nose: sinusitis and loss of smell
- Mouth and throat: sore throats, bad breath, loss of taste, and changes in vocal tone
- Respiratory tract: bronchitis, pneumonia, cough, abnormal airway secretions, chronic obstructive pulmonary disease, and emphysema
- Cardiovascular: atherosclerosis, heart attack, congestive heart failure, hypertension, heart rhythm problems
- Gastrointestinal: increase in acid production, gastroesophageal reflux, and ulcers
- Genitourinary: impotence
- Musculoskeletal: osteoporosis
- Neurological: stroke and vascular dementia
- Financial: Life insurance quotes from a major life insurance company for a $250,000 policy for a 50-year-old male are more than double for smokers as compared with their non-smoking counterparts (broken down monthly, this means $75.68 vs. $33.25).
- Psychiatric: pre-existing disease (you have to be crazy to smoke!)

Benefits when Smokers Quit

When a smoker stops smoking, tobacco's detrimental effects begin to reverse almost immediately, with continued improvement the longer the smoker refrains from smoking. To give you an idea of how these benefits increase with the passage of time, consider the following timeline adapted from the American Cancer Society and the U.S. Surgeon General's reports on smoking:

Within...	A former smoker's...
20 minutes	Blood pressure, heart rate, and temperature in the hands and feet normalize (this occurs as the chemical effects of nicotine wear off)
8 hours	Carbon monoxide level in the bloodstream drops to normal as the oxygen level in the bloodstream increases to normal
24 hours	Chance of heart attack decreases
48 hours	Smell and taste improve and nerve endings start to grow back
2 to 12 weeks	Circulation improves, walking is easier, lung function increases; cough may increase as the cleansing system of the lung begins to function again
1 to 9 months	Cough, sinus congestion, fatigue, and shortness of breath decrease; new cilia grow in airways; ability to eliminate mucus increases; infection rate is reduced; overall energy increases
1 year	Risk of heart disease is one-half that of a continuing smoker
5 years	Lung cancer death rate decreases by 50 percent, as does the death rate for cancers of the mouth, throat, and esophagus
5 to 15 years	Stroke risk is reduced to that of a nonsmoker
10 years	Lung cancer death rate is similar to nonsmokers; precancerous cells in the airway have been replaced by normal tissue; risk of cancer of the mouth, throat, esophagus, bladder, kidney, and pancreas continue to decrease
15 years	Risk of heart disease is now that of a nonsmoker

* Printed with permission from the American Cancer Society

How to Stop Smoking

Ready to stop smoking? Great! Along with my best wishes, I offer these tips:

- Motivation must come from within; no one can do this for you.
- Set a target date to stop smoking and tell everyone what you will be doing.
- Before stopping, switch to a brand of cigarettes that you don't like.
- Draw a line halfway down the cigarette and only smoke to this line. This reduces your tobacco use and adds half a cigarette's worth of tobacco as a filter for smoke to pass through before it reaches you.

- For seven days, keep a diary of when, where, and with what you smoke. Use this to identify your patterns and what circumstances prompt you to smoke. Try to disrupt these associated routines when you stop. If you smoke with coffee, switch to tea; if you smoke with beer, switch to wine; if you smoke on the phone, move its location; if you smoke on the road, switch cars with your spouse or friend for a while.
- When you reach your target date, discard all cigarettes and ashtrays in your home and office.
- Consider a formal tobacco cessation course through the American Cancer Society or the American Lung Association.
- For six weeks, put aside the money that you would have spent smoking, and treat yourself with it.
- If you get the urge to smoke and somehow get a cigarette in your hand, force yourself to wait an additional 15 minutes before lighting it.
- Nicotine replacement options (gums, inhalers, patches) can help break the chemical addiction to tobacco. When you smoke, the nicotine stimulates an addiction center in your brain and satisfies the craving. When you stop smoking, this center screams at you for a cigarette. Nicotine replacement helps quiet this craving. I prefer the 24-hour patches; they provide just enough nicotine to satisfy the craving, but since the nicotine levels in your body are constant when wearing the patch, your brain doesn't see the high and low levels and the addiction doesn't seem to be as reinforced. After several weeks, the patch size is slowly decreased, sneaking the nicotine out of your system without waking the addiction center back up.
- Bupropion (Zyban) is a prescription product available for tobacco cessation. It is a new name for Wellbutrin, a drug available for years for the treatment of depression. It affects norepinephrine (associated with withdrawal symptoms) and dopamine (associated with the rewarding effects of addicting substances) in the brain. When combined with nicotine replacement, Bupropion doubles the short-term success rate for tobacco cessation. Unfortunately, many patients who use this drug resume smoking at a later date. Bupropion does have significant side effects, including seizures in 0.1 percent of users. Use of this drug should be discussed with your doctor.

Alcohol

S tatistics tell me that one in seven of my patients will suffer from an alcohol use disorder at some point in their lives. Ninety percent of Americans drink alcohol. Research suggests that 10 to 20 percent of men and 3 to 10 percent of women either abuse or become dependent on alcohol. Five percent of all deaths in the United States can be directly related to alcohol abuse and dependence. Because of the size of this epidemic, I spend considerable effort trying to identify patients who have problems with alcohol. I routinely ask about drinking habits. I ask patients to specify the type and amount of alcohol that they consume during each physical exam. Despite all of the attention I place on this issue, I suspect that I miss more than 90 percent of the alcohol-related problems in my patients. Alcohol abuse is carefully hidden and denied; most times, the signs are very subtle or non-existent until major complications force their recognition. I wish that I could do a better job in identifying and addressing this condition before these complications occur.

What is Considered "A Drink?"

A drink is equivalent to one 12-ounce beer or wine cooler, one 4-ounce glass of wine, or 1.5 ounces of 80-proof liquor.

Be wary of large wine glasses and shots poured directly from the bottle to the glass; most serving portions are greatly in excess of these "one drink" measurements.

How Much is Too Much?

Moderate drinking is two or fewer drinks a day for a man and one or fewer drinks a day for a woman. You cannot "bank" these quotas for the weekend; each 24 hours starts anew. Because of changes in body composition and metabolism that occur with aging, patients over age 65 are more affected by the same amount of alcohol that they consumed as younger adults. How much they should reduce their consumption is controversial and depends on the individual patient's overall health and the concurrent use of medications that may interact with alcohol.

Heavy drinking means 14 to 20 drinks a week for a man and 7 to 13 drinks a week for a woman. With this frequency, the risk for adverse health consequences starts to rise.

Hazardous drinking means 21 or more drinks a week for a man and 14 or more drinks a week for a woman. Adverse health events become inevitable at this level.

Harmful drinking means drinking at any level (moderate, heavy, or hazardous) where the use of alcohol has actually caused physical or psychological harm.

Alcohol abuse is defined as having one or more of the following alcohol-related problems in the past year: alcohol use that has consistently interfered with work duties or personal obligations, recurrent use in hazardous situations (driving), legal difficulties related to alcohol use, and continued drinking in spite of obvious harm to self or relationships.

Alcohol dependence is defined as having three or more of the following alcohol-related problems in the past year: A need for increased amounts of alcohol to achieve the desired effect, withdrawal symptoms when drinking is interrupted (or drinking alcohol purposefully to avoid these symptoms), unsuccessful attempts to quit or cut down, an inability to control the amount of alcohol consumed in a specified period, a loss of significant leisure or employment activities due to alcohol, or continued drinking despite an awareness of ongoing physical or psychological harm from its use.

The Benefits of Moderate Alcohol Use

Although some acknowledged health benefits are associated with moderate alcohol use, I never encourage patients to drink alcohol for these benefits. It is simply too hard for me to know who the current and potential problem drinkers are. Encouraging a problem drinker to drink alcohol "in moderation" for its health benefits is in my mind akin to instructing a patient who is phobic of handguns to keep a loaded pistol on their bedside to get used to it—just too dangerous.

That said, let's examine these perceived benefits. Several studies suggest that moderate drinkers live longer than those who don't drink at all, primarily due to a reduction in deaths from cardiovascular disease and certain kinds of cancer. There appears to be a narrow therapeutic range of alcohol intake; drinking above the moderate level actually increases the death rate in those same diseases that small amounts of alcohol seemed to help. Several chemical effects of alcohol have been noted to account for its health benefits:

- Alcohol serves as a vasodilator, increasing the size of arteries and improving blood flow.
- Certain alcohols boost the level of HDL ("good") cholesterol.
- Compounds in red wines called *polyphenols* limit the oxidation of LDL ("bad") cholesterol, a process that otherwise would lead to cholesterol deposits and inflammation within the walls of arteries.
- The antioxidants found in some alcohols reduce the growth rate of certain cancer cells.
- Recent studies suggest that women who drink a glass of wine a day have higher bone densities than those who don't.

The Chemistry of Alcohol

Alcohol is broken down by the enzyme alcohol dehydogenase (ADH) into acetaldehyde. This enzyme is present in the liver. It is also present in the lining of the stomach in men in a much greater concentration than in women, which helps explain why men have a greater tolerance to alcohol than women. The enzyme ADH requires other substances to do its job. The depletion of these substances interferes with other chemical processes in the liver that also require them. This can lead to a build-up of lactic acid (causing acidosis, which can suppress heart function and result in irregular heartbeat and changes in brain or muscle function) and uric acid (which causes gout), interfere with the liver's ability to manufacture glucose (leading to hypoglycemia), or interfere with the liver's ability to oxidize fats (leading to fatty accumulation in the liver, causing localized liver damage and dysfunction).

The second chemical in the pathway of alcohol metabolism, acetaldehyde, has noxious properties and is responsible for many of the adverse side effects of alcohol use, including flushing, dizziness, and nausea. Acetaldehyde is broken down into acetate by acetaldehyde dehydrogenase (ALDH). Some ethnic groups have lower levels of ALDH and are therefore more sensitive to these noxious effects of alcohol use.

Medical Problems Related to Alcohol Abuse

Medical problems related to alcohol are caused by the direct effects of alcohol on the different tissues and metabolic processes of the body and the indirect effects of the malnutrition that often accompanies alcohol abuse, including protein malnutrition and vitamin deficiencies. Alcoholics on average live 10 to 12 years less than their non-alcoholic counterparts. One-fourth of all suicides occur in alcoholics; two-thirds of all murders involve the use of alcohol.

Effects on the Brain and Nervous System

In the brain and nervous system, chronic alcohol abuse can affect many parts and functions of the nervous system:

- Cerebellar degeneration, leading to loss of coordination and balance
- Cerebral atrophy, leading to dementia and memory loss
- Frontal lobe dysfunction, leading to emotional and thought disorders
- Neuropathy, causing altered sensations and loss of motor control in the extremities

Alcohol use impairs judgment and coordination. Studies show that an alcohol level of 0.02 will significantly affect driving skills such as steering and response time to sudden changes in driving conditions. Drivers under the influence of small amounts of alcohol knock down more cones on a driving course than drivers who have consumed no alcohol; these drivers were also unable to avoid sudden obstacles in their path. (This effect is intensified when alcohol is mixed with medications that have similar effects, such as common off-the-shelf antihistamines.) Most states don't consider a driver to be driving under the influence of alcohol until his or her alcohol level reaches 0.08, or four times this amount. For reference, the average adult male will have an alcohol level of 0.04 one hour after he drinks two beers.

The effects of alcohol on the brain's chemistry are responsible for its addictive nature. Alcohol causes both release of—and increased sensitivity to—chemical messengers in the brain that are associated with the sensation of pleasure, including dopamine, serotonin, GABA (Gamma-aminobutyric acid), and the opioid peptides. Over time, heavy drinking depletes the brain of these same chemicals. When a drinker stops drinking, these changes in the brain's chemistry produce unpleasant and painful side effects. When the brain runs out of GABA, the electrical activity increases. As the brain becomes more excited, adrenaline-like and steroid hormone-like substances increase, further heightening the unpleasant over-excitation of the brain. In trying to restore its equilibrium, the brain begins to scream at you to take another drink.

Effects on the Gastrointestinal Tract

In the gastrointestinal tract, alcohol effects are most commonly seen in the liver, upper portions of the gastrointestinal tract, and pancreas. The liver becomes choked with fatty deposits resulting from changes in metabolism caused by the liver's attempts to break down alcohol. Alcoholic hepatitis is an acute inflammation of the liver related to the toxic effects of alcohol. Significant alcoholic hepatitis carries a 25 percent risk of death. Symptoms include fever, abdominal pain, jaundice (a yellow color to the skin and whites of the eyes), dark urine, and light colored stools. Cirrhosis refers to the scarring of the liver that can occur over time in 10 to 20 percent of heavy drinkers. As the liver scars it is less able carry out its normal functions. Hypoglycemia can occur as the liver becomes less able to produce glucose while the body is fasting; in addition, the production of blood clotting proteins declines, which increases the risk of bleeding. In a healthy body, almost all blood flow to the intestines passes through the liver to be processed before it returns to the heart. As the liver scars, pressure builds up in the blood circulation between the liver and intestines that leads to dilated veins or "varices" in the lining of the gastrointestinal tract and elsewhere. Bleeding from the rupture of one of these plump varices can be devastating.

Chemical irritation from the effects of alcohol can lead to inflammation of the lining throughout the gastrointestinal tract, including the esophagus, the stomach, and the first part of the small intestine. The inflammation may be associated with ulceration of the wall of the gastrointestinal tract and/or gastrointestinal bleeding. Bleeding from the upper gastrointestinal tract may produce symptoms such as weakness, dizziness with standing, abdominal cramping, and black tarry stools (caused by the bacteria in the gut oxidizing the iron in blood cells, which turns the red blood dark as it flows through the intestines). Forceful vomiting and retching from an inflamed stomach can rip the lining at the juncture of the esophagus and stomach (called a Mallory-Weiss tear), causing heavy internal bleeding.

The pancreas is responsible for two separate functions: the production of insulin to regulate blood sugar and the production of enzymes that aid in the digestion of certain foods. Alcohol abuse is a common cause of pancreatitis, or inflammation of the pancreas. In this condition, the digestive juices stored in the pancreas are activated and released in the pancreatic tissue, prompting the pancreas to try to digest itself. This condition causes severe abdominal pain and vomiting in a very ill patient. Repeated bouts of pancreatitis can destroy the pancreas enough so that it cannot perform its roles, resulting in diabetes and digestive problems.

Chronic diarrhea in alcoholics is common, often relating to protein and vitamin deficiencies, previous pancreatitis, and difficulties in absorbing food in the intestine.

Effects on the Cardiovascular System

Alcohol has negative effects on the cardiovascular system. Heavy drinking (two or more drinks a day in men and one or more drinks a day in women) can significantly elevate blood pressure and interfere with the beneficial effects of blood pressure medications. Alcohol and nutritional deficiencies associated with its use (low potassium and magnesium levels) can lead to serious disturbances in the electrical rhythm of the heart muscle. While small amounts of alcohol seem helpful in raising HDL and preventing heart disease, larger amounts can have a direct toxic effect on heart muscle, leading to a dilated baggy heart that doesn't contract well. Small amounts of alcohol use may reduce the risk for stroke, but larger amounts are associated with an increased risk of hemorrhagic stroke, a particularly deadly form of stroke involving bleeding into the brain. The amount of alcohol consumption in any individual patient that will cross this line between help and harm is impossible to predict.

Effects on Bone Marrow

The bone marrow is affected by alcohol, both through a direct toxic effect of alcohol on the cells that produce new blood cells and other blood components and the indirect effects of vitamin deficiencies associated with alcohol abuse. The production of platelets (components which help form blood clots), white blood cells (infection fighting cells), and red blood cells can fall simultaneously or separately.

Effects on Immune Function

Chronic alcohol use affects immune function. Alcoholics are at higher risk for certain infections and adverse outcomes from those infections. The immune system is also responsible for detection and elimination of cancerous cells. Alcoholics are ten times more likely to develop cancer than the general population. Common cancers in alcoholics include those in the mouth, throat, voice box, esophagus, liver, breast, colon, and rectum. It is felt that these increased cancer rates occur both from alcohol's suppression of the immune system and direct toxic effects of alcohol on tissues that may induce changes leading to more cancerous cells.

Effects on Metabolism and Hormones

Metabolic and hormonal effects of chronic alcohol abuse are numerous. Chronic alcohol abuse is associated with lower testosterone levels, higher estrogen levels, osteoporosis, hypoglycemia, gout, and disturbances in the metabolism of electrolytes such as calcium, magnesium, potassium, and phosphate. Alcohol has a profound effect on reproduction. Women who drink have higher rates of miscarriages and low birth weight babies. Fetal alcohol syndrome, associated with mental and growth retardation, is a devastating consequence of excessive alcohol use during pregnancy. How much alcohol must be consumed to increase the risk for this syndrome is unknown and seems to vary from woman to woman.

Effects on Nutrition

Nutritional deficiencies are common in alcoholics and have significant medical consequences:

- Niacin deficiency, resulting in dermatitis, diarrhea, and dementia
- Thiamine deficiency, resulting in visual disturbance, cranial nerve palsy, and cardiovascular collapse
- Riboflavin deficiency, resulting in dermatitis and mucous membrane (mouth) inflammation
- Folic acid and vitamin B deficiencies, resulting in anemia
- Vitamin C deficiency, resulting in bleeding
- Calcium deficiency, resulting in osteoporosis and muscle dysfunction

Recognizing Alcohol Abuse Disorders

The recognition of an alcohol abuse disorder in a patient, loved one, or associate is not an easy task. Denial by the patient and those around him block recognition of the symptoms. The public regard of alcoholism as a personal failing rather than a medical addiction creates a stigma that prevents many from seeking help for themselves or those they care about. Most chronic alcoholics do stop drinking for extended periods from time to time. The fact that someone can temporarily stop their alcohol intake does not mean that they can control their addiction.

Several researchers and therapists have designed screening tools that use certain key questions to identify signs of alcohol abuse disorders:

- Have you ever felt that you should cut down on your drinking?
- Have people annoyed you by criticizing your drinking?
- Have you ever felt bad or guilty about your drinking?
- Have you ever taken a drink first thing in the morning to steady your nerves or get rid of a hangover?
- Does it take more than three drinks to make you feel high?

These questions are simply screening tools. A single "yes" answer should prompt further discussion with your physician.

Other signs of alcohol abuse disorders include the following:

- Drinking alone
- Starting alcohol intake early in the day
- Periodically quitting drinking, or purposefully switching the type of alcohol consumed
- A history of accidents and marital and work conflicts
- Violence and abuse of spouse and children
- A preoccupation with drinking
- Little control over the quantity or duration of drinking episodes
- The development of tolerance to the effects of alcohol
- Blackouts and hangovers after drinking
- Continued drinking despite a recognition of current problems associated with it
- Experiencing alcohol withdrawal symptoms after a period of abstinence
- A family history of alcohol abuse
- Problem drinking which begins in adolescence
- A history of anxiety or depression with attempts to self-medicate through alcohol
- Impulsive, excitable, novelty-seeking personalities

Alcohol Withdrawal

As I mentioned, alcohol's general effect is to inhibit brain activity; when the regular consumption of alcohol is suddenly stopped, the brain becomes overexcited. This leads to many of the symptoms of alcohol withdrawal: fever, accelerated heart rate, blood pressure fluctuations, aggressive behavior, hallucinations, seizures, and delirium tremens.

Heavy drinkers who suddenly stop drinking may experience withdrawal symptoms. This includes generalized trembling 8 to 24 hours after the last drink, followed by hallucinations 24 hours after the last drink. Alcoholics in withdrawal often talk back to their hallucinations and become agitated. Up to 20 percent of these people experience seizures from the surge of brain excitement in alcohol withdrawal.

The syndrome of delirium tremens is a life-threatening complication of chronic alcohol abuse associated with a 20 percent mortality rate. This syndrome may occur on average one to three days after a person abruptly ceases his or her alcohol intake. Patients experiencing this syndrome are hyperactive, tremulous, combative, disoriented, and confused. Activation of the autonomic nervous system produces dilated pupils, sweating, increase in heart rate and breathing, and fever. Repetitive seizures may occur. Delirium tremens is a medical emergency, and may last from one to six days.

Treatment of the above conditions primarily includes supportive medical care including monitoring, correcting fluid and electrolyte imbalances, and treating seizures. Medications such as benzodiazepines are commonly prescribed to lessen the activity of the central nervous system.

Treatment of Alcohol Abuse Disorders

The goal for treatment of a patient with an alcohol abuse disorder is total abstinence—the complete cessation of alcohol use and the lifestyle associated with it. Of all people treated for an alcohol abuse disorder, 80 to 90 percent will relapse. Relapse is more common in patients who are frustrated or angry, who have social pressures to drink ("All my friendships center around drinking."), who are exposed to temptation, and who are deprived of sleep for any reason. Thus treatment of the patient with an alcohol abuse disorder must include a plan for long-term follow-up and support to promote recovery from the relapses.

To help a person with an alcohol abuse disorder recognize the need for treatment and remain willing to pursue treatment, his or her family, friends, and professional associates must strongly and consistently offer their support and encouragement. Members of this supportive team must be aware of the local resources that exist to help this person address his or her addiction and be prepared to participate in formal, moderated intervention sessions with that person. Inpatient treatment may be suggested for patients with coexisting medical or psychiatric problems, those at risk of harming themselves or others, those with a disruptive home environment, or those who have failed other approaches. Other community-based programs, such as the 12-step program through Alcoholics Anonymous, offer a strong network of support in a well-established framework of care.

Medications are currently available and on the horizon to address alcohol abuse disorders, including:

- Opioid antagonists such as naltrixone reduce the intoxicating effects of alcohol and the urge to drink.
- Aversion medications, such as disulfiram, interact with alcohol to produce distressing side effects if alcohol is consumed, such as flushing, headaches, and gastrointestinal distress.
- Newer medical approaches are addressing the chemical messengers in the brain relayed to alcohol addiction, such as GABA, dopamine, serotonin, and norepinephrine. These may offer novel approaches to the treatment and prevention of alcohol abuse disorders in the future.

CHAPTER 9

Cancer

Life begins as a single cell. This cell contains 26 chromosomes, which include all of the needed information for the cell to grow, multiply, and eventually differentiate—that is, become specialized to the functions and shapes of various body parts. Some cells become eye cells, some become heart cells, and some become toenails; however, they all started from the same cell. They do this by turning on or off portions of the chromosomes (genes) that instruct the cell how to develop. The fact that the billions of cells can do this correctly in the formation of a human body is nothing short of miraculous.

Once the body is formed, this process doesn't stop. Most cells have a limited life span and must renew themselves, replacing themselves with exact copies. The selected information encoded on the chromosomes is again used to perform this feat. Some cells, such as stem cells in the bone marrow, retain the ability to make many different types of cells. Other cells, such as skin cells, are fully differentiated into their special function and can only form new skin cells.

When cells make copies, mistakes happen. Imagine trying to match up tens of thousands of chemicals correctly every time over a life span of 75 years. There is a role for mistakes; this is how the evolution of a species occurs. The chemical duplicating machinery of some viruses makes millions of mistakes each generation on purpose in the hope of the random chance of making a new virus that is better, stronger, or more resistant to the attacks of the host's immune system. Changes in the eagle's eye helped it to better see prey on the desert floor; changes in muscle made a kangaroo's hind legs stronger; changes in humans help make a brilliant scientist, a talented musician, or a skilled athlete.

Some mistakes lead to cancer. If the error involves a gene coding for differentiation, the new cell may not precisely resemble its source. If the error involves a gene coding for growth, the new cell may grow more rapidly or spread from its initial location. If this cell looks different enough, divides fast enough, and ignores the signals from those around it, a cancer is formed.

Most times, the body's immune system looks for cells that have made these programming errors and destroys them. Cancer occurs when this surveillance system fails. This may happen when the new cell looks enough like the old cell that the immune system does not recognize it as different or when the immune system itself has failed in its function.

Many factors play a role in this process. There are inherited tendencies for certain tissues to make more mistakes, perhaps explaining the increase in breast and colon cancer in those patients whose relatives have had the disease. Aging plays a role, probably because more cell divisions have occurred over time—which increases the cumulative number of mistakes—and because the immune system's surveillance function does not work as well. Environment clearly plays a role in causing tissue damage and genetic changes, such as demonstrated in the relationship between tobacco smoke and lung cancer. Some viruses attack cells and become part of the chromosomes, disrupting the information encoded there and promoting cancer.

Most cancerous tissues' cells divide faster than normal cells because of a change in the cells' ability to regulate growth. Many cancer therapies take advantage of this fact. Radiation therapy and some chemotherapy simply kill dividing cells; since cancer cells divide more often than regular cells, the chemotherapy causes more selective damage to the cancer. This also explains many side effects of cancer chemotherapies, particularly their toxic effects on normal cells that divide rapidly, such as those that produce hair or those that line the gastrointestinal tract.

Recent chemotherapies have become more tissue selective. All cells have proteins on their surface that serve as identification and often function as holes or passageways into the cell. Chemotherapeutic agents can be designed that seek out particular surface proteins on the cancer cells, entering and limiting their damage to them.

A cure for cancer? This will be difficult. Cancer is a process that is somewhat different in each patient because of his or her individual makeup and biology. The greatest hope for the next generation of cancer therapies lies in a better understanding of the process of cell differentiation, how to turn on and off select portions of DNA within cancer cells, and how to get the immune cells to recognize and destroy cancerous tissue.

Approach to Evaluating and Treating Cancer

Each cancer may go through several stages: 1) *initiation*, where the initial tissue damage and genetic changes occur; 2) *precancer*, where the tissue is abnormal but not cancerous (such as dysplasia on a Pap smear); and 3) *clinical* or *invasive* cancer.

Five Most Common Causes of Cancer Deaths

According to data from the American Cancer society in 2001, the five most common causes of cancer death in the United States were:
1. Lung (158,500 deaths)
2. Colorectal (57,200 deaths)
3. Breast (40,600 deaths)
4. Prostate (31,500 deaths)
5. Pancreas (28,900 deaths)

Medical evaluation of cancer involves:

1   Diagnosis (finding the cancer and determining its type)
2   Staging (determining how far it has spread)
3   Local and regional control (evaluating whether it can be removed, killed, or slowed down)
4   Systemic adjuvant therapy (seeking therapies that can be given to the entire body to promote healing or prevent relapse)

Therapeutic plans must balance toxic effects on the body with effectiveness in eradicating the cancer, quality of life versus chance for cure. This requires a close, collaborative working relationship with the patient's personal physician, a team of cancer specialists, and an understanding of the patient's values and priorities. Specific cancer therapies are beyond the scope of this book.

Screening for Cancer

To understand various screening techniques for cancer, it is important to keep in mind the following timeline:

HEALTH

Health is the disease free state.

INITIATION

Initiation is when the process of change to cancerous tissue begins.

DIAGNOSIS by SCREENING

Diagnosis by screening is when a diagnostic test (screening test) is able to find the cancer.

DIAGNOSIS by SYMPTOMS

Diagnosis by symptoms is when the cancer would become obvious by noticeable changes in the patient.

OUTCOME

Outcome refers to death or organ loss from the cancer.

At some point along this timeline, each cancer reaches a point of irreversibility (PI), where the outcome is inevitable regardless of what treatment is given. This point is very important. If the PI occurs soon after initiation, then screening does not affect outcome and is of no benefit. (It doesn't often help to find a cancer earlier if there is no effective treatment for it.) If the PI occurs between when the diagnosis can be made by screening and when symptoms would be expected, then screening may be the only way to detect the disease in time to make a difference. Waiting for symptoms would be too late. If the PI occurs well after symptoms occur, then screening may not offer any benefit to the patient; we could wait for symptoms and treat it then.

Primary prevention includes avoiding the initiation of cancer. This can involve changes in lifestyles to avoid cancer-associated habits and exposures (smoking cessation or reduction of occupational exposures to cancer-causing chemicals) or chemoprevention, the use of chemicals to reduce cancer risks (for example, vitamin A to reduce head and neck cancer recurrences, oral contraceptives to reduce ovarian cancer, synthetic estrogen receptor modulators to reduce breast cancer, and aspirin to reduce colon cancer).

Deciding to screen for a disease requires several considerations:

- Is the condition worth screening for? That is, how severe is the medical condition in regard to mortality or suffering, and does an effective treatment exist if the condition is found early?
- How should the screening be conducted? If the test is to be applied to a large number of people it must be simple, of reasonable cost, very safe, and acceptable to patients and doctors.
- The test must do what we are asking of it—that is, finding the condition in a reliable way.

Screening for Skin Cancer

Skin cancer is screened for by visual examination, noting the asymmetry of the lesion, whether its border is irregular, and the color and size of the lesion.

Self-exams are useful; most of my patients identify their own skin cancers. Physician exams should occur with the periodic physical. Patients with risks for skin cancer (a previous skin cancer, fair complexion, a history of heavy sun exposure, or a family history of skin cancer) should be followed more closely.

See *Skin Cancer* on page 118 for more information about the different types of skin lesions that may turn cancerous.

Screening for Mouth Cancer

Most mouth cancers occur in smokers, oral tobacco users, and those with a history of alcohol abuse. They appear as a sore, irritation, or white patch that does not heal with time. Regular dental checkups are effective screening tools.

Screening for Lung Cancer

Lung cancer is the most common cause of cancer death. Large trials of routine chest x-rays in smokers have been conducted and showed no survival advantage of screening chest x-rays. Frequently, by the time a lung cancer is big enough to see on a chest x-ray, it often has already spread. The lack of effective treatment for many lung cancers also reduces the benefit of screening. Additionally, there is the concern that smokers who are told that they have a normal chest x-ray may be falsely reassured and have less motivation to stop smoking.

A study published in the July 1999 issue of *The Lancet* investigated the use of special screening CT (computed tomography) scans for the detection of lung cancer in high-risk individuals. These were patients 60 years of age or older who had smoked 1 pack per day or more for at least 10 years (referred to as having a "10 pack year history"), or patients 50 years or older with a 20 to 30 pack year history. The CT scanning techniques were more effective in detecting early lung cancers in time for a surgical cure. Well-designed studies and trials are needed to confirm the findings of these early reports.

Screening for Breast Cancer

I recommend annual mammograms for all my female patients age 40 and above.

Although excellent data exists to support the recommendation for those 50 and above, fewer facts are available to guide physicians in advising women ages 40 to 50. We do encourage women with a personal or family history of breast cancer to start annual mammograms sooner. Physicians have dropped the recommendation for women age 35 to have a baseline mammogram; we have learned that younger breasts are denser and the views we obtain are often unsatisfactory with current techniques. Furthermore, under the older recommendations, the burden on younger women of investigating suspicious mammograms at this age (additional studies, biopsies, and breast surgeries) did not appear justified by the number of cancers found. Finally, breast cancer in younger women seems to be biologically more aggressive, and mammograms didn't clearly affect the death rate.

Adult women of all ages should examine their own breasts monthly and have their physician examine them during their annual gynecological visit. Though the data regarding the effectiveness of such exams is somewhat sketchy, these exams are low cost, safe, and acceptable to most patients.

Screening for Gastrointestinal Cancer

CANCER OF THE ESOPHAGUS

Much cancer of the esophagus is related to the effects of smoking and alcohol abuse. Screening tests traditionally have not been effective and—as discussed in *Screening for Lung Cancer* on page 53—the disease usually becomes apparent beyond the point of irreversibility.

Recently, a new appreciation has grown of the relationship between the chronic reflux of stomach acid into the esophagus and esophageal cancer. Chronic acid reflux can cause precancerous changes to the lining of the esophagus, called *Barrett's esophagus*. Studies by Swedish researchers in patients with chronic acid reflux showed that patients who had symptoms at least once a week had 8 times the normal risk for esophageal cancer, 11 times if reflux occurred at night. If patients experienced symptoms of reflux longer than 20 years, their risk was increased 44 times. Barrett's esophagus can be detected by examination of the esophagus through a lighted fiberoptic tube called an endoscope. This requires sedation and is done in an outpatient setting. Endoscopy should be considered for anyone who has daily heartburn despite treatment for greater than one month, heartburn at least two times a week for one year, or heartburn once a week for five years. Caucasian males over 40 are at additional risk for esophageal cancer.

CANCER OF THE PANCREAS

Despite pancreatic cancer being the number five cause of cancer death in the United States, there are no effective screening techniques for it at this time.

CANCER OF THE COLON

Screening for colorectal cancer is more effective than that of most other cancers. Most patients who get screened and follow through on results essentially eliminate their chance of dying with this cancer. The lifetime risk for colon cancer is 6 percent. If a family member had colon cancer after age 50, the lifetime risk for other family members is 12 percent; before age 50, the risk for other family members rises to greater than 20 percent. Colon cancer screening is one of the few techniques that both prevent and detect cancer; this technique both detects and removes intestinal polyps—tiny mushroom-like growths on the inside of the colon that are precursors of colon cancer.

I follow the current screening options as outlined by the American Cancer Society, American Gastroenterology, and the United States Preventive Services Task Force. These options are discussed in more detail in *Chapter 23: The Gastrointestinal System* on page 217.

- Patients should see their physicians annually for a digital rectal examination. During this exam, the physician will insert his or her finger into the rectum and feel for polyps or unusual growths. In addition, patients should seek one of the following:
  — Annual fecal occult blood test to detect microscopic traces of blood in the stool and—every five years—a flexible sigmoidoscopy. This remains the only method of screening backed by research showing a reduction in total deaths from colorectal cancer by two-thirds.
  — A complete colonoscopy at age 50, repeated—if normal—every ten years. Polyps are thought to take 10 to 15 years to develop and turn cancerous.

Colonoscopy is a more thorough test than flexible sigmoidoscopy—the flexible sigmoidoscope inspects the lower half of the colon, where roughly half of cancer begins, while the colonoscope is capable of reaching the entire colon. However, colonoscopy has a higher rate of complications, including bleeding and perforation of the colon. Some insurance companies are less likely to pay for screening colonoscopy in patients who are not at high risk for cancer. The procedure requires referral to a gastroenterologist, is done in the hospital's outpatient setting, and requires a 24-hour preparation of a liquid diet plus repeated laxatives. Intravenous sedation is needed. Flexible sigmoidoscopy can be done in the physician's office, requires minimum preparation and no sedation, and is less than one-tenth the cost of a colonoscopy.

- Patients at high risk of cancer because of family history or a personal history of previous polyps require special consideration in screening and should discuss this with their doctor. In those with a family history, screening should begin at least ten years before the age of the youngest family member diagnosed with colorectal cancer. If a mother, father, sister, or brother had colon cancer, I would recommend the first colonoscopy by age 40.

(The recommendations for colorectal cancer screening from the U.S. Preventive Services Task Force were published in the July 2002 issue of the *Annals of Internal Medicine*. These recommendations provided additional validation that either the flexible sigmoidoscopy and stool occult blood testing approach or the colonoscopy approach to colorectal cancer screening is acceptable. In the summary of recommendations, the authors stated, "It is unclear whether the increased accuracy of colonoscopy compared with alternative screening methods... offsets the procedure's additional complications, inconvenience, and cost.").

Screening for Urinary Tract Cancer

Accepted guidelines do not yet exist for the detection of cancers of the urinary tract (kidneys, ureters, and bladder). These are usually discovered as blood in the urine noticed by the patient or during a routine laboratory examination.

Screening for Reproductive Organ Cancer

CANCER OF THE CERVIX

Most cases of cervical cancer are related to infection with the human papilloma virus (HPV), which is sexually transmitted. The Pap smear examines cells from the surface of the cervix for abnormalities that may suggest precancerous changes. Pap smears should begin in all women at age 18 or at the onset of sexual activity, whichever comes first. After two normal Pap smears one year apart, Pap smears are advised every one to three years based on the discretion of the woman and her physician.

CANCER OF THE UTERUS

Physicians who detect abnormalities while feeling (palpating) the uterus during a pelvic examination and who evaluate abnormal bleeding patterns may order further screening tests for uterine cancer. These tests include endometrial biopsies (an in-office procedure somewhat similar to a Pap smear) and ultrasound images of the thickness of the lining of the uterus.

CANCER OF THE OVARIES

No accepted screening tests currently exist for the early diagnosis of ovarian cancer. Palpation of the ovaries during pelvic examination has proven ineffective in the early detection of ovarian cancer. Some ovarian cancers are associated with high levels of the protein CA-125. Monitoring the blood concentration of the CA-125 protein has proven effective in evaluating patients with a known history of ovarian cancer to measure their response to therapy or monitor them for recurrence. It has not proven effective as a screening test for the early detection of ovarian cancer in patients not previously known to have it. Many other benign processes can cause the CA-125 level to rise significantly. Any attempt to use CA-125 levels to screen a large number of asymptomatic women for ovarian cancer would detect a number of women with elevated CA-125 levels who didn't really have ovarian cancer, but would now need to go through a variety of other procedures (such as surgical removal of the ovaries), including their costs and complications, to prove that the blood test was wrong. Current studies show that the benefit of CA-125 testing in screening the general adult female population is outweighed by the cost and complications of the secondary testing required on women who really didn't have ovarian cancer after all. Special protocols are available for high-risk women with certain genetic syndromes or strong family histories of ovarian cancer.

CANCER OF THE TESTICLES

Testicular cancer occurs most commonly in men ages 15 to 30, though it can occur at any age. Men in the at-risk age group should perform testicular self-examinations monthly, with periodic examinations performed by their physician.

CANCER OF THE PROSTATE

I recommend that all my male patients have an annual rectal/prostate exam beginning at age 40 and an annual prostate-specific antigen (PSA) blood test beginning at age 50. Exceptions would include patients with advanced age or other diseases who do not have a reasonable chance of living another ten years or high-risk patients—including African American men and men with a family history of prostate cancer—should start PSA testing earlier. These recommendations are controversial; for further discussion of prostate cancer, see the *Prostate Cancer* section in *Chapter 27: Men's Health Issues.*

CHAPTER 10

Vaccinations and Associated Diseases

Vaccinations are tools to prime the immune system to respond faster to certain infections. This is accomplished by exposing the body to a piece of the infectious organism (such as part of the outer shell of the pneumococcal bacteria) or a weak or inactivated form of the organism (such as that found in the flu vaccine). The immune system then develops a memory for this organism and attacks it much more quickly if re-exposed. This attack can eliminate the organism before an infection develops or result in a much less serious form of the infection if it occurs. This chapter describes the diseases for which vaccinations prove beneficial and discusses when vaccinations are indicated.

> **For more information about diseases for which you might be at risk while traveling, and possible vaccinations that might be available to prevent them, see *Chapter 11, Travel Health*.**

Dead or Synthetic Vaccines

Some vaccines are created using dead infectious organisms, inert portions of the organism, or synthetic materials modeled after the organism. These include the Pneumococcal pneumonia, influenza, tetanus–diphtheria, hepatitis, meningococcal meningitis, and Lyme disease vaccines.

Pneumovax Vaccine

Pneumonia is an infectious disease of the lungs that is usually caused by viruses or bacteria. Pneumococcal pneumonia is a serious type of pneumonia that kills thousands of people in the United States each year. *Pneumococcal pneumonia* spreads relatively quickly to the bloodstream, a condition called *bacteremia*. Five out of every 100 people with Pneumococcal pneumonia die despite appropriate antibiotic therapy. The risk is doubled in those with a history of alcoholism, certain heart or lung diseases, kidney failure, diabetes, and some cancers. Of those over age 65 that get pneumococcal pneumonia, 20 to 30 percent develop bacteremia; 20 percent of those with bacteremia die, even with antibiotics.

Increased resistance of this type of pneumonia to antibiotic therapy has made the treatment of pneumococcal pneumonia much more difficult, increasing the importance of vaccination against it. Pneumovax is a vaccine made from part of the shell of the bacteria. It does not contain the whole bacteria and cannot cause infection. The present vaccination covers 23 different types of the pneumococci that account for 85 to 90 percent of illness. While the vaccination doesn't eliminate the chance of pneumonia, it does reduce the rate of infection, bacteremia, and death. The vaccine is up to 80 percent effective in preventing pneumococcal bacteremia.

Current guidelines recommend Pneumovax for all patients age 65 and older and also younger patients with chronic illness such as heart or lung disease, diabetes, or a weak immune system (those with kidney disease, cancer, or other diseases). Some doctors recommend use of this vaccine for any patient over the age of 50. This sounds like a reasonable recommendation to me. Side effects are minor and include swelling and soreness at the injection site. Less than 1 percent of patients experience fever or a muscular pain after the vaccine. Revaccination is usually recommended after five to seven years.

Influenza Vaccine

Influenza ("the flu") is a viral infection of the respiratory tract caused by the influenza virus. It occurs in epidemics in winter months, peaking between December and early March in the United States. It is spread by airborne transmission, such as sneezing, which produces microscopic droplets that suspend in the air and are breathed in by the next victim. Symptoms include headache, fever, chills, muscle aches, and coughing. Most patients simply feel miserable. Influenza typically has an abrupt beginning and lasts about a week.

The influenza vaccine is made from inactivated virus grown in chicken eggs. Each year, vaccine developers examine strains of virus prevalent in other portions of the world and make a new vaccine based on the best guess of what flu strains will affect the United States the following season. The flu shot begins to provide protection one to two weeks after injection. The protection begins to drop off four to six months after vaccination.

Flu vaccinations are recommended annually for all patients 65 and older. I advise them for all patients over 50. Flu shots should also be given to other high-risk patients and their close contacts that could bring the influenza virus to them. High-risk patients include:

- Residents of nursing homes and other chronic care facilities
- Patients with chronic lung or heart disease
- Patients infected with HIV
- Patients that require regular medical attention due to chronic metabolic diseases (diabetes), kidney failure, sickle cell anemia, or the use of drugs that suppress the immune system
- Children and teenagers on long-term aspirin therapy

- Women who will be in their second or third trimester of pregnancy during flu season
- Travelers
- Any person wishing to reduce their likelihood of becoming ill with influenza.

Health-care personnel are vaccinated given their heavy exposure to influenza during flu season and their compromised productivity if this disease were transmitted to them.

All other individuals should consider a flu vaccination. Vaccination of healthy working adults has been shown to reduce absenteeism. Vaccinations are particularly important in persons who live in close quarters where flu is passed rapidly, such as college dorms, military barracks, or other institutional settings.

The flu vaccine *cannot* cause influenza. This is a common misconception. The flu vaccine can cause soreness at the injection site. Fever, muscle aches, and fatigue may occur for one or two days, usually in those with no previous exposure to influenza. People who should *not* receive the flu vaccine include those with a history of a severe reaction to eggs, a history of a hypersensitivity reaction to previous flu vaccines, or an illness with fever at the time of vaccination. Vaccination is 70 to 90 percent effective in healthy, young adults and less effective in the elderly and those with compromised immune systems.

Tetanus–Diphtheria Vaccine

Tetanus is a disease that is acquired from contaminated wounds. *Diphtheria* is a respiratory disease that is transmitted from person to person; diphtheria epidemics have occurred in Eastern Europe the past few years. Tetanus and diphtheria vaccinations cover these different and unrelated diseases. They are given together since they follow the same dosing schedule: a primary series of at least three injections and booster shots every ten years. Patients commonly experience local soreness at the injection site for one or two days; other side effects are rare. It is especially important to update this vaccination before travel to remote areas, where medical assistance may not be close by.

Hepatitis Vaccines

Hepatitis is a viral infection of the liver and is classified into types. The most common types are hepatitis A and hepatitis B. Hepatitis B was identified in the 1960s; it is transmitted by blood and body fluids from person to person, including sexual transmission (responsible for at least 50 percent of cases), shared infected needles (drug addiction, tattooing, or body piercing without proper sterilization of equipment), or infected blood. Hepatitis A was identified in the 1980s; it is transmitted from person to person by ingestion of contaminated food or bodily secretions. It is present in shellfish from contaminated waters and found in areas of poor sanitation where the food or water supply can be contaminated by human waste, including child day-care centers and throughout third-world countries. Many other types of hepatitis exist, but only A and B have vaccines at this time.

HEPATITIS B VACCINE

The Hepatitis B vaccine is given as a series of three injections over six months. Most people tolerate it well, rarely experiencing significant side effects other than local irritation. The hepatitis B vaccine is currently part of the routine childhood immunization series. It is also recommended for patients at risk for hepatitis B, including:

- Heterosexuals with greater than one sexual partner in the past six months
- Men who have sex with men
- People with a sexually transmitted disease or who have ever had a sexually transmitted disease
- Sex partners and household contacts of those with hepatitis B
- Illicit drug users and sex partners of illicit drug users
- Health-care and emergency response personnel with risk of blood exposure

It is currently unknown whether booster shots are required over time to retain protective immunity.

HEPATITIS A VACCINE

The hepatitis A vaccine is given as two injections, six months apart. The first vaccination provides protection within two weeks of administration; the second is felt to help promote long-term immunity. The hepatitis A vaccine is recommended for persons traveling to or working in countries with a high rate of hepatitis A, children in communities with a high rate of hepatitis A, men who have sex with men, illicit drug users, and those with chronic liver disease such as hepatitis C—another type of viral hepatitis often associated with chronic infections (see *Chapter 23: The Gastrointestinal System* on page 201 for more information). Travelers going outside of the United States, Western Europe, Canada, Australia, or Japan should receive hepatitis A vaccinations.

Meningococcal Vaccine

This vaccination protects against meningococcal meningitis. This disease begins as a flu-like illness that progresses rapidly to a life-threatening illness. Tourists traveling to areas where epidemics are occurring should receive this vaccination. Although typically found abroad, a few outbreaks of this disease have recently occurred in college campuses in the U.S., so vaccination is also a good idea for college students who live in dorms where diseases are easily spread. Approximately 175 cases of meningococcal meningitis occur per year, with 15 to 20 deaths. Meningococcal meningitis is highly contagious. Three primary types of the meningococcal bacteria have been identified; unfortunately, the current vaccination only covers types A and C, not type B, and therefore misses about 30 percent of serotypes of meningococci. The vaccination is felt to provide protective immunity for at least three years.

Lyme Disease Vaccine

As of February 25, 2002 the manufacturer of the Lyme disease vaccine (LYMErix by GlaxoSmithKline) announced that the vaccine would no longer be available. Their application to market a pediatric version of the vaccine was withdrawn, and apparently all funded research at the company for Lyme disease vaccine development has been halted. The given reason for pulling the vaccine was economic: high costs and poor sales. The following information about Lyme disease and the previous vaccine is supplied for reference.

Lyme disease is transmitted by infected ticks. Greater than 90 percent of cases occur in the Northeast, Middle Atlantic area, and upper Midwest. People who live and work in grassy or wooded areas where exposure to ticks is common are at risk for this disease.

Lyme disease usually appears as a reddish skin lesion where the tick was attached, 3 to 30 days after the tick bite. This lesion expands slowly over days to weeks and may develop some central clearing (giving it the classic appearance of a "bull's eye" or target). Most studies suggest that the tick must be attached for greater than 12 hours to transmit this disease. People who notice a skin lesion may also experience flu-like symptoms, headache, and enlarged lymph nodes. Antibiotics cure 90 percent of Lyme disease if it is recognized and treated early. If the disease is not detected or treated in time, late effects of the disease involve problems with the musculoskeletal system, brain, and heart.

The vaccination was made from recombinant surface proteins and did not involve use of the infectious organism. This vaccine was given as a series of three injections over 6 or 12 months. It has been shown to be 76 percent effective in preventing Lyme disease. Side effects include soreness at the injection site, muscle pain, and flu-like symptoms. The long-term safety of this vaccine has not been evaluated, and the length of protection provided by the vaccination is also unknown.

Live Vaccines

Three vaccinations involve the use of live viruses that have been weakened so as not to cause infection in most individuals. These include the MMR (measles, mumps, and rubella), the OPV (oral polio), and the Varicella (chicken pox) vaccines.

Measles, Mumps, Rubella (MMR)

Adults born in 1957 or later should receive a first dose after their first birthday. Adults born before 1957 most likely had these diseases and do not need vaccination. A second dose is given for high-risk persons, such as health-care workers, college students, or international travelers. This vaccination cannot be given to a woman who is pregnant or plans to become pregnant within three months, or to certain patients with compromised immune systems.

Polio

For adults, controversy exists as to whether the risk of vaccine related polio is higher than the risk of acquiring the disease by exposure to an infected source. The oral vaccine (OPV) is a live vaccine, carrying a risk of polio and associated paralysis in one case per 2.6 million doses in those receiving the vaccine or their household contacts. The injected vaccine (IPV) is made from inactivated virus and does not carry this risk. Those patients considering the polio vaccine should discuss it with their doctor.

Varicella

The chicken pox vaccine is now routinely given as part of the childhood vaccination series. It can also be offered to adults who have no history of chicken pox and negative blood test for antibodies to chicken pox. Current research is evaluating whether giving the chicken pox vaccine as a booster at age 50 or 60 will reduce the risk for shingles, the late complication of this infection.

CHAPTER 11

Travel Health

International travel has certainly become more commonplace among my patients, and with it has come exposure to a variety of adverse health circumstances and exotic diseases. This chapter will relate some common sense recommendations for international travelers and outline the basic vaccinations frequently needed.

Studies show that 1 to 5 percent of international travelers must seek medical attention during their trip, some with serious enough problems to need medical evacuation. Most deaths from international travel are from cardiovascular disease (heart attack and stroke). Second—at 25 percent of deaths—is trauma, which is the leading cause of the death and disability for younger travelers. Infectious diseases are more likely to cause misery than death, but are a risk.

Most international travel involves commercial airline flights at high altitudes. Despite the partial cabin pressurization, the atmospheric pressure in airplane cabins on international flights is similar to that at 10,000 feet in the mountains. Oxygen levels fall considerably at this pressure, and patients with pre-existing lung or heart disease may not be able to extract enough oxygen from the cabin air for safe travel. Patients with heart or lung disease who are planning flights should discuss this problem with their doctor and make appropriate arrangements.

Travelers planning international travel should see their doctor at least two months before the trip to discuss needed vaccinations and other health precautions. Many vaccinations take weeks until they protect the body from disease and the trip to the doctor should take early priority in vacation planning. A pre-trip physical and dental checkup should be considered if you are due for these examinations or if your trip is exotic or prolonged. Medical attention should be sought after the trip if any flu-like or other unusual symptoms develop.

Tips for Staying Healthy while Traveling

- **Avoid unprotected sex.** Realize that condoms frequently fail. HIV, hepatitis B, and other sexually transmitted diseases occur frequently in high-risk populations overseas. These are not souvenirs that you wish to bring home.

- **Avoid mosquito bites.** Mosquitoes frequently transmit exotic diseases. Wear protective clothing that minimizes skin exposure and use extreme caution at dawn and dusk when mosquitoes are most active. Sleep safe with either mosquito netting or in an appropriate environment. Use insect repellent with 30 percent or greater DEET.
- **Wear shoes.** Many tropical parasitic diseases are transmitted through tiny puncture wounds in the soles of the feet.
- **Avoid swimming in non-chlorinated fresh water.** Non-chlorinated fresh water in tropical regions of the world may contain parasites. These organisms can enter the body of a swimmer through the ears, eyes, nose, mouth, genitals, anus, or other breaks in the skin and cause disease. When traveling in these regions, it is wise to swim only in salt water or treated water and not rivers, lakes, or other enclosed bodies of water.
- **Take precautions when preparing food and water.** Adopt the mantra "Cook it, peel it, boil it, or forget it." Avoid tap water, including ice cubes made from tap water; drink only purified, treated water instead. Do not eat food offered by street vendors; these vendors face too many challenges in keeping their areas clean and their food at proper temperatures. Eat well-cooked food that is served hot. Avoid raw fruits unless you peel them yourself. Be especially cautious with lettuce and other vegetables that may have been rinsed in contaminated water. The fact that residents can eat or drink local food or water does not imply that you can; they may have built up tolerance or immunity over time.
- **Avoid excessive physical activity in areas of heavy air pollution.** Inhaling polluted air at the volume and rate required during exertion exposes you unnecessarily to breathing-related problems.
- **Take care on the road.** Avoid driving at night. Wear seat belts. Avoid mopeds and motorcycles; many serious travel-related injuries involve them. Do you really want to be driving at high speed with no protection around you in a country where traffic laws are non-existent and the blood transfusion supply for those with serious injuries is questionable at best?
- **Avoid skin-perforating procedures.** Wait until you get home before you go to an acupuncturist, pierce anything, get a tattoo, or have blood drawn.
- **Avoid dehydration.** Drink enough fluid.
- **Be familiar with your medical insurance coverage overseas.** Purchase additional insurance if you need it. (Medicare provides no coverage outside the United States.)
- **Be informed about political and criminal problem areas in your planned travel regions.** Investigate the consular section of the government web site **http://travel.state.gov** for up-to-date information.
- **Pack a travel medicine kit.** See *What Should a Travel Medicine Kit Include?* for a list of prescription and nonprescription items to pack.

What Should a Travel Medicine Kit Include?

Nonprescription items:
- Pain killer (ibuprofen or acetaminophen)
- Antibiotic ointment or cream
- Bandages, gauze pads, mole skin for blisters
- Oral thermometer
- Insect repellent with 30 percent or greater DEET
- Sunscreen with an SPF of 30 or greater
- Cough suppressant
- Decongestants and antihistamines
- Long-acting decongestant nasal spray for congestion or nosebleeds
- Diarrhea relief (Imodium in tablet form)
- Hydrocortisone 1% cream for skin irritation and insect bites
- Tweezers for splinter removal
- Saline eyedrops or eye wash
- Pre-moisturized towelettes for washing
- Water purification tablets or filter
- Motion sickness medications

Prescription items:
- Prescription medications require special attention. Drug safety and supplies are not as certain as they are in the United States. You do not want to have to take time from your travels to try to hunt down reliable medication. I advise my patients to carry a double supply of all their medications and divide them between carry-on and checked baggage or—better yet—have a friend carry the duplicate supply. Carry all drugs in their original containers to avoid problems with customs. Carry new written prescriptions for your medication with generic names in case you need to replace them.
- Carry extra glasses or contact lenses.
- Carry an emergency supply of antibiotics to treat traveler's diarrhea (significant diarrhea associated with sensation of ill health and a fever). Do not, however, take them to try to ward off an infection; the risk of side effects is greater than the odds of benefit, and studies suggest that those taking antibiotics in this manner have a false sense of security and take unnecessary chances. Ciprofloxacin twice daily for three days is sufficient for most treatable causes of traveler's diarrhea.

Travel Vaccinations

The following is a list of common travel vaccinations for adults. Women who are pregnant, or may become pregnant within three months, should consult their physicians about special needs.

Disease	Cause	How Transmitted	At-risk Areas	Incubation Period	Symptoms	Treatment	Prevention	Vaccination Recommended?
Cholera	Microscopic organism Vibrio cholerae	Contaminated water, milk, or food, especially shellfish	Asia, Africa, South and Central America, India, Bangladesh	1 to 3 days	Watery diarrhea, stomach cramps, vomiting which may lead to dehydration and loss of electrolytes, with symptoms usually lasting 2 to 5 days; if untreated, severe cases are associated with 50 percent mortality	Fluid and electrolyte replacement, 3 days of oral antibiotics	Avoid uncooked or poorly prepared food, especially seafood. Peel fruit. Avoid local unprocessed water. "Cook it, peel it, boil it, or forget it."	No. Currently available vaccines are only 50 percent effective and are associated with significant side effects, such as pain at the injection site, fever, headache, and fatigue.
Hepatitis A (See Chapter 10 for more information about the hepatitis A vaccine.)	Virus	Food contaminated with fecal material from infected individuals; uncooked fruits and vegetables, shellfish, and water	Areas of poor sanitation	2 to 7 weeks	Flu-like symptoms with muscle aches, headache, fever, and fatigue	None	Hand washing, better sanitation. "Cook it, peel it, boil it, or forget it," and vaccination	Yes. The first injection is administered at least 2 weeks before departure, providing protection for at least a year. A second injection is given 6 months later, extending the protection to at least 10 years. Although more serious reactions have been reported, typically patients only experience soreness at the injection site.
Hepatitis B (See Chapter 10 for more information about the hepatitis B vaccine.)	Virus	Human blood and body fluids (medical personnel handling these fluids, medical or dental procedures, tattooing, body piercing or sexual contact)	Southeast Asia or sub-Saharan Africa	4 weeks to 6 months	Fever, fatigue, loss of appetite, nausea and vomiting, jaundice (yellow skin and membranes)	Being developed	Avoid exposure to blood or body fluids; vaccination	Yes, if you anticipate medical or dental care, a prolonged stay in a high-risk area, sexual exposure or occupational exposure to blood and body fluids. Vaccination given as 3 shots over 6 months. Adverse effects include mild local reactions at the injection site.

Disease	Cause	How Transmitted	At-risk Areas	Incubation Period	Symptoms	Treatment	Prevention	Vaccination Recommended?
Influenza (See Chapter 10 for more information about the influenza vaccine.)	Virus	Respiratory secretions from infected persons, passed via direct contact or as droplets suspended in the air from a cough or sneeze	Crowded environments such as public transportation or gathering spots during "flu season"	1 to 5 days	Headache, fever, chills, muscle aches, coughing	Antiviral medication if started within the first 48 hours of onset of symptoms may reduce the severity and shorten the duration of symptoms	Vaccination	Yes. One shot is administered annually from that season's vaccine. The flu shot begins to provide protection after 1 to 2 weeks and lasts for 4 to 6 months. Some patients experience soreness at the injection site and fever, muscle aches, and fatigue for 1 or 2 days.
Malaria	Parasite	The bite of an infected mosquito	The tropics and subtropics, particularly tropic Africa south of the Sahara	Varies from 6 days to months	A shaking chill followed by fever and fatigue, which can occur in cycles of 48 to 72 hours; anemia is common	Anti-parasite medication	Prevention of mosquito bites; preventive medication selected according to the pattern of drug resistance seen in the malaria species in the planned area of travel. Medication must be started one week before travel, taken weekly during the trip, and continued for 4 weeks after returning from the area of risk.	No vaccine available.

Disease	Cause	How Transmitted	At-risk Areas	Incubation Period	Symptoms	Treatment	Prevention	Vaccination Recommended?
Measles	Virus	Direct contact with an infected person, or airborne transmission of droplets of respiratory secretions from an infected person	Schools and households with unvaccinated individuals	10 to 14 days	High fever, fatigue, cough, runny nose, and tearing for 2 to 4 days, followed by a red raised rash beginning on the face and torso, spreading to the extremities; in adults, gastrointestinal symptoms (abdominal pain, vomiting, and diarrhea) are common, as are muscle and joint pain. More serious complications can occur, including secondary infections (such as pneumonia) or infection of the central nervous system (encephalitis, manifested as headache, seizures, alteration in awareness)	Supportive care	Vaccination	Vaccination is usually given as part of the childhood vaccination series, including 2 doses after age 1. Adults born after 1956 who have received only 1 dose should have a second dose before traveling, usually given as the combined MMR (Measles, Mumps, and Rubella). About 5 percent of vaccinated patients experience fever and rash.
Meningococcal disease (See Chapter 10 for more information about the meningococcal vaccine.)	Bacteria	Respiratory droplets from infected individuals	Can occur anywhere, but especially in crowded living quarters such as in military barracks or college dormitories; outbreaks also occur throughout Africa	A few days	A rapidly progressive illness that spreads through the bloodstream; infected persons may go from normal health to irreversible shock and death within hours. Symptoms begin as flu-like chills and muscle aches with a fever greater than 102 degrees Fahrenheit. A rash develops, especially over the torso, and tiny areas of bleeding develop within the skin and rapidly enlarge. Symptoms also include headache, neck soreness and stiffness confusion, and coma.	High-dose penicillin and supportive care in a hospital's intensive care unit	Antibiotics supplied to those who have been in close contact with suspected cases; vaccination	Yes, if traveling to areas where epidemics are occurring. A single injection is given; protection begins in 2 weeks and lasts at least 3 years. The current vaccine covers only types A and B, but provides no protection from type C (which makes up 30 percent of cases).

Disease	Cause	How Transmitted	At-risk Areas	Incubation Period	Symptoms	Treatment	Prevention	Vaccination Recommended?
Polio	Virus	Food or liquid contaminated with fecal material from an infected person	Tropical or developing countries outside of the Western Hemisphere	On average, 9 to 12 days for onset of symptoms, 11 to 17 days until onset of paralysis	Range from a mild infection producing no symptoms to a flu-like illness with fever, headache, sore throat, and vomiting to a major illness with muscle pain, meningitis, and paralysis	Supportive care	Vaccination	This vaccine is administered as part of the routine childhood vaccination series. Travelers who received their initial series and have never had a booster, or are traveling to an area of the world with polio, should receive a booster shot. Given by mouth, in one case per 2.6 million doses, the polio vaccine can cause polio and paralysis in those receiving the vaccine or in their non-immune household contacts. This adverse effect is not reported when the vaccine is injected.
Tetanus–Diphtheria (See Chapter 10 for more information about the tetanus and diphtheria vaccines.)	Bacteria	Tetanus: through spores entering an open wound Diphtheria: through respiratory droplets from an infected person	Tetanus: worldwide Diphtheria: recent outbreaks in Russia and the Ukraine	Tetanus: 3 to 21 days Diphtheria: 2 to 5 days	Tetanus: painful and sustained muscle spasms Diphtheria: fever, sore throat, painful swallowing, blockage of airway with respiratory distress	Tetanus: human tetanus immunoglobulin and antibiotics Diphtheria: antitoxin and antibiotics	Vaccination	Tetanus-diphtheria vaccines are given to adults every 10 years. Patients with severe wounds will receive a booster sooner if their last booster was given more than 5 years before the injury. Adverse effects include pain at the injection site, drowsiness, and—rarely—allergic reaction.

Disease	Cause	How Transmitted	At-risk Areas	Incubation Period	Symptoms	Treatment	Prevention	Vaccination Recommended?
Typhoid fever	Bacteria Salmonella typhi	Food or liquid contaminated with fecal material from an infected person	South and East Asia, Africa, Latin America, and areas of poor sanitation	1 to 3 weeks	Fever, often higher than 103 degrees Fahrenheit, weakness, headache, stomach pain, and loss of appetite	Antibiotics and supportive care	"Cook it, peel it, boil it, or forget it;" vaccination	Yes, if traveling to these areas. The oral vaccine (Vivotif Berna) requires 4 doses given over 7 days and provides protection 2 weeks after the regimen is completed. It lasts for 5 years, but has recently been unavailable from the manufacturer. The shot (Typhim Vi) is given at least 2 weeks before travel and lasts for 2 years. Patients usually tolerate both forms of the vaccine well, although some do experience nausea, vomiting, and abdominal pain.
Yellow fever	Virus	The bite of an infected mosquito	The equatorial forests of South America, Panama, Trinidad, and Africa	3 to 6 days	Varies from flu-like symptoms to a severe illness characterized by high fever, headaches, muscle pain, nausea and vomiting, and bleeding gums and nose followed by a second phase with fever, vomiting, bleeding, liver and kidney dysfunction; mortality is 5 percent overall	Supportive care	Prevention of mosquito bites, vaccination	Yes, if traveling to the areas mentioned. This vaccination is available in the United States only at centers designated by state health departments. One injection is given 10 days before travel, with booster shots administered every 10 years. Of those receiving the vaccine, 2 to 5 percent will develop headache, fatigue, and muscle aches.

Despite all of the above concerns, foreign travel can be safe and rewarding. Plan ahead to optimize your chances for a successful trip with no unwanted souvenirs. Visit your doctor well in advance of your travels—preferably months ahead—so that needed vaccinations can be researched and provided.

Bon voyage!

CHAPTER 12

Herbals, Vitamins, and Other Nutritional Supplements

Herbals, vitamins, and other nutritional supplements: my patients take them, and there are more questions than answers regarding their use. The market for nutritional supplements tops $15 billion a year. One in three adults in the U.S. takes supplements; of these, only one in three tells his or her doctor about them. In surveys, those who take supplements take an average of approximately six different compounds. The chemistry of mixing this many chemicals together is complex and completely unexplored.

My Personal Bias

I must truthfully admit my bias before going further. My patients who take mega doses of multiple herbal and vitamin supplements either humor or frustrate me, depending on my mood that day. I have two major concerns.

First, herbal medicine has its roots in long established tradition, dating centuries before western medicine began. As with any large body of knowledge, it takes years of education, supervised training, and practice to master the fundamentals and intricacies of herbal medicine. In addition to knowledge of the properties of the herbs themselves, the conditions under which an herb is grown, harvested, and stored are essential in determining its medicinal activity. This information simply is not available for most commercially prepared products. My average patient who takes herbs relies solely on word of mouth or product advertising, with no formal training in the subtleties of herbal practice. The idea that a lay person can practice herbal medicine safely and effectively makes as much sense to me as giving a cancer patient a drug book and turning them loose in a pharmacy, with the lights off, to design their own chemotherapy.

Second, many of my patients have told me that they prefer herbal products to drugs because they don't want to put "chemicals" in their bodies. Our bodies are chemical soups. Everything that we ingest is a chemical, be it food, drink, the air we breathe, herbal products, or pharmaceuticals. The idea that a substance—taken from a portion of a plant, ground up and processed in large vats in a chemical factory, concentrated hundreds or thousands of times beyond its natural potency, and combined with numerous and often unknown additives and fillers—will retain its wholesome goodness and benefit as a "natural product" is laughable. I don't think that it is fair for herbalists to try to have it both ways, to insist that their products are safe and natural substances yet claim medicinal benefits for them. Herbal products are chemicals, plain and simple.

While some objective evidence exists for herbal product use in some conditions, this evidence is generally incomplete and preliminary only. Accurate information about short- and long-term toxicity and side effects is scanty. It is impossible at present to separate evidence of biological effectiveness from advertising, and current applicable laws encourage this confusion.

A Legal History

In 1989, over 150 patients were documented to have developed the painful immunologic disease Eosinophilia Myalgia Syndrome from ingestion of the nutritional supplement L-tryptophan. This substance had been marketed for muscle building, weight loss, and sleep benefits and was the catalyst for much legislative attention to nutritional supplements. As a result, most physicians expected stronger regulation of this industry. Unfortunately, after an intense period of lobbying by the involved industries and popular support at that time for deregulation, instead of the regulation we had hoped for all we received was the 1994 Dietary Supplement Health and Education Act.

This act allowed the marketing and sale of products claimed to "affect the structure and function of the body" as "dietary supplements," without the evaluation or approval of any government agency (that is, the Food and Drug Administration in the U.S.), as long as the product labeling made two points: 1) a disclaimer saying that the product has not been evaluated by the FDA and 2) a statement that the product is not intended to diagnose, treat, or prevent any disease. The 1994 act further put the burden of proof for safety concerns on the FDA, not the manufacturer. No proof of safety is required to market the product. Worse, manufacturers are not required to report claims of adverse effects that they receive. Thus, the FDA only investigates if it directly receives a significant number of reported problems from the public or medical providers.

Since March of 1999, the FDA has required that dietary supplements contain a label similar to that on processed foods that specifies the type and quantity of ingredients contained in it. This official-looking label has caused some confusion about product safety and purity. It does not imply that the FDA or anyone else has actually looked at the product or approved it. Study after study has proven that the contents of vitamin and herbal supplements, including the "active ingredients," vary widely from brand to brand, and even from pill to pill within the same brand. The purity and potency of products sold in the United States are simply unknown.

Our current laws also hurt consumers in regards to their attempts to responsibly use these products. The manufacturer can't legally be specific enough on the label to completely describe what the herb is for, how it works, how to safely adjust the dose, who should use it and who shouldn't, or what drugs it may interact with. Providing these specifics would run the risk of crossing the line between drug and nutritional

> ## How Safe are Dietary Supplements?
>
> Some dietary supplements do offer benefit. However, keep in mind that although the Food and Drug Administration (FDA) requires manufacturers to list the type and quantity of ingredients in a supplement, manufacturers are not required to conduct formal safety tests on these substances or report what seem to be isolated problems when they occur. Current regulations do not evaluate products on the shelf to see if their contents maintain consistency from one batch or brand to another.
>
> Read labels, and be an educated consumer!

supplement, and possibly lead to action by the FDA. Consumers are left to outside sources for this information and may not receive reliable, factual information pertinent to their needs. These substances are currently marketed with only vague claims for effectiveness accompanied by a nod and a wink. I believe that it is time to revisit the laws governing dietary supplements and provide greater protection and information for those who choose to use them.

Common Sense Advice

What to do in the meantime? If you choose to use supplements, I would offer the following suggestions:

- **Discuss your plans with your doctor.** Your doctor should be able to help with basic questions about product safety and potential drug interactions, and can help you weigh the risks and benefits of supplements.
- **Get a diagnostic evaluation.** If you plan to use a supplement to treat a medical condition, get a proper diagnostic evaluation first. Any supplement or alternative medicine approach that delays the diagnosis of an underlying medical condition with known effective therapy creates the potential for harm by omission of that therapy.
- **Be a skeptic.** Use common sense—if it sounds too good to be true, it probably is. Glowing personal testimonials to the benefits of a product are advertising, not evidence of effectiveness.
- **Conduct your own study.** If you are considering a supplement to address specific symptoms, perform your own therapeutic trial. Carefully document—in writing, as studies show that memory is unreliable—your symptoms for two or three weeks before using the supplement. This gives you a chance to note the natural variability of symptoms that you experience. Do the same thing after starting the supplement. If you note an improvement, stop the supplement and see if your symptoms return. If they do, and vanish yet again when you restart the supplement, you probably

have a winner. Know how long to give a supplement to work; some take months to show an effect.

- **Once you begin, stick with the same brand.** This is not the time to shop in the bargain basement. I strongly recommend U.S.-based manufacturers for a greater chance of purity and safety. Because it is easier to sue a U.S.-based firm, these firms are more motivated to do things right. Tougher environmental laws here also reduce the chance for inadvertent exposure to pesticides and toxic chemicals (lead, mercury, arsenic) in herbal products. Tougher drug laws make it less likely that an herbal product will be spiked with controlled substances, such as steroids or mood altering medications. Unfortunately, analysis shows that even products marketed in the United States have huge variations in the concentrations of their active ingredients from brand to brand, and even from batch to batch within the same brand.

- **Be knowledgeable about the herbs you take.** Different parts of the plant have different effects, some helpful and some toxic; products may differ in what part of the plant they use. Different forms of a product may have different potencies. A pill may deliver a large amount of the product to your body, but a tea made from the same substance may deliver none if the substance doesn't dissolve in water. Growing conditions, soil richness, and harvesting and storing techniques can all affect the strength of a product. Recent trends have seen the marketing of nutritional supplements in snacks and candies at the supermarket checkout lane. These chemicals are too serious to be treated in such a fashion.

- **Be alert for side effects.** All botanical products have a risk of causing an allergic reaction that may appear as a rash, stomach upset, joint pain, or other change in bodily function.

- **Be aware that serious consequences of herbal therapy may not show up for decades.** For example, cancer-promoting effects of borage, clotsfoot, comfrey, and sassafras took decades to see; 40 percent of tested patients who took aristolochic acid (a component of a weight loss regimen using Chinese herbs) ten years ago are now developing bladder cancer. While this risk of unknown long-term consequences is also true for controlled medications, the intense scrutiny that these drugs receive from the FDA at least gives hope that their problems will be actively looked for and disclosed when found. Remember, manufacturers of "nutritional supplements" are not required by law to disclose problems with their products when they are discovered.

- **Keep in mind that "natural" does not always mean safe.** Some of our most potent chemotherapies and toxic poison come from "natural" substances. Just ask Socrates about hemlock.

- **Stop supplements before surgery.** If you are scheduled for surgery or an invasive procedure, stop all supplements at least three weeks in advance. Many drug and herbal interactions are unknown, and the midst of surgery is not the time to find out about them.

Common Dietary Supplements

Let's review some dietary supplements (herbals, vitamins, minerals). On the next few pages, I list some common supplements in alphabetical order and briefly discuss their properties and areas of medical concern.

Aloe

Topical aloe products promote superficial wound healing and are used in the treatment of burns and frostbite. No side effects are reported from the aloe, but these products are frequently combined with other substances. Avoid combination products with topical analgesics (pain killers) due to the risk of reactions to the analgesic. Aloe deteriorates over time; use a fresh product.

Oral aloe is a strong cathartic (digestive system cleanser), inducing side effects such as cramps, diarrhea, potassium and other electrolyte loss, and pregnancy loss. I do not recommend its use.

Antioxidants

At the tiniest level, all substances are made of atoms. Atoms are made of a central core of protons and neutrons, surrounded by a cloud of electrons. Electrons like to exist in pairs for stability. Atoms that lose an electron in a chemical reaction are called free radicals. These free radicals then seek to steal another electron from surrounding molecules to regain their stability.

The body uses oxygen to convert foods into energy. During this process, some oxygen molecules lose an electron, becoming free radicals. These attack other chemicals and cells to steal an electron back, leading to damage to cells and their DNA. Aging cells are more vulnerable to damage. Free radical production increases with smoking, alcohol, and high-fat diets.

Antioxidants are chemicals that "mop up" free radicals by giving them extra electrons, in theory before they have a chance to cause much damage. Antioxidant-rich diets with fruits, vegetables, whole grains, and fish seem to limit free radical damage. Studies suggest that a good diet provides enough of these nutrients (with the exception of Vitamin E) to provide maximum protection without additional supplements. Although plenty of evidence exists to support a good diet, no good evidence exists that similar benefits can be obtained from pills. Spend your resources on improving your diet, not popping pills, until more information is available.

Androstenedione

Androstenedione is a testosterone precursor that can increase strength and muscle mass. However, users of this drug face the same problems as those from other anabolic steroids: acne, mood swings, liver toxicity, heart disease, premature closing of the growth plates with stunted growth in teens, and possibly an increased risk of prostate cancer.

The brain monitors and regulates the amount of androgens in the body. Taking this substance by mouth causes the body to produce less of its own testosterone. Women who use this supplement experience the side effects of male sexual hormones: deeper voice, acne, facial hair, male-pattern baldness and coarsening of skin. These side effects are often irreversible.

In a study of patients who took an over-the-counter androstenedione supplement reported in the November 2000 *Journal of the American Medical Association*, sophisticated urine testing showed that *all* of these supplements were contaminated with other steroids.

I do not recommend this supplement.

Bearberry

Bearberry is used as a short-term urinary tract antibacterial. Its side effects include stomach upset with nausea and vomiting. This product loses its effect in acidic urine, so it shouldn't be combined with cranberry juice.

Beta-Carotene and Vitamin A

See *Vitamin A* and *Beta-Carotene*.

Black Cohosh

Black cohosh is used to treat premenstrual discomfort and painful menstruation. It affects communication between the hypothalamus and the pituitary in the brain, leading to a decrease in luteinizing hormone (LH) production. Studies suggest that this substance can help decrease hot flashes and menstrual pain.

Common side effects can include stomach upset and lower blood pressure. Long-term effects are not well documented. Black cohosh does not seem to provide the same benefits as estrogen supplements in regards to bone, heart, and brain function or in the maintenance of estrogen sensitive tissues (skin, vagina, bladder support). Be well educated and use this supplement with caution and in consultation with your doctor.

Calcium

Calcium is crucial to the development and maintenance of a healthy skeleton. The skeleton develops in childhood and soon after, reaching a peak in density in the mid-twenties. Inadequate calcium in adolescents can mean that the expected peak skeletal density is never reached. This is particularly a concern as body conscious adolescent girls switch from dairy products to diet sodas. The phosphates in these carbonated beverages actually promote calcium loss from bone.

Children and adolescents should consume at least 1,000 milligrams (mg) of calcium a day. Women need 1,000 mg daily before menopause. Postmenopausal women on bone stimulating medications and men ages 50 to 65 need 1,200 mg daily. There seems to be little need for calcium supplements in men younger than 50. Postmenopausal women not on bone stimulating medications and men over 65 need 1,500 mg daily.

Calcium is obtained from the diet in dairy products. The average dairy serving (8 ounces of milk or a slice of cheese) has 250 mg calcium. Calcium supplements can make up the difference. Calcium carbonate is inexpensive and has the most calcium per tablet; however, it dissolves less well and requires acid in the stomach to be absorbed. Calcium carbonate products are best taken with meals. Calcium citrate products are more easily absorbed and stomach acid is not essential. They are more expensive, but best for the elderly or those on acid-reducing drugs.

For best absorption, don't take more than 500 mg of calcium at once. Avoid taking calcium products with other drugs or vitamins; calcium can complex with these other chemicals and block their absorption. Do, however, supplement the calcium with 400 to 600 IU (International Units—how vitamin quantities are measured) of Vitamin D daily to help your body absorb the calcium.

Capsicum

Small nerve fibers communicate pain signals through the use of "substance P," a chemical messenger. Capsicum is a topical compound that depletes the nerve endings of substance P and can decrease the perception of pain. It is useful for some cases of arthritis, shingles, trigeminal neuralgia, and diabetic neuropathies.

Capsicum initially increases the sensation of pain for days before it begins to work. This painful period may be too difficult to work through for some patients. It must be applied topically over the painful region four to five times daily, and can take up to four weeks to reach full benefit.

Cascara

Cascara is a stimulant laxative for occasional use. It is moderately effective. Pregnant or nursing women cannot use this supplement. If the cascara is too fresh, it can induce severe vomiting. Chronic use of stimulant laxatives can cause metabolic problems (loss of potassium and other electrolytes), pigmentation of the lining of the colon, and dependence on stimulants for any bowel activity, leading to chronic bowel problems.

Cellasene

Cellasene is promoted to get rid of cellulite. It contains a multitude of substances: ginkgo, bladder wrack, sweet clover, grape seed extract, borage seed oil, fish oil, and lecithin. Claims are made that it increases circulation, decreases excess fluid, and makes skin look smoother, but there is no scientific evidence that it works. This substance can cost more than $200 for an eight-week course. It contains a large amount of iodine, which places those with thyroid disorders at risk. Increased bleeding tendencies have also been reported with this substance. I do not recommend the use of this supplement.

Chamomile

Chamomile is a substance that has a variety of effects on the gastrointestinal tract. It has properties that reduce spasm and inflammation and is active against some infectious agents. It has been promoted to treat peptic ulcers, spasm of the gastrointestinal tract, and inflammation of mouth and gums.

Chamomile preparations are also used topically to treat inflamed membranes brought on by conditions such as eczema or wounds.

Side effects are rare and mostly limited to allergic reactions. Taking chamomile in large amounts can upset the gastrointestinal tract. Some physicians feel chamomile significantly interacts with blood thinners.

Chaste Tree Berry

Chaste Tree Berry is used to treat menstrual disorders (PMS, breast pain, and menopausal symptoms). It binds to dopamine receptors in the brain, inhibiting prolactin release and increasing the relative concentration of progesterone to estrogen in the body. Rare side effects include gastrointestinal upset, menstrual changes, and drug interactions. I do not have any experience with this supplement.

Cholestin

As of this writing, Cholestin is no longer available from U.S. manufacturers, but may be imported from foreign sources. Cholestin is a yeast byproduct that lowers cholesterol. It is not as effective as prescription drug therapy, and at $1.00 a day is not a low-cost alternative to traditional therapy. Given the well-documented safety and efficacy of the statin class of cholesterol-lowering medications, I do not see a role for this supplement in those patients who need cholesterol reduction.

Coenzyme Q-10

Coenzyme Q-10 plays a biological role in the production of energy in every cell. It is necessary in the production of ATP, which is an energy source for chemical activity in the cell. High levels of Coenzyme Q-10 are present in heart muscle, the liver, kidney, and pancreas. Levels tend to fall with aging, and low levels are found in patients with certain types of cancer. As a supplement, Coenzyme Q-10 is touted to help cells produce energy, protect and improve heart function, act as an antioxidant, and stimulate the immune system. Published studies show a correlation between the use of this supplement and fewer complications from congestive heart failure. A 1999 study showed a favorable effect on lowering blood pressure in patients with hypertension and heart disease. Some cancer trials suggest a benefit from Coenzyme Q-10 coupled with certain chemotherapies.

The American Heart Association's current position is that the trials presently available for review involved too few patients and did not follow these patients long enough to make any generalizable observations about the benefits of Coenzyme Q-10. Two recent studies showed no benefit when Coenzyme Q-10 was administered to patients who already had congestive heart failure. Supporters of this supplement state that it was added too late for these patients to benefit and that the doses given were too low. The statin drugs, commonly used to treat elevated cholesterol levels, reduce Coenzyme Q-10 production in cells; current studies are looking at the use of Coenzyme Q-10 supplements with cholesterol-lowering medication to negate this effect. I don't argue with my patients who take statin drugs who choose to take extra Coenzyme Q-10.

No serious toxicity has been reported from Coenzyme Q-10 use. Reported side effects include insomnia, rash, nausea, abdominal discomfort, dizziness, sensitivity to light, irritability, and headache.

Cranberry

The ingestion of cranberry products produces an acidic urine that inhibits micro-organisms from attaching to the urinary tract, thus helping to prevent and treat bladder infections. It also reduces urinary odor.

Large amounts of cranberry may cause diarrhea. Commercial preparations made with lots of sugar are of questionable benefit.

Creatine

Creatine is an extremely popular supplement among athletes to boost performance. This substance is present in meat and fish, and made in the liver. Muscle cells use creatine to generate energy. Studies show that while creatine supplements may help for short bursts of energy, no benefit is seen for endurance exercises. Body builders commonly load 20 grams a day for five days, and then continue with 2 to 5 grams a day. Creatine seems to increase body mass due to fluid retention.

Doses greater than 40 milligrams (mg) a day can cause toxicity to the kidneys and liver. Deaths have been reported in young athletes using high doses of creatine without adequate fluid intake. Those who take creatine will affect the results of blood tests commonly used to measure kidney function (creatinine). I do not recommend the use of this supplement.

DHEA

DHEA is a steroid hormone produced by the adrenal gland and metabolized in the body to androgens (male sexual hormones) and estrogens (female sexual hormones). Normally, DHEA levels in the bloodstream peak at 20, then decrease progressively with age. This fact has led to theories that replacing DHEA may help inhibit the aging process. Sexual hormones also are known to help mood, and DHEA has been tried for the treatment of mood disorders including depression.

Adverse effects are plentiful. Women may experience acne, hair loss from scalp, growth of facial hair, and voice deepening. These effects may be irreversible. When men take DHEA, their bodies automatically reduce their own production of natural testosterone. This leads to a net increase in estrogen levels in men from DHEA, and breast development may occur. Since DHEA is converted into testosterone and estrogen, the risk of hormone-sensitive tumors of the breast, uterus, and prostate may increase. Other side effects on mood have included aggression, mania, and psychosis.

Since there is no convincing evidence that DHEA has any beneficial effect on aging or any disease, given the potential side effects, I advise my patients not to take it.

Dong Quai

Dong quai is used for hot flashes and other menopausal symptoms, frequently taken in an effort to stimulate normal menstrual flow and prevent cramping. Its effectiveness is controversial.

Dong quai inhibits blood clotting, and can cause serious problems when combined with blood thinners. Sun-induced rashes can occur from using this compound. A component of Dong quai is an essential oil that contains safrole, a known cancer-causing substance. In herbal preparations, Dong quai is frequently mixed with other substances. I do not advise the use of products containing this substance.

Echinacea

Echinacea is thought to boost the immune system's response. Studies in people do show increased activity of white blood cells after exposure to echinacea. This may be a good thing if the white blood cells are fighting infection, but a bad thing if autoimmune disease is present and the white blood cells are attacking the body.

Echinacea doesn't prevent colds, but its use at the first sign of a cold may shorten the duration of symptoms by one or two days. Long-term use of echinacea over stimulates the immune system and increases the risk of infection. Its use should be limited to no more than six weeks at a time, preferably much shorter.

Echinacea does share allergic responses with other plants in its group, including ragweed, daisies, and chrysanthemums. Don't use it if you are allergic to these plants.

Ephedrine (Constituent of Ma Huang)

Ephedrine is promoted as a "natural" herbal stimulant and weight loss promoter. I advise against its use. Side effects include insomnia, tremor, hypertension, glaucoma, urination difficulties, and elevated blood sugar. At the time of this writing, due to the increased numbers of strokes in individuals who use ephedrine-like products, closer regulation of its use is being proposed. Some states have already imposed a ban on sales except by pharmacists. Phenylpropanolamine, a similar drug used for decongestants, is linked with hemorrhagic strokes in women and has been pulled from the market.

Erythropoietin

Erythropoietin is a biological product that increases the production of red blood cells. Some athletes use this supplement to improve the oxygen-carrying capacity of the blood and to enhance endurance. However, a greater concentration of red blood cells makes the blood thicker, which can lead to blood clots, heart attack, and stroke.

Feverfew

Feverfew is used to prevent migraine headaches, treat fever, and alleviate menstrual discomfort. It inhibits the production of prostaglandins, which are chemicals involved in these problems. It also affects the action of serotonin, a chemical in the brain related to mood and behavior.

Pregnant women cannot use feverfew as it may induce a miscarriage. I also advise caution in using feverfew in combination with blood thinners. Gastrointestinal side effects may occur. Fresh leaves can cause mouth ulcers. Some users experience headache, sleep disturbance, and/or muscle and joint pains when they stop using feverfew.

Flax Seed

Flax seed contains omega-3 fatty acids. Evidence shows that these substances lower cholesterol and inhibit blood clotting. Flax seed is useful as a bulk-forming laxative.

Folate

Folate is obtained from meat, dark-green leafy vegetables, and fortified foods. As of January 1998, all enriched cereal grains sold in the United States contain folate. Higher levels of folate prevent neural tube defects in pregnancy. Folate also lowers homocysteine levels in the body, and is felt to lower the risk of cardiovascular disease and stroke.

Garlic

Garlic may help with lipids (cholesterol and triglycerides) and heart disease, but there are no well-controlled medical studies supporting its use. Of the available smaller studies, two separate sets of reviewers found no evidence of benefit from garlic.

Garlic compounds inhibit platelet function and may reduce blood clotting. However, garlic may interact with blood thinners and seems to raise insulin levels, which is associated with an increased risk for heart disease. In rare cases, users may develop an allergic reaction. Stomach acid destroys many of the active ingredients in garlic; therefore, garlic tablets may be rendered largely useless before the body can absorb them.

Ginger

Ginger is used to treat motion sickness and nausea. It also has anti-inflammatory effects that may be useful in the treatment of arthritis. Ginger also interacts with platelets, which may prolong bleeding.

Ginkgo Biloba

Ginkgo biloba is prepared from an extract from a tree. It has chemical effects that dilate blood vessels and increase blood flow. Over 40 medical trials in Europe have shown this supplement to be effective in treating mild to moderate cerebral insufficiency (decreased blood flow to the brain) and intermittent claudication (decreased blood flow to the legs). It has also been used to treat dementia, vertigo, tinnitus (ringing of the ears), and sexual dysfunction related to antidepressant medications, with variable response.

There is little evidence that Ginkgo biloba can boost memory in normal people or that it will slow the natural decline in short-term memory with aging. One study suggested modest improvement in the mental functioning of demented patients who took it.

Ginkgo biloba interferes with clotting and interacts with blood thinners. It may interfere with the metabolism of other drugs and has been suspected of inducing hypoglycemia. Occasional problems with stomach upset, headaches, allergic reactions, and dizziness have been reported. Use this supplement with caution.

Ginseng

Ginseng is marketed as an energy booster to treat fatigue, counter stress, and enhance mental and physical performance. Its effectiveness is poorly supported; a few studies outside of the United States report a benefit in effects that are hard to measure, such as quality of life and vigor.

Side effects include increased nervousness and excitation, headache, insomnia, and interruption in heart rhythm. It can raise blood pressure and affect the potency of diabetes medications to lower blood sugar. Estrogen-like effects may cause vaginal bleeding and breast stimulation. Ginseng may interact with monoamine oxidase inhibitors that some patients use to treat depression. Ginseng also affects the action of blood thinners and should not be mixed with them.

Be cautious in taking ginseng and design your own trial as discussed in the introduction.

Goldenseal

Goldenseal is used to treat inflammation of the mouth and mucous membranes, including gastritis. Its effectiveness is poorly supported by any medical data.

Side effects include nausea, vomiting, diarrhea, stimulation of the nervous system, and reactions in the upper airway and respiratory tract.

Glucosamine and Chondroitin

Glucosamine and chondroitin sulfate are naturally occurring compounds that the body uses to build cartilage. Over 30 published trials suggest that they relieve pain and improve mobility better than placebo, but most studies were too small, too short, or had problems in their research design. In a three-year study of 212 patients in Belgium, patients on these supplements reported fewer symptoms and x-rays suggested less ongoing cartilage loss than those on placebo. Scientists speculate that these substances may inhibit the enzymes that break down cartilage in diseased joints, may stimulate joint repair, and may make the joint fluid more protective.

In general, most people tolerate these supplements well and experience few side effects. Some animal studies suggest that they can increase blood sugar by increasing insulin resistance. Other side effects are rare. Unfortunately, a year's supply of medication can cost from $300 to $750. Since profit is to be made, many companies have begun to market these products. In a study at the University of Maryland, 30 different products were analyzed. Several contained significantly different amounts of glucosamine or chondroitin from what the label claimed, while a few contained none at all.

If you wish to try these supplements, stick with a reputable brand and design your own trial over a few months as suggested in the introduction to see if you benefit enough to justify the expense. The recommended daily dose is 1,500 milligrams (mg) of glucosamine and 1,200 mg of chondroitin.

Grapeseed Extract

Grapeseed extract is an antioxidant used to treat and prevent atherosclerosis and its complications. Theoretical support exists for using antioxidants in this regard, but little factual data. No adverse reactions are reported.

Guarana

Guarana is a plant-derived source of caffeine. It is marketed as a stimulant. Side effects include hypertension, anxiety, interruption in heart rhythm, and interference with the blood clotting action of platelets. I do not advise the use of this supplement.

Hawthorn

Hawthorn dilates blood vessels, including those in the heart. It is used to treat heart disease, angina, and some sleep disorders.

Hawthorn interacts with other blood pressure and heart medications. At higher doses it can cause sedation and low blood pressure.

Given the seriousness of the medical conditions that it is said to treat and the safety and effectiveness of prescription drugs for these conditions, I advise my patients against the use of this substance.

Horse Chestnut

Horse chestnut is used in the treatment of varicose veins. Its effectiveness is controversial.

Horse chestnut is unsafe if not properly prepared. Deaths have been reported from its misuse. It is associated with allergic reactions, including contact dermatitis, and contains substances known to cause cancer. I do not recommend the use of this supplement.

Human Growth Hormone

There is a natural decline in the blood levels of Human Growth Hormone with aging, which may contribute to the decrease in muscle and bone and increase in body fat experienced as people grow older. Supplemental growth hormone has been used to try to prevent or restore these changes.

Most studies in humans with normal or moderately reduced growth hormone levels have shown no significant benefit to using supplements. Some research suggests that extra growth hormone increases the risk of colon cancer, diabetes, heart failure, hypertension, and prostate cancer. Growth hormone also stimulates excessive bone growth, principally in the hands, feet, and facial bones.

I strongly advise against the illicit use of this substance.

Kava-Kava

Kava-kava is marketed as a substance to reduce anxiety and aid sleep without the sedation, lethargy, and addiction risk associated with anti-anxiety medications. It is derived from the root of a plant in the pepper family. The best of a handful of clinical studies in Germany suggest that it is helpful for some, but provides no benefit in one-third of users and only mild benefit in a second third.

Kava-kava can impair coordination or blur vision. Long-term use has resulted in psychological addiction, yellow skin, skin lesions, and muscle weakness. Pregnant women should not use this supplement. It should not be combined with alcohol or—because of its interaction with the drugs commonly used to treat these diseases—used by patients being treated for Parkinson's disease, anxiety, and depression.

Lemon Balm

Lemon balm has been used to treat sleep disorders and functional gastrointestinal disorders such as irritable bowel. Topical preparations are used for Herpes simplex lesions. Although no side effects are reported, little is known about the effectiveness of these compounds.

Licorice

Licorice has been used to treat peptic ulcers and as an expectorant. Higher doses of licorice are unsafe and increase blood pressure, cause water retention, and create potassium loss. Licorice should not be taken by pregnant women, patients with liver disorders, or patients taking diuretics and certain heart medications.

L-Arginine

L-arginine is promoted for sexual dysfunction as the "Natural Viagra." This chemical is a precursor to nitric oxide, which acts locally in the penis and other areas to regulate blood flow. Some evidence exists that extra L-arginine improves blood flow and lowers blood pressure.

However, researchers studying the effect of L-arginine have had to use very high doses (3 to 6 grams a day) over several weeks before they see an improvement, if one occurs. This is a much higher dose than the advertised supplements offer. Effects from single doses are generally not measurable. Since there is such a strong response to placebo for sexual dysfunction (men think the drug will help, so it does), the actual benefit of this supplement is questionable.

Avoid mixing L-arginine with other substances that lower blood pressure, such as Viagra, nitrates, or blood pressure medications. This could dangerously lower blood pressure.

Lutein

Diets high in lutein are associated with a lower risk of cataracts and macular degeneration. Dark green and yellow vegetables (kale, spinach, broccoli, yellow squash) are the highest in lutein. This yellow pigment is concentrated in the macula (the area responsible for finest vision) and filters out blue light, which can damage the retina.

Whether lutein in pill form has the same benefits as that in fruits and vegetables remains unproven. We don't know whether it is the lutein itself that provides the benefit or whether its benefits lie in something else associated with plants that contain it.

Lycopene

Lycopene is the pigment that gives tomatoes and some fruits their red color. It is an antioxidant. Diets high in lycopene seem to lower the risk of prostate, lung, and gastric cancer.

Whether lycopene in pill form has the same attributes as that in fruits and vegetables remains unproven. We don't know whether it is the lycopene itself that provides the benefit or whether its benefits lie in something else associated with plants that contain it.

Ma Huang

Ma Huang is an herbal source for ephedrine. It is marketed for bronchial asthma, as a stimulant, and is a common ingredient in weight loss products. See *Ephedrine* for further details.

Side effects include insomnia, nervousness, palpitations, tremor, hypertension, glaucoma, urination difficulties, and elevated blood sugar. Ma Huang is not felt to be safe or effective for weight loss, although it is a commonly used for this purpose.

I advise against the use of Ma Huang. At the time of this writing, due to the increased numbers of strokes in individuals who use ephedrine-like products, some similar substances are being pulled from the market.

Melatonin

Melatonin is a hormone secreted by the pineal gland in the brain that helps set the body's clock. Melatonin has been promoted as a cure for jet lag. The scientific data about melatonin's effect on sleep is contradictory. It may simply help shift the phase of sleep rather than be a true sedative. It is hard to know how to advise a patient to use it properly in regards to timing and amount.

It is also promoted as an agent to slow the aging process, although this is controversial and an answer won't be available for years.

Melatonin is another profitable product manufactured by many companies. The strength and purity of different preparations vary considerably.

Metabolism Enhancers

Metabolism enhancers are marketed to promote weight loss. These products contain ephedrine and caffeine, derived from herbs (Ma Huang and guarana). The recommended dose exceeds the FDA's proposed limit for ephedrine. See *Ephedrine* for details.

I do not recommend the use of these products.

MSM

MSM (methylsulfonylmethane) is promoted to provide arthritis relief by reducing pain and inflammation. This chemical is a metabolite of dimethylsulfoxide (DMSO), without the fishy/garlic odor. MSM's claims arise from testimonials, not from good scientific data.

Reported side effects include nausea, diarrhea, and headaches.

Nettle

Nettle has different properties depending on the portion of the plant used. The sap acts as a diuretic. The root is used to relieve the symptoms of an enlarged prostate gland. The potential for error is obvious. A man with an enlarged prostate who has to urinate frequently hears that "nettle" will help, but buys a product made from sap instead of root. His urinary frequency worsens rather than improves.

The root compounds do seem to reduce inflammation in the prostate and may affect the prostate's response to hormones. Side effects are few. Rare allergies have been reported. People with impaired heart or kidney function should not use nettle.

Phytoestrogens

Phytoestrogens are plant compounds that are converted to estrogens in the gastrointestinal tract. They are promoted as "natural" estrogen substitutes. Common varieties include isoflavones (soybeans), lignans (flax seed), black cohosh, and red clover. These compounds generally act as weak estrogens, but may have anti-estrogen effects (they occupy the estrogen receptor on a cell, but don't fully stimulate it, thereby blocking the receptor from stimulation by estrogen).

Evidence of benefit mostly comes from observing women with a high amount of phytoestrogens in their diet (for example, the traditional Asian diet). They seem to have fewer hot flashes and a reduced severity of menopausal symptoms. Some women who eat soy have a lower incidence of breast cancer. Eating soy can also lower cholesterol.

A word of caution: Phytoestrogens are hormonally active products and as such may cause a variety of effects, from helpful to harmful. Widespread belief in the goodness of these products has far outstripped the existing research and our scientific understanding of their actions. Promotion of these products is heavily driven by marketing forces and influenced by prejudice against traditional estrogen replacement therapies. Be wary.

Pau D'Arco

Pau D'Arco is claimed as an anticancer and anti-inflammatory agent. Studies at the National Cancer Institute show no benefit from its use.

Peppermint

Peppermint decreases muscular contractions of the gastrointestinal tract and relieves some abdominal pain.

Overuse can cause excessive relaxation of lower esophageal sphincter, leading to acid washing up into the esophagus and heartburn. Only adults should use peppermint medicinally; in children, peppermint can cause laryngeal and bronchial spasms. Allergic reactions can occur.

Primrose (Evening)

Evening primrose slightly lowers serum cholesterol and is used to treat atopic eczema. No adverse reactions or toxicity have been reported in its use. Due to the safety and effectiveness of the statin class of drugs for elevated cholesterol, patients with a medical need for cholesterol reduction are advised to discuss statin therapy with their physician.

Psyllium

Psyllium is a bulk-forming laxative used for constipation and irritable bowel. It also slightly lowers cholesterol.

Psyllium can interfere with absorption of other drugs. Adequate liquid must be taken with psyllium products to prevent obstructions caused by the collection of psyllium in the gastrointestinal tract.

Pyruvate

Pyruvate products are promoted to enhance fat loss and improve endurance. The claim is that they increase glucose uptake into muscle, which leads to a protein-sparing effect during weight loss.

Studies only show enhancement of weight loss when exceedingly large amounts are consumed as part of a low-calorie diet. These research doses were much higher than doses you can obtain from supplements. Smaller doses appear to have no measurable effect. I do not recommend the use of this supplement.

SAM-e

SAM-e (S-adenosylmethionine) was originally promoted in the 1950s as an antide-pressant. It has recently been promoted for a variety of conditions, including arthritis, fibromyalgia, and neurological diseases. European studies suggest that when administered intravenously, SAM-e is an effective aide to the treatment of depression and may relieve arthritis pain comparably to some arthritis medications (NSAIDs). Some lab research data suggests that SAM-e may affect the production of components of cartilage.

Unfortunately, when taken by mouth, only 1 percent of the drug is absorbed into the system; the rest is destroyed by stomach acid or in the liver. Of the effectiveness studies referred to by the promoters of this substance, 35 of the 40 trials were done with intravenous therapy. All five trials done with pills had serious flaws in their design and gave unimpressive results.

Reported side effects in the trials included mild gastrointestinal distress, skin rashes, mania, pressured speech, and grandiose ideas in 5 to 30 percent of subjects.

An expensive supplement when taken at the recommended dose, this substance is not recommended.

Saw Palmetto

Saw palmetto is a fruit extract that is fairly effective for treatment of benign prostatic hypertrophy (BPH). It has anti-inflammatory properties and blocks the effects of testosterone on the prostate gland. It doesn't shrink the prostate, but it does relieve symptoms. In a trial of 300 patients, 88 percent noted benefit.

Rare side effects include gastrointestinal upset, headache, and diarrhea.

Selenium

Selenium is promoted for the prevention of prostate cancer and some indirect evidence exists in support of its benefit. In a study at Harvard, selenium intake was calculated by the concentration of selenium in toenail clippings. The risk of advanced prostate cancer was two-thirds less in men with highest selenium levels. This is obviously not overwhelming proof of benefit, but it is interesting.

Selenium is available in many foods; the amount in a particular food varies based on soil content of selenium where it was grown. The recommended daily allowance for selenium is 70 micrograms (mcg) per day; the dose studied was from 150 to 200 mcg a day. Greater amounts of selenium are toxic, leading to weak fingernails, hair loss, and fatigue.

Senna

Senna is a stimulant laxative used for constipation. It is moderately effective. Its chronic use can result in an electrolyte imbalance, potassium loss, discoloration of the wall of the colon, and damage to the nerves and muscles that are responsible for normal colon function. It should be used infrequently. Patients who feel that they need a stimulant laxative more than once or twice a month should discuss their bowel problems with their doctor.

St. John's Wort

St. John's Wort is used for depression, bladder and skin problems, and—in Germany—for anxiety and sleep disorders. St. John's Wort affects the brain's concentration of multiple neurotransmitters, chemicals used to communicate between nerve cells. The active constituents of St John's Wort involve ten or more chemical components, whose roles in this supplement's effect are not known. Most studies compare St. John's Wort with older antidepressants; its effectiveness appears to be modest in comparison to these medications. The newer antidepressant medications, more effective and with fewer side effects, have not been studied head-to-head with St. John's Wort.

Side effects of St. John's Wort can include dry mouth, dizziness, confusion, constipation, headache, nausea, and excessive sensitivity to sunlight. It affects blood levels when taken in conjunction with a variety of prescription drugs, including medications for asthma, congestive heart failure, HIV infection, oral contraceptives, cholesterol medications, and birth control pills. St. John's Wort accumulates in the lens of the eye, interacts with ultraviolet light, and may contribute to cataracts.

I do not recommend this supplement since more effective and safer medications for depression are available.

Valerian

Valerian is promoted for the treatment of mild insomnia. It stimulates the release of the neurotransmitter GABA, which is involved in sleep.

Side effects include increased drowsiness the next morning. Drug interactions have not been studied.

Vitamin A and Beta-Carotene

While convincing evidence exists that a diet rich in vitamin A and beta-carotene is healthy, current studies show essentially no benefit—and a potential for harm—to taking supplements of these same substances. Good dietary sources for vitamin A and beta-carotene include meats, fish, fish oil, dairy products, and deep yellow and deep green vegetables. Diets rich in these foods seem to reduce the risk for cardiovascular disease and lung cancer.

A 12-year randomized study of 22,000 men found no benefit on cancer rates or heart disease from the use of these supplements. A Finnish study actually showed an increase in cancer deaths in those taking beta-carotene. What could explain this? There are over 50 naturally occurring carotenoids; supplementing one of them might cause the body to absorb less of the others. If the right ones weren't selected for inclusion in the supplement, your body would actually take in less than what it needs of the beneficial type of carotene from other dietary sources.

Vitamin B₁₂

Vitamin B_{12} is abundant in meat, fish, and dairy products. It cannot be directly absorbed into the body, but requires a carrier protein called Intrinsic Factor to latch onto it in the gut and pull it through the lining of the intestine to the bloodstream. Vitamin B_{12} is important for healthy nerve and brain function and for proper blood cell development.

Vitamin B_{12} may be poorly absorbed in some elderly patients who no longer make Intrinsic Factor and in those with little stomach acid, including those on long-term acid suppressing medication. Of the people in the United States over age 60, 10 to 30 percent are deficient in B_{12}. All adults over age 50 should take a multivitamin or vitamin B supplement, and be monitored for signs of deficiency during their regular examinations.

Vitamin C

Vitamin C owes its fame to the Nobel Laureate, Linus Pauling. Many of the benefits attributed to high-dose vitamin C have been soundly disproved, but continue to live on—firmly entrenched in medical folklore.

Studies at the National Institutes of Health show that high-dose vitamin C is generally useless since the body only absorbs a limited amount. Studies of blood saturation with vitamin C show that the body's tissues hold as much vitamin C as they can at a dose of 200 milligrams (mg) a day. While this is more than most people consume, it is easily obtainable from the diet. Eating the recommended 5 to 9 servings of fruits and vegetables daily will supply 200 to 350 mg of vitamin C, enough to completely saturate the blood.

What about taking vitamin C for colds? Contrary to firm and fixed belief, there is no evidence that high-dose vitamin C helps prevent or ward off colds. Proposed in the 1960s, multiple placebo-controlled studies show that it is ineffective, convincing even most of the original researchers. There may be a minor benefit in those with low vitamin C levels to begin with.

Excessive doses of vitamin C can cause harm. The excess pours into the kidneys and intestines for elimination, resulting in gas and diarrhea and increasing the building blocks of kidney stones. New research reported at an American Heart Association meeting suggested that those patients who took more than 500 mg of vitamin C daily had a higher risk of thickening of the carotid (neck artery) walls. In a controversial article in the journal *Nature* in 1997, it was reported that vitamin C in large doses functions as a pro-oxidant, not anti-oxidant, providing the opposite effect desired. To add to the confusion, a study reported this year suggested that supplemental vitamin C doses blunted the beneficial effects of cholesterol medications. The healthy HDL cholesterol subcomponent did not go up as much as expected in patients on cholesterol medications if they were also taking vitamin C.

Warnings of excessive intake and disclaimers of effectiveness against colds aside, a diet adequate in vitamin C is essential. Extra vitamin C has been shown to boost healthy HDL cholesterol levels in those whose blood was less than 70 percent saturated with vitamin C beforehand. Observational studies of over 7,000 Americans showed that cardiovascular death rates were a third higher in those with the lowest vitamin C levels than in those with higher levels. Thirty-six of forty-eight observational studies showed that people with the most dietary vitamin C had the lowest incidences of cancer of the gastrointestinal and respiratory tracts.

My recommendations? Eat a diet rich in vitamin C by consuming the 5 to 9 servings of fruits and vegetables recommended daily. If you must take a supplement, take no more than 500 mg.

Vitamin D

Vitamin D helps the body absorb calcium. At least 400 IU—but no more than 1000 IU—per day are required, especially elderly men and women who typically are deficient in this vitamin. Sources of vitamin D include meat, fatty fish, fortified milk, and sunlight. If you are not sure how much of this vitamin to supplement, ask your doctor to check your blood to determine how deficient you are in this vitamin.

Vitamin E

The oxidation of LDL-cholesterol is an important step in the development and progression of atherosclerosis. Vitamin E is an antioxidant. Although studies have shown that people who eat fruits, vegetables, and other foods high in vitamin E have a reduced risk of heart disease, the studies can't tell us whether the reduction is due to the vitamin E in the diet or to other contributing factors such as exercise or a different substance also found in vitamin E-rich foods.

Studies of vitamin E supplements are controversial. In patients at high risk for cardiovascular disease, a study published in the *New England Journal of Medicine* in 2000 found that treatment with vitamin E for a mean of 4.5 years had no apparent effect on cardiovascular outcomes. However, a British study of 2000 patients found a reduced risk of heart disease in those who took vitamin E. Studies based on questionnaires found that in 85,000 nurses followed over eight years, those with the highest vitamin E intake had the lowest risk of heart disease. Similar findings were noted in a study of 40,000 men.

To add to the confusion, a study reported this year suggested that supplemental vitamin E doses blunted the beneficial effects of cholesterol medications. The healthy HDL cholesterol subcomponent did not go up as much as expected in patients on cholesterol medications if they were also taking vitamin E.

While I do not argue with patients who wish to take 400 to 800 IU of vitamin E a day, I no longer recommend it to my patients.

White Willow

White willow is an analgesic (pain killer). It is converted to salicylic acid (aspirin) in the body, usually below therapeutic doses. It has the same side effects as aspirin with no net advantages. I do not recommend taking this supplement.

Yohimbine

Yohimbine is promoted to treat impotence. It affects nerve signals to blood vessels that affect blood flow. It may provide a mild benefit for erectile function in men;

however, it has many side effects. It stimulates the central nervous system, can affect blood pressure, and causes excessively rapid heartbeat, nausea, and occasional psychosis.

Due to a high risk-to-benefit ratio, I do not recommend this supplement.

Sources for Additional Information

Food and Drug Administration
http://www.fda.gov

American Association of Poison Control Centers
http://www.aapcc.org

Natural Medicines Comprehensive Database
http://www.naturaldatabase.com

Herb Research Foundation
http://www.herg.org

American Botanical Council
http://www.herbalgram.org

CHAPTER 13

Health Assessment

Much of my day in the office is spent performing physical examinations (PEs). I encourage patients to schedule these comprehensive visits periodically until age 40, annually thereafter. I have included a copy of my standard PE format at the end of this section to give you an idea of how thorough a PE should be. For a PE, I review the patient's chart ahead of time. I note their past history and habits and decide what screening tests they should consider. During their visit, we review basic information about their past and present health status, update issues regarding their family history and lifestyles, and perform an age appropriate hands-on examination. After we discuss the patient's desires for testing, we draw appropriate laboratory tests and plan any needed procedures. After all results are in, I provide my patients with a comprehensive review of their health status and make recommendations to foster future good health.

This all sounds good, and I truly believe that I am helping my patients reach better health by this approach, but what is the actual evidence that periodic physical examinations and testing leads to better health outcomes? Despite good intentions, for the majority of testing that physicians do, the evidence for a benefit to the patient is quite slim.

I originally began this chapter writing about concepts and lessons from epidemiology with discussions about how clinical trials are developed, how medical knowledge is gained, and what makes up a good test. I quickly became mired in the statistical concepts of sensitivity, specificity, prevalence, incidence, reliability, and bias and could not find a way to explain the science of health assessment in a way that would encourage patients to read past the first paragraph. The fact of the matter is that there is tremendous disagreement among health experts in what tests to perform for preventive health. Groups such as the United States Preventive Services Task Force, similar agencies in Canada and the United Kingdom, the American Cancer Society, many professional organizations, and many more disease interest groups all publish their own guidelines. Their recommendations are somewhat grounded in science, but are often political.

To remain honest, I've decided simply to tell you what I do after 15 years of practicing medicine.

1. I review the medical record in detail with the patient to be sure that what I think I know about him or her, including medical and family history, is accurate. In this

process, I commonly find errors in my own medical records, acquired during previous miscommunications with the patient. Having correct information is essential to giving good advice.

2. I allow the patient to express any specific issues that he or she is concerned about. In the interest of time, I ask everyone to do this in writing before the visit. In this way, I can quickly identify issues that may be of crucial importance in health.

3. We discuss all medications, supplements, and herbal products being used to look for problem interactions and unnecessary practices that may affect health. I also review drug allergies for accuracy.

4. We discuss family and social support issues. These human connections are essential to understanding a person's current health and future resources if assistance is needed.

5. We review habits such as smoking, alcohol or drug use, exercise, safety issues, sleep, sex, and diet.

6. I examine the patient's vaccination history and recent testing.

7. I ask the patient to review a comprehensive checklist of questions about every organ system in an attempt to tease out other health concerns.

8. I then perform a hands-on physical examination. Then—and only then—do we discuss and consider laboratory tests and procedures. With rare exceptions, if I don't suspect a problem by this time in the exam, I rarely find one from all the money spent on lab tests and procedures.

Recommended Tests, Procedures, and Vaccinations

In this section, I summarize the laboratory tests, procedures, and vaccinations I recommend to my patients.

Laboratory Tests

- **Automated laboratory profile to measure electrolytes, blood sugar, kidney function, proteins, and liver chemistries.** Not much data exists to support a blood panel of this size, but it is relatively cheap and easy to do. It is actually less expensive in our lab to order the big panel than to tease out the few tests a patient really needs. Normal test results are defined as a range of results into which 95 percent of a healthy population would fall. Based on pure statistics, when a large panel of labs are drawn, some will return outside of the normal range. It is up to the physician to determine which abnormalities are significant enough to pursue. If labs show minor abnormalities in a pattern that does not suggest disease, I may choose not to pursue them.

- **Cholesterol profile.** Conducting this profile every 3 to 5 years is adequate if previous profiles have been normal. Patients frequently insist that this be checked annually.

- **Urinalysis.** This test should be performed with each physical.

- **Complete blood count.** This test should be performed with each physical.
- **Prostate-specific antigen.** Men age 50 and up should be tested annually, earlier if risk factors for prostate cancer exist. I begin at 40 in those with a family history of prostate cancer or of African American heritage.
- **Thyroid function.** Women over 30 should be tested every 5 years or if fatigue or other suggestive symptoms are reported.

Procedures

- **Mammography.** Women age 40 to 49 should have a mammogram every one to two years, annually after age 49.
- **Pap smear.** Begin at age 18 or earlier if sexually active. After two normal examinations one year apart, schedule routine exams every one to three years at your physician's discretion. Exams are advised more frequently in females who are of high risk (early age of onset sexual activity, multiple partners, or abnormalities on previous Pap smears). I do not do pelvic exams in women who have had hysterectomies; there is nothing to check and, unfortunately, studies show no ability to pick up ovarian cancer in time to alter its outcome by doing a pelvic exam.
- **Stool for occult blood.** I recommend an annual set of three beginning at age 50 in those patients who are not receiving colonoscopies.
- **Flexible sigmoidoscopy or colonoscopy.** I recommend one every five years after age 50. See *Chapter 23: The Gastrointestinal System* on page 201 for more information.
- **Cardiac stress test.** I recommend this test at age 45 and periodically thereafter in those with four or more risk factors for cardiovascular disease (age, male gender or postmenopausal status without estrogens, tobacco use, hypertension, hypercholesterolemia, diabetes, family history of premature cardiovascular events), those who would endanger the public safety should they experience sudden cardiovascular events, or sedentary patients with risk factors planning a new, rigorous exercise program. See *Chapter 21: The Heart and Cardiovascular System* on page 180 for more information.
- **Pulmonary function testing.** I recommend this test every two years in smokers over age 40, mainly so that I can detect the early signs of emphysema and push these patients harder to stop smoking.
- **Bone density measurement.** All postmenopausal women who either decline or do not qualify for estrogen replacement therapy should receive this test, with periodic follow-up testing. I also check women on hormone replacement therapy after ten years of use (15 percent will develop osteoporosis despite hormones), earlier in those with a family history of osteoporosis.
- **EKG.** I recommend a baseline at 40 (for men) and 50 (for women). I often repeat the EKG at least every five years. Thirty percent of heart attacks are said to be silent (no chest pain, no symptoms), and I know of no other way to pick these up.
- **Chest x-ray.** I do not recommend chest x-rays as a screening test. Multiple studies have shown no statistical ability to detect early disease (including cancer) in a way

that would improve the health outcome. CT scans of the chest are being promoted for lung cancer screening in smokers who don't exhibit symptoms. Little data exists to support the cost of such as expensive screening program, and patients who obtain these scans are exposed to a significant amount of radiation during them, as well as possible invasive procedures to investigate suspicious—but ultimately benign—abnormalities seen. I do not recommend screening CT scans to my patients.

- **Vision and glaucoma screening.** Performed by an eye care professional, I recommend this screening at least every few years after age 40.
- **Audiogram.** I refer my patients for this test if they are experiencing significant symptoms. I do not do random screenings. Patients aren't often interested in hearing evaluation and hearing aides unless they themselves sense a problem.

Vaccinations

- **Tetanus/diphtheria.** I recommend this vaccination every ten years.
- **Influenza.** I recommend this vaccination annually for patients over the age of 65 or at high risk (heart, lung, kidney disease, sickle cell disease, diabetes, immune dysfunction). I also recommend this vaccination for any patient who desires a flu shot.
- **Pneumococcal pneumonia.** I recommend this vaccination for high-risk patients and those over age 65, repeated every five to seven years. I think this shot is probably a good idea for everyone over 50 given the increasing resistance of this type of bacterial infection to antibiotics.
- **Hepatitis B.** I recommend this vaccination for health-care workers, intravenous drug users, sexually active adults with multiple partners, dialysis patients, and household contacts of hepatitis B patients. I also routinely vaccinate adolescents who missed the vaccine as a child.
- **MMR (Measles, Mumps, Rubella).** I recommend two vaccinations after the age of 1.

> For more information on these and other vaccinations, see
> *Chapter 10: Vaccinations and Associated Diseases*
> and *Chapter 11: Travel Health*

Charlotte Medical Clinic—Complete History and Physical Examination

Name: _____

Age: _____

In order for us to provide you with the most effective health care, we need to have some basic information about your past and present health. We also need to ask about your lifestyle because it directly affects your physical and emotional well-being. Information provided to your physician is confidential.

Note any specific issues that you would like to discuss with the doctor:

_____

_____

_____

_____

_____

_____

Past Surgical History: _____

_____

Past Medical History: _____

_____

Medications: Please review the attached list and make corrections and additions.
(A list is inserted)

Please list all other medications that you're taking with the dose and frequency. Be sure to include all over-the-counter drugs, vitamins, birth control pills, herbal remedies, and others:

_____

_____

_____

Drug Allergies:

Family History: as of (date)
Father (known history inserted)
Mother (known history inserted)
Siblings (known history inserted)

Please pay particular attention to list those diseases that are inherited, such as Diabetes, Hypertension, Cancer, Heart disease before age 65, Thyroid disease, Depression, Cholesterol disorders, or Genetic diseases

Updates: _____

_____

_____

_____

Social History:
Marital status: _____

Children: _____

Education: _____

Occupation: _____

Spouse's occupation: _____

Habits:
Have you ever smoked? Yes_____ No_____ (if no, skip to the next section)

#pack/day_____ # years smoked_____

Ever wanted to quit? Yes_____ No_____

Do you smoke now? Yes_____ No_____   Year stopped:_____

Are you exposed to secondhand smoke at home? Yes_____ No_____ At work? Yes_____ No_____

Do you drink alcoholic beverages? Yes/No

#drinks/day < 1   1   2   3   4   5   > 5

(A drink = 12 oz beer, 4 oz wine, or 1 1/2 oz liquor)

Do you currently use drugs for other than medical reasons? Yes_____ No_____

Have you ever used nonprescription drugs injected with a needle? Yes_____ No_____

Do you exercise? Yes_____ No_____ What type and how often:

_____

Please rate the quality of your sleep: good   fair   poor   #hours/night _____

Do you wear seat belts: 0%   25%   50%   75%   100%

Are you at risk for sexually transmitted disease? Yes_____ No_____

(Risk = unprotected intercourse other than with your lifetime partner, sexual contact with > 3 partners in the last two years, nonmonogamous homosexual intercourse, sexual contact with partners with prior homosexual relations or prior use of IV drugs)

Have you made any significant changes in your diet over the past year? Yes_____ No_____

Health Maintenance:

___**Tetanus/diphtheria:** every 10 years

___**Influenza:** annually if over 65 or with heart, lung, kidney disease, diabetes, or immune deficiency

___**Pneumococcal pneumonia:** at age 65, then every seven years. Earlier if at high risk due to diabetes, chronic lung, heart, kidney, liver, or neurologic disease.

___**Hepatitis B:** health care workers, sexually active adults with multiple partners, dialysis patients, children, young adults.

Please list the last year for procedures that you have had:

_____ Mammogram   _____ Pap Smear
_____ Stool Series for a Occult Blood
_____ Sigmoidoscopy Exam or Colonoscopy
_____ Cardiac Treadmill Stress Test   _____ Bone Density Test
_____ EKG   _____ Chest X-ray
_____ Vision and Glaucoma Screening

Circle other problems you are having:

General: weight gain   weight loss   lack of appetite   well-being   insomnia   fatigue
exhaustion   feel blue   irritable   frequent tears   anxious   can't relax   worrying

Skin: psoriasis   eczema   skin cancer   rosacea   rashes   dry skin   dandruff   bruises
excessive sweating   itching   nail problems   hair loss   hives   abnormal mole   persistent sore

Glandular: diabetes   hypoglycemia   thyroid disease   gout   cholesterol   osteoporosis
excessive thirst   excessive urination   sudden change in vision   numbness in feet

Blood: anemia   enlarged lymph nodes   bleeding disorder   leukemia   lymphoma
history of cancer   blood clot in vein or lung   frequent infections

Eyes: cataracts   glaucoma   recent vision change   red eyes   wear glasses   wear contacts
eye pain

Nose and mouth: allergies   nasal congestion   sinus disease   nosebleeds   sore throat
hoarseness   taste change   tonsillitis   gum disease   dental problems

Lungs: asthma   emphysema   pneumonia   short of breath   chronic cough   excessive phlegm
frequent bronchitis   cough of blood   wheezing   tuberculosis exposure

Heart: heart attack   angina   chest pain   heart failure   swollen ankles   heart murmur
take antibiotics for dental work   wake up short of breath   heart rhythm problems
irregular pulse   high blood pressure   history of rheumatic fever   mitral valve prolapse
leg cramps when walking   varicose veins   must prop up to breathe at night   pacemaker

Musculoskeletal: joint pain   swelling   redness   warmth   stiffness   arthritis
rheumatoid arthritis   lupus   fractures   muscle pain   weakness   back pain   bursitis
fibromyalgia

Gastrointestinal: ulcer   gastrointestinal bleeding   rectal pain   irritable bowel/spastic colon
Crohn's disease   constipation   ulcerative colitis   diverticulosis   hepatitis   cirrhosis   gallstones
pancreatitis   hiatal hernia   heartburn   indigestion   jaundice   difficulty swallowing
stomach pain   nausea/vomiting   gas   diarrhea   hemorrhoids   blood in stool
change in bowel habits

Urinary: kidney disease   kidney stones   bladder infections   difficulty passing urine   burning
itching   frequency   urgency   urinate frequently at night (# of times _____)   incontinence
blood in urine

Infectious disease: HIV infection   AIDS   herpes   syphilis   sexually transmitted disease
tuberculosis   history of IV drugs   history of blood transfusions   hepatitis C
multiple sexual partners.

Neurologic: stroke   transient ischemic attack (TIA)   migraine headaches   seizures
sleep apnea   headaches   dizziness   blackouts   fainting   paralysis   incoordination
head trauma   frequent falls   confusion

Psychiatric: anxiety   depression   drug addiction   alcoholism

Females Only: changes in period length, frequency, flow   excessive bleeding
excessive cramping   vaginal discharge   2 vaginal itching   breast lump   breast discharge
breast pain   fibrocystic breast disease   discomfort with intercourse   infertility
Length of periods: _____ Frequency of periods: _____ Menopause? (Year: _____)
Do you perform breast self exams? Yes ___ No ___ How often? _____
Are you using contraception? Yes ___ No _____ Type _____
Problems with pregnancies? Yes ___ No ___ Type _____
Are you currently planning a pregnancy? Yes ___ No ___

Males Only: prostate difficulties   discharge from penis   impotence
pain/lump/swelling in the scrotum   rash   ulcers   blisters   trouble starting your urine stream
frequent urination at night (# times in average night ___)
weak or interrupted urine stream   feeling of incomplete bladder emptying with urination

CHAPTER 14

How to Get What You Want from Your Office Visit

D octor's offices are very busy places these days. Because of changes in insurance practices, most doctors are working harder, seeing more patients, and making less money than they did 5 to 10 years ago. In addition, the office staff has changed. Most staffs are bigger in order to handle the paperwork and phone requirements of Managed Care. The use of physician extenders (Physician Assistants and Nurse Practitioners) has mushroomed, and many offices have reduced their dependence on Registered Nurses by hiring more affordable but less knowledgeable Medical Office Assistants and clerical staff. In today's tight job market, support staff for a doctor's office is much harder to recruit and maintain, and those individuals answering the phone, dealing with insurance, and assisting patients and staff are generally less well-trained and experienced than in past years.

So, how should you watch out for your own health concerns in this environment? Be prepared!

- **Know your doctor.** The time to choose your physician is not when you are acutely ill and in need of urgent attention. Make a well visit to get a feel for the doctor, office, and staff—and to let them get to know you. Ask questions up front about how acute-care health needs are handled in the practice. Learn the tricks to make the office work for you.
- **Be clear about what type of appointment you need.** Specify whether you need a complete physical, specific attention for a complex problem, or a brief visit for a simple issue. This will help ensure that you get adequate time for your visit.
- **Write down your list of concerns in their order of priority.** Review your issues quickly, and then spend time on the ones that concern you. Most experienced physicians and extenders are very efficient in addressing multiple concerns when necessary, as long as you are well organized and clear.
- **Rehearse your story.** Telling an understandable story about how your symptoms have progressed will greatly assist your doctor in logically interpreting them and helping you. If the doctor doesn't have to spend most of your visit piecing your story together in a coherent fashion, more time can be spent on thinking and developing solutions.

- **Don't minimize your symptoms, or your doctor may be led to also.** A visit with your doctor is not the time to act heroic or shy. Tell it like it is.
- **Be honest about your concerns.** I have had elderly women not tell me about breast lumps that they have found. They either don't want to admit a problem, or feel if it is really an important issue that I will discover it myself. I frequently have men see me for a well check-up with no concerns, only to have their irate wives call back the next day with a half-dozen issues that their husbands "forgot" to bring up. Would you take your car in for a tune-up without telling the mechanic what kind of problems you were experiencing? Don't keep your doctor in the dark; your care will suffer and you will both seem stupid.
- **Listen to your doctor's responses.** I find nothing as irritating as a patient who has clearly moved on to thinking about how to ask the next question without waiting for the answer to the last one.
- **Keep a list of current drugs, supplements, and adverse medication reactions with you.** This will save significant time and go a long way toward preventing adverse drug reactions.
- **Build a relationship with your doctor.** Understand that in a busy primary care office, your relationship with your doctor and your overall health assessment and care is a process that builds through a series of visits over time. One stop, all-issues-on-the-table visits will frustrate both of you and will lead to inferior care. If you raise ten issues during our visit, I will drown in information overload and lose all sight of their relative importance in the overall scheme of your health.
- **If you don't understand something, ask again.** If you still don't get satisfaction, ask for a call back after hours when the doctor can sit down in relative quiet and discuss matters with you.
- **Choose a primary care MD to coordinate all of your medical care.** Be sure that all other physicians, therapists, and alternative health care providers keep your doctor up to date with what they are doing. Dividing your care among many providers is an invitation to disaster. I have witnessed this time and time again with drug interactions, duplicate testing, and unnecessary health expenditures.
- **Know how your doctor's office will communicate test results to you.** Refuse to accept "If you don't hear from us, everything is ok." Reports get misplaced. Don't risk this happening to you.
- **Know what to do and expect if you have an emergency after hours.** Know who to call and where you might need to travel for emergency care.
- **Thoroughly understand your insurance plan.** Know what is covered, when referrals are required, what co-payments are, and what your drug plan is like. In my office, we deal with over 200 different insurance plans, including plans that have slightly different versions contracted individually with each employer. We cannot possibly be as expert as we would like to be on your individual policy. Do your homework!
- **Be alert for trouble at the office.** Watch for signs that indicate you may receive more attentive care elsewhere:

> — Routinely experiencing long waits to be seen
> — Frequent interruptions during your visit
> — Calls that are not returned
> — Differences in philosophy towards care
> — Your general sense of trust in your doctor and his advice

- **Keep new events in your family history up to date in your file.** New health issues experienced by family members may help plan your future health care.

- **Keep your address and phone numbers current.** Make it easy for your doctor to contact you with test results or other health information he or she may want to share with you.

- **Discuss any end-of-life wishes that you have with your doctor.** If you have a Living Will, give a copy to your doctor. To be assured that your wishes will be followed if you are incapacitated, be familiar with your state laws and prepare a Health Care Power of Attorney document if you need one. If you would refuse a blood transfusion under any circumstances due to religious or other beliefs, notify your doctor in writing. If you have decided not to undergo life support (mechanical ventilation or cardiac resuscitation), let your family members and your doctor know of your decision.

- **Be aware that, like marriages, not all doctor-patient relationships work out.** Every year I see a few new patients that I know need a doctor with a different style than my own. Our approaches to medical care, philosophies toward life, and/or general style of communication are simply not compatible, and the difference is not fixable. When this happens (and it will since humans are involved), it is best simply for both parties to recognize the incompatibility and move on. I don't want or expect to be everyone's favorite doctor.

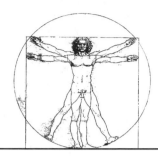

Body Systems—
How They Work and What
to Do When They Don't

In Part II, we will explore the major body systems, from head to toe, and some common things that can go wrong within these systems.

CHAPTER 15

The Skin

The skin, when considered as a single unit, is the largest organ in the body. It includes the epidermis (outermost layer), the dermis (the living, most active portion), and several embedded structures such as hair follicles, sweat glands, and sebaceous glands.

The skin has three distinct functions:

- **Protection.** The skin is a tough covering that protects the body, resisting tears and cuts. It also protects the body as the immune system's first line of defense against invaders, such as splinters, bacteria, and other infectious agents.
- **Preservation.** The skin provides an envelope that helps protect the body from loss of fluid. The skin also helps preserve the body's desired temperature. If the body is too hot, blood vessels just underneath the skin dilate and transfer heat to it, and sweat glands activate causing the body to cool as moisture evaporates from the skin. If the body is cold, blood vessels beneath the skin constrict, reducing blood flow to the skin and therefore reducing heat loss.
- **Presentation.** The skin and its appendages (hair and nails) help create our appearance, playing an important role in how others view us and how we view ourselves.

Numerous diseases and processes affect the skin. This chapter will review skin problems we see most often in the primary care office setting: acne, rosacea, contact dermatitis, seborrheic dermatitis, atopic dermatitis and eczema, psoriasis, tinea versicolor, skin infections, hair (to little and too much), photoaging, and skin cancer.

Acne

Acne is a chronic infectious and inflammatory disorder of the skin that typically waxes and wanes over time. It is not caused by poor hygiene; in fact, excessive scrubbing can worsen the underlying inflammation and worsen the acne. Acne affects 80 percent or more of the population ages 12 through 25, but can occur at any age. It affects the sweat and oil glands of the face, chest, and back, and is painful both physically and psychologically.

Sebaceous glands are larger structures in the skin that produce sebum, a lipid mixture important in maintaining hydration of the skin. Several factors lead to the development

of acne. During adolescence, the surge of androgen hormones stimulates an excess production of sebum. The sebaceous gland becomes blocked by some of the excess material
it is producing. It continues to produce more sebum and keratin, leading to whiteheads
or blackheads. Propionibacterium acnes, bacteria that reside in the follicles, begin to
grow in number. This creates inflammation, both as the body's immune system attacks
the bacteria and as the bacteria produce fatty acids that irritate the wall of the follicle.
The sebum leaks from the irritated follicle into the surrounding dermis, further worsening the inflammation.

The goal for therapy in acne is to reduce the severity and frequency of outbreaks,
lessen discomfort from inflamed lesions, improve appearance, and prevent or minimize
scarring. Most adolescents want immediate gratification from their efforts. I warn my
patients right from the beginning that it usually takes six weeks before we begin to see
the benefit of a treatment for acne, and that our ultimate goal is for the control of acne,
not cure.

To successfully treat acne, both the infectious and inflammatory portions of the disease must be addressed. Treatment programs are designed to kill or greatly reduce the
number of bacteria and to prevent inflammation. Killing the bacteria takes time. Even
when the bacteria are dead, their bodies continue to stimulate the immune system until
they are naturally washed out of the glands, a process which takes four to six weeks.
Medications must be taken regularly to be effective, and topical therapies must be applied to whole regions of skin, not just individual pimples. Oil-based cosmetics and
moisturizers can plug up sebaceous glands, thereby worsening acne. Picking, popping,
or excessive scrubbing irritates the skin and increases the likelihood of inflammation and
scarring. Despite popular belief, diet does not seem to play much of a role in acne and
numerous trials of rigid dietary restrictions have not proven beneficial in acne
management.

The following common therapies are used to control acne:

- **Benzoyl Peroxide.** This common, over-the-counter and prescription acne treatment improves acne by killing the acne bacteria. It also dries and promotes skin
  peeling, which helps clear blocked follicles. Little evidence exists that 10 percent
  benzoyl peroxide is any better than lower concentrations, and it is certainly more
  irritating. In general, gels are more effective. I usually prescribe a thin film of a 5
  percent gel twice daily.
- **Tretinoins (Retin-A).** This topical therapy works to prevent formation of
  whiteheads and blackheads and resolve those already present. It stimulates the turnover of new cells within the sebaceous gland; because of this, acne may initially
  worsen before it improves. Depending on the dose, the skin may look more red
  and scaly for two to four weeks; for this reason, therapy is started at the lowest dose
  and slowly increased. These products are inactivated by sunlight, so they are best
  applied at bedtime. They are also inactivated by benzoyl peroxide; therefore, these
  two products cannot be applied at the same time.
- **Antibiotics.** These work by killing or inhibiting the growth of the acne bacteria.
  Most studies show that topical antibiotics are quite close in effectiveness to

antibiotics by mouth. I generally leave this to the patient's preferred choice. While swallowing a pill is easier than cleansing the skin and smearing a cream on twice a day, pills can have other, unpleasant side effects.

- **Accutane.** This is a powerful drug, and is the only drug that actually alters the natural history of acne. Accutane causes sebaceous glands to shrink and become much less active; it lowers the number of bacteria in the gland, changes the type of sebum produced, and also directly reduces inflammation. Of patients with severe acne, 90 percent have complete or almost complete clearing of their acne with a 16-week course of therapy, and this improvement can last a long time. Unfortunately, the drug can have severe side effects—including irritation of the lining of the mouth, eyelids, and nose; sensitivity to sunlight; joint and muscle pains; headaches; hair loss; loss of night vision; adverse effects on triglycerides and cholesterol; liver and bone marrow problems; severe birth defects when taken soon before or during pregnancy, and psychological effects—and is therefore recommended only for patients with severe cystic and scarring acne. Accutane should be prescribed by a physician well familiar with its use.
- **Hormone therapy.** The use of birth control pills increases the blood level of a protein that binds hormones. This protein binds the androgens, reducing their level in the bloodstream and thereby reducing the excessive stimulation for sebum production.

Effective treatment of acne requires a good level of cooperation between patient and physician and knowledge about the nature of acne and its therapies.

Rosacea

Rosacea is an acne-like condition of the skin that usually begins in middle-aged adults. It is characterized by tiny bumps and pustules on the cheeks, chin, nose, and forehead, excessive flushing, and the development of tiny superficial blood vessels. The nose can develop a characteristic appearance with overgrowth of connective tissue and sebaceous glands (the W.C. Fields nose). Rosacea is worsened by consumption of hot liquids such as coffee and tea, alcohol, some spicy foods, and sunlight.

Rosacea is the result of a superficial, slow-growing infection of the skin in susceptible patients. It is treated with antibiotic therapy, including oral tetracycline and topical antibiotics. Treatment must often be prolonged to be effective, and must continue at a low dose to prevent relapse. The development of superficial blood vessels and nose changes can be minimized or avoided altogether if the condition is recognized early and treated. If the superficial blood vessels are large or numerous, laser therapy may be needed for improvement.

Contact Dermatitis

Contact dermatitis is an inflammatory reaction of the skin to a substance that it has been in contact with. Two types of contact dermatitis exist: *Irritant dermatitis*, which is caused by exposure to substances that chemically irritate the skin (such as acid or paint removers) and *allergic dermatitis*, which results from exposure to substances that the body has previously seen (such as plants, cosmetics, or topical antibiotics).

Often, the cause of the rash is obvious based on recent exposures and the distribution of the dermatitis on the skin. If the cause of the reaction is not known, dermatologists may perform patch tests by applying small quantities of likely substances to see what the skin reacts to. Heat, sweating, friction, or preexisting skin disease generally worsen reactions.

Plant dermatitis (reaction to contact with Poison Ivy, Oak, and Sumac) is particularly a problem in our region of North Carolina. The sap on the leaves and vines can invoke severe allergic reactions. "Leaves of three, let it be" is a good rule of thumb in avoiding the poison ivy plant and its subsequent irritation. Unfortunately, the sap can also cause reactions when the vines are barren of leaves, so try to avoid touching the plant even in winter when its leaves have fallen off. Also remember that sap on gloves and clothing retains its ability to cause reactions for weeks unless the articles are washed in hot, soapy water and that pets can bring the sap to owners on their coats. When you touch one of these plants, the sap physically imbeds itself in skin; after a few minutes, you cannot wash or scrub it off.

Plant dermatitis causes an inflammatory reaction to the skin, characterized by red, warm, swollen patches that develop superficial blisters filled with clear fluid. Contrary to popular belief, poison ivy does not "spread." Areas with the heaviest exposure of the most sensitive skin break out first, followed within a day or two by areas with lighter exposure. Sometimes, exposure to poison ivy triggers a generalized immune response, causing rashes to erupt on skin that was not exposed to the plant.

Often, topical therapies are insufficient for the treatment of poison ivy and steroid injections or oral steroids must be used. As with any severe skin inflammation, the possibility of a secondary bacterial infection of the open skin exists; skin that is not improving with therapy must be reevaluated for possible infection.

The best treatment is knowledge of—and avoidance of—the irritants. Consider wearing barrier creams and gloves to protect from further exposure. If you have already come in contact with an irritant, use cold compresses or oatmeal baths to help relieve inflamed skin. To help relieve the itching, try older, over-the-counter antihistamines (the newer "nonsedating" antihistamines don't seem to work as well for this problem). Avoid scratching and rubbing the skin or exposing irritated skin to heat, which increases the level of histamine in the skin and worsens the itching. If your reaction is severe, your doctor may prescribe topical or oral steroids.

Seborrheic Dermatitis

Like acne, seborrheic dermatitis is a chronic inflammatory disorder that affects areas where sebaceous glands are most prominent—the scalp (dandruff), eyebrows and lashes, mustache and beard, forehead, ear canals, chest, and body folds. Seborrheic dermatitis appears as red and itchy areas with white, fine scales on a greasy base. It is usually symmetric on the body. This condition occurs in 3 percent of the population, affecting men slightly more than women.

Although the cause of seborrheic dermatitis is not precisely known, it is associated with yeast infections and responds to topical antifungal medications. Hygiene is important; frequent cleansing with soap removes excess oils and improves the appearance. Antifungal preparations, such as dandruff shampoos and prescription alternatives, along with anti-inflammatory creams (steroid creams) form the bulk of most therapies. Sunlight does help reduce the severity of the condition.

Atopic Dermatitis and Eczema

Atopic dermatitis and eczema are also chronic, inflammatory conditions of the skin. They occur in 5 to 10 percent of children and 1 percent of adults; because most patients get atopic dermatitis before age five, this condition is usually diagnosed by pediatricians. Atopic dermatitis often is a marker for patients who will develop problems with allergies and asthma later in life.

Whereas contact dermatitis typically resolves in days to weeks, atopic dermatitis and eczema last from months to a lifetime. These conditions appear as red, shallow erosions in the skin and tiny blisters filled with clear fluid. Intense itching leads to red, scratched, thickened areas, skin dryness, and changes in skin pigmentation. Affected areas typically involve the neck, creases of the elbows and knees, wrists and ankles, and hands and feet. Atopic dermatitis is worsened by certain foods (including eggs, peanuts, milk, wheat and soy products, and fish), allergy-inducing substances in the air (including pollen and mold), animal dander, heat, irritation (such as wool fabrics), sweating, infection, and stress. These associations suggest that these diseases are associated with a general activation of the immune system. In 90 percent of atopic dermatitis lesions, the bacterium Staphylococcus aureus exists and secretes toxins that activate the immune response in the skin; in some cases, the skin can improve with medication to treat these bacteria.

Atopic dermatitis is a chronic disease that cannot be cured but can be managed by identifying and removing the factors that worsen it. This includes receiving an allergy evaluation and removing those factors such as foods, irritants, stress, and infectious agents. It is important to keep the skin moisturized and hydrated; soaking in a bath for 10 to 20 minutes and applying oil to seal in the moisture helps. Itching is controlled with antihistamines. Typically, the older, more sedating antihistamines work better than the newer, non-sedating agents. Topical steroids and other medications are used to control the inflammation. In general, treatment is started with mild preparations and increased in strength over time as needed.

Psoriasis

Psoriasis is a chronic skin disease that usually occurs in young adults and affects between 1.5 and 2 percent of the U.S. population. Inflamed, raised areas of silvery, scaly skin on the scalp, elbows, and knees characterize this disease.

Skin cells are constantly shed from the topmost layer of skin and replaced with new skin cells. New skin cells form in the deepest portions of the skin and slowly mature as they head toward the surface, a process that normally takes about 14 days to complete. With psoriasis, the cell turnover is greatly accelerated and the entire process occurs in as little as 2 days. Cells cannot fully mature in this short life cycle, altering their appearance into the scaly patches characteristic of psoriasis lesions. We do not know what causes this accelerated turnover of skin cells, but there appears to be a strong genetic basis. Of patients with psoriasis, 5 to 10 percent also develop psoriatic arthritis. Psoriatic arthritis is an inflammatory type of arthritis characterized by involvement of the spine and the joints of the hands and feet. It is often associated with prolonged morning stiffness lasting more than 30 minutes, and begins with greatest frequency between ages 30 and 50.

Sunlight helps improve psoriasis. Other topical therapies include steroid creams and coal tar preparations. Drugs that affect cell turnover, such as the cancer drug methotrexate, are widely used for treatment. Some therapies combine the use of a drug that sensitizes the skin to light with controlled doses of ultraviolet light, and new therapies are continually becoming available. Most patients with moderate to severe psoriasis benefit from consultation with a dermatologist.

Tinea Versicolor

Tinea Versicolor is a superficial skin disease that usually affects the trunk and central portions of the extremities. It is characterized by circular areas of altered skin pigmentation; these areas do not become scaly unless they are scratched. This condition worsens with summer's heat and humidity. Tinea Versicolor typically does not itch and cannot be passed from one person to another.

A yeast called Pityrosporum orbiculare causes this condition. Although this yeast is found on everyone, patients who develop Tinea Versicolor may be genetically more susceptible to an immune system reaction to the yeast, causing the change in skin appearance.

Tinea Versicolor is treated with antifungal shampoos (dandruff shampoos such as selenium sulfide and ketoconazole) or with a short-term course of antifungal tablets. Some of these medications concentrate in sweat; this creates an ideal delivery mechanism—the patient takes a pill, waits 30 to 60 minutes, and then exercises, allowing the sweat to dry on the skin. Often, this condition must be retreated every summer season.

Skin Infections

Skin infections can be caused by bacteria, viruses, or fungi. Bacteria, most commonly Staphylococcus aureus or group A Streptococcus, can cause a skin infection called *cellulitis*. Viruses in the Herpes family can cause a skin infection called *shingles*. Fungi sometimes cause affect *fingernail* and *toenail infections*.

Cellulitis

Cellulitis is a bacterial infection that typically appears as a red, hot, painful swelling on the surface of the skin. Often spreading rapidly, cellulitis requires a physical crack or break in the skin for the bacteria to get around the skin's natural defenses and cause infection. In my practice, I most commonly see cellulitis of the foot and lower leg related to cracks between the toes from athletes' foot. Cellulitis must be treated promptly with antibiotics, and it is important for you to contact your physician at once if you suspect that you have it. Athletes' foot should be treated to prevent this complication.

Shingles

Shingles is a common viral infection of the skin seen in primary care offices. Shingles is caused by the Varicella-zoster virus in the Herpes family, a virus that is often acquired in childhood as chicken pox. It lives permanently in an inactive state in the roots of your spinal nerves. In approximately 20 percent of patients, the virus eventually reactivates and attacks one or more adjacent spinal nerves. This creates exquisite skin sensitivity in a band-like region on one side of the body, followed by pain that is often described as burning, intense itching, aching, or stinging. After about three days, this area of skin will break out in tiny white blisters that appear in clusters on a reddened base. The risk of shingles increases after age 50, most likely as a result of changes in how the immune system functions at that age.

If you have symptoms that you suspect relate to early shingles, it is important to see your physician promptly. Antiviral medications exist that can ease the pain of shingles, speed healing, and minimize chronic pain associated with this condition. However, to be effective, these medications must be started within 72 hours of the development of the rash. At times, I have started medication later than this and seen some benefit, but early treatment is certainly better.

The pain of shingles can be severe. When usual pain medications are ineffective, the patient can be referred to a pain specialist to have a nerve block performed. In a nerve block, the pain specialist identifies the nerve roots that are involved in the shingles outbreak and injects a long-acting anesthetic and other medications at the base of the nerve to deaden all sensation transmitted by the involved nerve. This exchanges the painful sensation for a numb one. Injections can be repeated if the pain returns when the initial injection wears off. Some patients with shingles will go on to develop post-herpetic neuralgia, a painful, disabling, and chronic pain along the nerve related to the shingles outbreak. Doctors are trying a variety of new treatments to try to provide relief to patients with post-herpetic neuralgia. Researchers are evaluating the use of the chicken pox vaccine in adults to reactivate the adult's immune system to respond to the virus before shingles occurs.

Fungal Nail Infections

Fungal nail infections are common infections that cause thickening and discoloration—progressing over many years—of fingernails and toenails. Because this infection involves the nail and nail bed itself, topical therapy is generally ineffective. A toenail takes 9 to 12 months to grow out; whatever therapy is chosen to treat the infection must provide adequate drug levels in the nail until this happens. For most patients, fungal nail infections are a cosmetic problem and do not lead to significant other medical problems or discomfort, and need not be treated.

In the past five years, new medications became available for treatment of this condition, including Lamisil and Sporonox. These antifungal medications reach high concentrations in the nail and are the most effective therapies available to date. Using these medications, treatment lasts 12 weeks for toenails and 6 for fingernails; the drug companies producing these medications claim a clinical cure rate (that is, the likelihood of restoring the nail to normal) of up to 38 percent for toenails and 60 percent for fingernails.

Unfortunately, some people experience adverse reactions to these medications. Mild and transient reactions include headaches, diarrhea, indigestion, rashes, and taste change. Rare but serious reactions include liver, skin, and bone marrow reactions. Use of these medications requires monitoring and laboratory tests by a physician. The drugs themselves are quite costly. Unless a patient is highly motivated to treat his or her nail condition, I have not found the expense and risk of therapy to be justified by the mediocre outcomes that most patients receive. Newer regiments for use of these drugs are being designed.

A promising therapy suggested by my patients involves the use of Vicks vapor rub applied on the nail twice daily. This can help thin the nail and improve appearance. Some clinical studies now in progress suggest that the chemicals in this substance may be effective in treating this condition.

Hair: Alopecia and Hirsutism

Hair grows in cycles that include a growth phase and a rest phase. Each cycle lasts approximately three months. When a hair follicle enters a growth phase, the new hair pushes the old hair out, resulting in an average hair loss of hundreds of hairs a day. Sometimes, hair loss is temporarily increased after a major illness, life stress, or pregnancy. This increased hair loss is usually a sign that hair growth had decreased for a while and new hairs are beginning to grow. Two common hair problems are *alopecia* (too little hair) and *hirsutism* (too much hair).

Alopecia

Alopecia affects one of two men by age 50, and is a complaint of 1 of every 20 women in surveys. This is generally a cosmetic problem only, and no treatment is needed unless the patient desires it. Topical therapies include Minoxidil, which is now available without prescription. We do not know for sure how this drug works, but it appears to have a direct effect on hair follicles, which increase in size with treatment, and also on the number of hairs in the scalp. When the drug is stopped, all newly regrown hair falls out. Side effects include local irritation, scalp dryness, and redness. The 2 percent solution is almost as good as the 5 percent solution in long-term studies, is less costly, and has fewer side effects.

Considerable interest has been generated in a new medication, finasteride (Propecia), for hair loss in men. This drug affects the metabolism of testosterone, blocking the enzyme that converts testosterone to dihydrotestosterone (DHT). DHT shortens the growth phase of the hair follicle, and reducing the amount of DHT can be of benefit. Of patients who use this drug, 80 percent see a reduction in hair loss and 60 percent see regrowth of some hair. This expensive drug must be used at least six months for full effect. In the original drug trials, side effects were significant enough for 1.4 percent of the patients to stop taking the drug. Reported side effects include decreased libido, changes in erections and ejaculation, breast tenderness and enlargement in men, and allergic reactions including rashes and hives. In these trials, 50 percent of those taking the drug for 24 months felt that their appearance was improved by this medication; however, keep in mind that in the same study, 30 percent of those using placebo—that is, no active medication—also felt their appearance was improved. The long-term effects of interfering with the metabolism of testosterone are unknown, and this medication must be taken forever in order to maintain its benefit. Because of its expense and the uncertainties of long-term treatment, I have agreed to prescribe this drug only on a very limited basis. Unfortunately, not many options currently exist for women with alopecia, other than excluding common scalp disorders that may be causing it.

Hirsutism

Hirsutism refers to excessive growth of facial and bodily hair. It can be inherited or caused by diseases such as polycystic ovarian disease or other conditions in which an excess of androgen is produced. Women with this condition should seek a medical evaluation to ensure that it is not a sign of underlying disease. One treatment option involves the use of the diuretic spironolactone, which reduces the sensitivity of hair follicles in skin to androgen stimulation. Another option is laser therapy reduction, with a minimum of six treatments; this therapy can be quite effective and less painful than electrolysis but carries the risk of pigmentary changes, especially in darker toned people. A third option includes a new prescription cream for women with excessive facial hair called Eflornithine HCl cream (Vaniqa), which became available in 2000. This cream blocks an enzyme related to hair follicle stimulation and effectively stops facial hair growth in 35 percent of women who used it for 24 weeks. Reported side effects include stinging, burning, and acne. At greater than $40 per tube, and with most patients averaging two tubes a month for treatment, this drug is for treatment of women with excessive hair growth, not for "prevention" of problems in women without a history of excessive facial hair.

Photoaging

Skin's texture and elasticity is affected naturally through the normal aging process. This process is accelerated by *photoaging*, the process of affecting skin structure through chronic ultraviolet irradiation (that is, sustained sun exposure). Photoaging leads to thickened, pebbly, coarse skin with prominent wrinkles and irregular pigmentation, eventual loss of skin thickness, development of superficial blood vessels on the skin, easily bruised skin, and skin cancer. You can best prevent photoaging by avoiding excessive sun exposure, particularly in childhood and early adult years. When you do venture out into the sun for long periods (such as an excursion to the beach on a sunny—or cloudy—day), use a sunscreen with an SPF of 30 or greater, and reapply it often.

Sunscreens: What is SPF?

Sunscreens are rated using a Skin Protection Factor (SPF) rating system. The SPF gives a ratio of how long skin can be exposed to the sun before burning while protected with the sunscreen, compared with unprotected skin. For example, an SPF of 15 means that average skin can be out in the sun 15 times longer before burning with the sunscreen on than without it. A sunscreen with an SPF rating of 30 or greater is recommended for partial protection from the sun's damaging ultraviolet-B (UVB) rays.

No rating system exists for ultraviolet-A (UVA) rays. Although UVA rays do not burn, they do penetrate the skin deeper and are suspected to be a significant contributor to skin cancer, skin damage, and wrinkling. Look for newer sun protection products that protect from both UVB and UVA rays.

One last thing… If you have any sunscreen products lying around the house from last summer, check the expiration date. If the date reminds you of happy childhood beach memories, throw the product away! The ingredients in sunscreen products lose their protective properties over time, and using sunscreens past their expiration dates protects nothing but your false sense of security.

Photoaging is treated using topical therapies such as topical tretinoin (Renova). This substance is a metabolite of vitamin A; it reduces the activity of certain enzymes that break down skin and increases the formation of collagen in the dermis. Using this cream in a 0.05 percent concentration for three to six months improves fine wrinkling, surface roughness, and pigmentary changes. Side effects can include redness, burning, itching, peeling, and dryness, side effects that can be tolerated over time. Tretinoin is inactivated by sunlight and should be applied at night. Some cosmetic products contain alpha-hydroxy acids, which—when used over a six-month period—can help thicken the skin and improve appearance; however, long-term studies are not available for these products.

Many other services are available through qualified specialists, including peeling of the skin (called dermabrasion) by an experienced provider, injecting collagen or fat to build up tissue below the skin, and injecting Botox to paralyze the fine muscles beneath the skin and reduce wrinkles. Before pursuing any of these treatment options, I recommend that you work with your primary care physician for referral to a specialist with adequate experience in these demanding procedures.

Skin Cancer

The primary risk of skin cancer correlates to excessive exposure to sunlight. A few serious sunburns in childhood or as a young adult significantly increase the future risk for skin cancer. It is crucially important to avoid excessive sun exposure, particularly during peak sun hours. As mentioned when we discussed photoaging, most sunscreens protect against UVB radiation (the cause of burns) but do not provide reliable protection for UVA radiation, which penetrates skin more deeply and may be more closely related to skin cancer.

Skin cancer can occur anywhere on the body, but is most common in areas heavily exposed to the sun such as the tops of the ears, cheeks, nose, back of the neck, and forearms. Your primary care physician should evaluate any lesion that appears to be changing over time or that won't heal. All patients should receive a complete skin survey during their periodic physical examination.

Common types of skin lesions that may turn cancerous include:

- **Dysplastic nevi:** Abnormal moles that have a higher risk of becoming cancerous. They are usually larger than a pencil eraser (6 mm) and have an ill-defined border.
- **Actinic keratosis:** Red, sandpaper-textured lesions that come and go. They frequently peel off and then grow again in the same spot. These are related to sun exposure and are felt to be precursors to squamous cell cancers—an invasive, aggressive form of cancer that can spread to other areas of the body.
- **Basal cell carcinoma:** A locally aggressive cancer that can appear as a pearl-like growth on the surface of the skin or a sore that does not heal, often on sun-exposed areas. The surface of this type of cancer commonly contains superficial blood vessels that bleed easily.
- **Melanoma:** A serious type of skin cancer that tends to spread to other body regions early and can be life threatening. Melanoma needs prompt identification and referral to a specialist for care.

The ABCDs of Melanoma

Recognize the signs of melanoma by remembering "ABCD":

Asymmetry, a frequent sign in all skin cancers

Border, which is often irregularly notched by the immune system in its failed attempt to destroy it

Color, which can be the red of inflammation, white from the loss of pigment, or a blue/black from excess production of pigmentation

Diameter (bigger than a pencil eraser)

CHAPTER 16

The Eye

An eye care specialist—an Optometrist or Ophthalmologist—provides the majority of eye care for most patients. The purpose of this chapter is to increase your awareness of some common conditions that affect the eye and vision so that you can seek appropriate attention if needed. This chapter will review those diseases that affect the structure or function of the eye: conjunctivitis, eyelid infections, subconjunctival hemorrhage, eye injury, cataracts, glaucoma, and macular degeneration.

The Eye

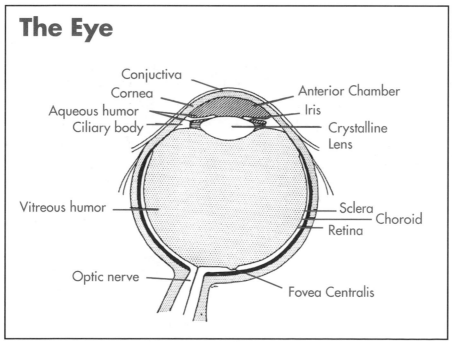

Conjuctiva
Cornea
Aqueous humor
Ciliary body
Anterior Chamber
Iris
Crystalline Lens
Vitreous humor
Sclera
Choroid
Retina
Optic nerve
Fovea Centralis

LifeArt, Lippincott Williams & Wilkins 2002

Conjunctivitis

Conjunctivitis is inflammation of the conjunctiva, the visible portion of the moist tissue surrounding the eyeball. In conjunctivitis, this tissue is red, swollen, and irritated and has a clear or discolored discharge. Conjunctivitis can be caused by infection stemming from a virus or bacteria, allergies, or other immune reactions. *Infectious conjunctivitis* is easily spread by touch from one eye to the other, or to another person. You can limit the spread of infection by washing your hands after touching the face and avoiding touching other people (shaking hands). It is difficult to tell on examination whether a virus or bacteria caused the infection, and as a result most patients are treated with antibiotic eye drops. As with any antibiotic, these must be used regularly and for the prescribed duration of treatment (typically seven days). Patients usually note improvement within 48 hours. Do not save or share antibiotic eye drops; the dropper tip often becomes contaminated by eye secretions and you can spread the infection by doing so. Some patients can develop an allergy to the eye drops; if your eye seems to worsen after two or three days of medicated drops, see your doctor again. Some infections benefit from steroid drops to reduce the inflammation. Given the potential for serious side effects of steroids in the eye, I recommend that only an eye specialist prescribe them.

Allergic conjunctivitis is usually diagnosed by its relation to allergen exposures and other allergy symptoms. A variety of topical medications are available, both with and without prescription. Oral antihistamines are typically ineffective for treatment of eye symptoms.

Eyelid Infections

A *stye*, or *hordeolum*, is a localized infection in the eyelid that may begin as a diffuse swelling and redness of the eyelid. Treatment consists of relieving the obstruction and improving drainage of the tiny glands near the eyelashes, reducing swelling and inflammation, and resolving the infection. A warm compress is held to the infected eye for five minutes. Then, the eyelid is gently scrubbed with a solution of 50 percent "no tears" baby shampoo in water on a cotton ball for several strokes. Antibiotic drops or ointment follows. The entire process is repeated four times daily. The role that the antibiotic plays in treating these types of infections is controversial; most of the benefit seems to come from the warm soaks and scrubs. Some patients have persistent or recurrent infections and need evaluation and possibly surgical drainage by a specialist.

Subconjunctival Hemorrhage

A *subconjunctival hemorrhage* appears as fresh blood covering a portion of the sclera (white part) of the eye. Although this is visually alarming and usually prompts an emergency call to the doctor, this condition is fortunately entirely benign. It is caused by rupture and bleeding of a tiny blood vessel on the surface of the sclera and is most likely due to minor trauma such as rubbing the eyeball. What would be an insignificant bruise anywhere else on the skin looks like a disaster on the eyeball because of the stark contrast of red blood on a white background. Unfortunately, it can take several days to weeks for the blood to be reabsorbed from the surface of the eye. A subconjunctival hemorrhage should not cause any pain or any change in vision; if these signs are present, seek medical attention.

Eye Injury

My advice in preventing eye injury consists of three words: wear protective lenses. If the instructions that accompany a machine or tool tell you to wear protective lenses, believe it. In our large primary care practice, we see patients weekly with eye injuries that could have been prevented by protective lenses. Once or twice a year, I must refer a patient with an injury that could potentially cause permanent vision loss. Any activity that has the potential for producing a projectile (small, flying object) should prompt you automatically to wear protective lenses. This includes common activities such as hammering a nail (small bits of metal may chip off the head and injure the eye) or using power lawn tools. Activities such as bicycle riding, motorcycle riding, and powerboat riding also call for sunglasses or other protective lenses. A bug in the eye at 20 mph can do a lot of damage.

Cataracts

The eye focuses light with a lens that is located immediately behind the pupil (the black circle in the center of the eye). A *cataract* is the result of clouding of the lens, caused when the proteins that make up the lens clump together. Proteins clump together when they are damaged by aging, the sun's ultraviolet rays, chemicals in cigarette smoke, and certain diseases and drugs (including steroids). The best ways to prevent cataracts are to avoid contact with cigarette smoke and to wear lenses with UV light protection when outside.

Some researchers believe that lens protein damage also occurs by a process of oxidation. The eye contains high levels of antioxidants, and studies suggest that individuals with a high amount of antioxidants in their diet have fewer cataracts. Whether taking supplemental antioxidant vitamins would help prevent cataracts is unproven.

Cataracts can be surgically repaired when the degree of clouding causes enough impairment of vision to prevent a patient from legally operating an automobile (that is, when the best-corrected vision is 20/50 or worse) or when it is bothersome enough to the patient to desire surgery. Cataract surgery involves making a tiny incision in the eye, pulverizing the lens with ultrasound, sucking the old lens fragments out, and implanting an artificial lens in its place. This surgery is performed under local anesthesia and most patients report only minor discomfort. Complications occur in 2 to 4 percent of cases and include temporary swelling, detachment of the retina, development of glaucoma, infection, or displacement of the lens. Half of all patients will experience a clouding of the back of the new lens over time, which can be cleared with laser surgery.

Glaucoma

The normal eyeball creates a constant supply of fluid that washes through the eye. If this fluid doesn't properly circulate, the build-up causes *glaucoma*, an increase in eye pressure. Two types of glaucoma exist:

- **Angle-closure glaucoma.** With this form of glaucoma, there is a sudden obstruction to fluid flow from the eye, often related to inherited anatomical characteristics of the eye. The patient will develop sudden and extreme eye pain and blurred vision, often accompanied by nausea and vomiting. Angle-closure glaucoma is a medical and surgical emergency in order to preserve sight.
- **Open-angle glaucoma.** More commonly, patients experience the open-angle glaucoma. In this disease, the extra pressure slowly damages the optic nerve (the large nerve in the back of the eye that transmits visual signals to the brain), eventually leading to progressive loss of vision and blindness. There are no warning signs for early open-angle glaucoma. Early detection requires regular examinations of the optic nerve and measurements of eye pressure. Studies show that at least 50 percent of patients with open-angle glaucoma don't know that they have it! Patients should receive routine exams every three to five years before age 45 and every one to three years after age 45. Those with additional risks for glaucoma—previous borderline elevations in eye pressure, African descent, family history of glaucoma, nearsightedness, diabetes, hypertension, and prolonged use of steroids—should be examined more often. Medical and surgical therapies are available for this disease.

Macular Degeneration

The retina, on the inside of the eyeball, collects visual images and transmits them as electrical signals along the optic nerve to the brain. The most precise area of vision is located in the macula, the center of the visual field. In this area, the concentrations of rods and cones (the receptors of light in the retina) are the highest. *Macular degeneration* is the breakdown of this crucial area of vision. This leads to loss of high definition vision, such as that used for reading, driving, watching television, and recognizing faces. While peripheral vision remains intact, the loss of central vision greatly affects daily activity and leads to reduced mobility and a greater number of falls and fractures.

Macular degeneration is the leading cause of severe vision loss in the elderly. In addition to age, risk factors include smoking—the risk of this disease triples in smokers—and race, with non-Hispanic whites at greatest risk. Studies show that individuals who have diets high in fruits and vegetables, such as green leafy spinach and kale, have less macular degeneration. There is no evidence that taking supplements helps prevent or treat this disease.

The disease is categorized as early or late. Early disease is only identified by an eye examination, where yellowish deposits are seen in the region of the macula just below the surface. In early disease, vision is usually stable for years and loss of vision is gradual.

Late disease is categorized into two types: *atrophic*, characterized by slow degeneration, and *exudative*, characterized by sudden degeneration. Most patients have the atrophic type. While no present therapy exists for this condition, it is important to have close follow-up with your eye physician to assess remaining vision and disability, recommend optical aides and devices, and provide training and suggestions to improve home safety. The exudative type of macular degeneration can be associated with sudden and severe visual loss from the development of fluid and tiny blood vessels beneath the retina. A small percentage of patients with this type of macular degeneration benefit from laser therapy, which reduces the risk of further visual loss.

CHAPTER 17

The Ear

The ear is responsible for two separate functions: hearing and balance. Issues related to malfunctions in balance are covered in *Chapter 28: The Neurological System*.

The ear is constructed of a large, fleshy external portion that helps capture sound from the environment and internal structures divided anatomically into different levels. Sound travels down the outer ear canal, which leads through the bone of the skull to the eardrum. The eardrum stretches across the base of the canal, completely closing it from the outside. The middle ear cavity is on the opposite side of the eardrum, and is connected to the back of the sinuses through a tiny tube called the eustachian tube. This tube functions to equalize pressure in the middle ear with the outside air. A series of three small bones connect the eardrum to the inner ear, the portion of the ear respon-

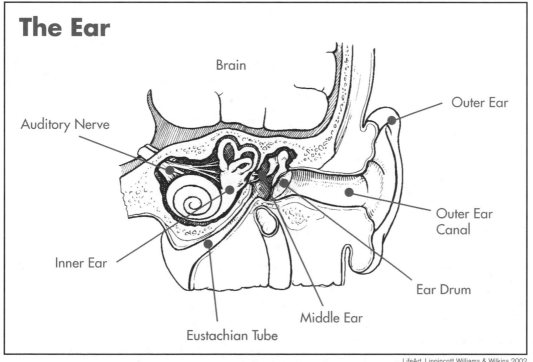

The Ear

Brain

Auditory Nerve

Outer Ear

Inner Ear

Outer Ear Canal

Eustachian Tube

Middle Ear

Ear Drum

LifeArt, Lippincott Williams & Wilkins 2002

sible for converting sound waves to electrical impulses transmitted to the brain for hearing. The portion of the ear associated with balance is also located in the inner ear.

This chapter will review those diseases that affect the structure or function of the ear: otitis externa ("swimmer's ear"), otitis media, ear wax impactions, and hearing loss.

Otitis Externa ("Swimmer's Ear")

Otitis externa ("swimmer's ear") is an infection of the outer ear canal between the outer ear and the eardrum. Patients suffering from this infection experience severe discomfort in the ear, which may be worsened by movement of the outer ear or chewing. The lining of the outer ear canal is stretched tightly over the bone of the skull, and there is not much room for swelling. Because of the intense swelling in this restricted space during an infection, this condition can be extremely painful. Usually, this infection is caused by a break in the lining of the membrane in the ear canal. This frequently occurs from trauma, such as the use of cotton swabs or other objects in the ear. The tip of the average cotton swab is larger than the diameter of the outer ear canal—pushing the swab in stretches and cracks the lining, allowing a door for bacteria and fungi to enter the tissue of the ear canal. Infections can also occur from breakdowns in the lining caused by chemical or water exposure, hence the name swimmer's ear.

You can prevent this infection by not placing any objects within the ear and by using prepared alcohol/acid drops after water exposure to dry the ear. As in all ear disorders, the diagnosis of otitis externa requires examination; many ear problems create the same type of pain and the diagnosis cannot be certain without inspection of the ear. Most outer ear infections are due to a combination of organisms (bacteria and fungi) and are complicated by the intense swelling which limits the ability to get medication to the site of infection. Prescription eardrops usually contain a combination of chemicals to treat these types of infection, as well as a steroid solution to reduce swelling. Occasionally, a cotton wick must be placed in the ear canal so that medication can reach all areas of infection.

Otitis Media

Otitis media involves infection of the middle portion of the ear. In adults, this frequently follows a nasal or sinus infection. When the nasal membrane is swollen, it can block the opening of the eustachian tube. This leads to accumulation of fluid in the middle ear cavity, which can become infected. Patients suffering from this infection experience severe pain, fever, and/or hearing loss and often describe that they are hearing in a drum or underwater. Physical examination can show an inflamed, bulging eardrum.

Treatment of otitis media involves treating the underlying infection and reducing its associated swelling. After these issues are addressed, the body will slowly reabsorb the extra fluid, sometimes taking weeks for hearing to be restored to normal. Doctors in the United States typically prescribe antibiotics for adults to clear the infection, selecting an antibiotic based on the most likely causes of infection and the characteristics of the patient (drug allergies and likely sensitivity to side effects). Because of the widespread used of antibiotics, greater than 50 percent of bacteria cultured from middle ear infections in research trials prove partially or totally resistant to the antibiotics that were used to successfully treat them. When the patient gets better on a drug that didn't cover the bacteria that caused the infection, the whole question about whether any antibiotic therapy was needed for the condition is raised. Doctors outside of the United States routinely prescribe fewer antibiotics for middle ear infections than we do. The patients in these countries seem to do just as well and experience fewer problems associated with excessive antibiotic usage. Current practice in the United States, however, has not yet been influenced by this observation.

Decongestants can help improve drainage and often the use of topical, long-acting nasal sprays for the first 48 to 72 hours can help relieve eustachian tube dysfunction. For patients with severe inflammation and pain, a dose of a short-acting steroid can help speed relief. Adequate pain medication—in most cases, ibuprofen or acetaminophen—is needed until the condition is controlled.

Ear Wax Impaction

Ear wax is constantly created in the outer ear canal. Its purpose is to moisturize the canal and to catch dust and other particles that make their way into the canal. The wax should flow slowly from the inside out, carrying debris with it as it gradually falls out of the ear canal. In many patients, the wax may be too dry, or the canal to small, for this system to function. Wax begins to accumulate and eventually can block the canal completely, resulting in discomfort and a significant drop in hearing.

Under no circumstances should anyone other than a trained professional place objects in the ear to attempt to remove the wax. The risks of damaging the ear canal or eardrum are simply too high. Doctors remove the wax using an instrument that gently scrapes or draws it out of the ear canal using suction; another technique involves washing it out with a stream of warm water and other chemicals. Once this is accomplished, the doctor teaches the patient how to flush the ear at home to prevent future impaction. For patients with significant and recurring ear wax impaction problems, I recommend they use a wax softener weekly and rinse their ears out with a special syringe, at least once a month, before they get completely blocked.

Hearing Loss

One out of every three people over age 65 has significant hearing loss. Most hearing loss relates to excessive noise exposure at a younger age. Once initial hearing loss occurs, the ear loses some of its protective reflexes, accelerating the risk of future hearing damage. It is extremely important to use hearing protection to prevent hearing loss when exposed to noise, including sound generated by high-pitched household appliances such as hair dryers and lawn tools. I advise my patients to purchase low-noise hair dryers and to use soft foam earplugs routinely when working with noisy tools and machinery or in other high-noise environments.

Symptoms of hearing loss include problems hearing normal conversation either over the phone or in settings with background noise, such as in restaurants, and difficulty hearing higher frequencies, such as the voices of women and children. Signs of hearing loss include playing the television or stereo too loudly, using an excessively loud voice, or misunderstanding speech leading to inappropriate responses.

While it is debatable whether routine hearing screening is warranted for adults other than for those in high-noise environments, anyone with a concern about their hearing should have a baseline hearing evaluation done and follow-up studies conducted as needed. Hearing aids, when appropriately prescribed, can be quite helpful. Unfortunately, most of the heavily advertised cheaper aids simply amplify all noise and do not help with the selective understanding of speech. Digital hearing aids have largely corrected this background noise problem, but these devices can be quite expensive. If you suspect you have a hearing problem and would like to seek professional help, I recommend obtaining a referral from your primary care physician to a reputable audiologist.

CHAPTER 18

The Nose and Sinuses

Why do we have noses? As a child with significant allergies and recurrent sinus infections, I vividly recall wanting to have my nose removed. My frequent trips to the doctor in childhood probably led to my own interest in medicine and my current profession.

The nose serves to warm and humidify the air before it reaches the lungs. It also acts as a rough filter, to help remove debris from the air. Additional functions include the sense of smell and performance as a resonating chamber for speech. The sinuses are air

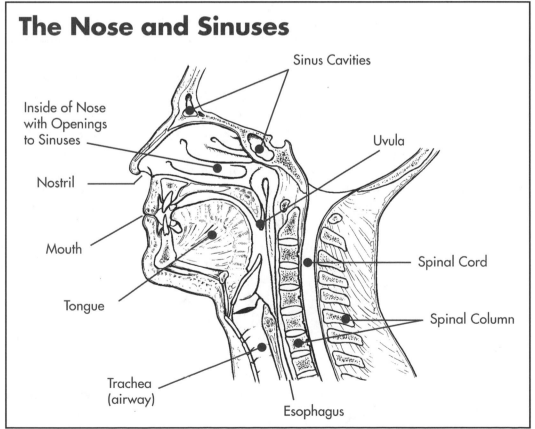

The Nose and Sinuses

Sinus Cavities

Inside of Nose with Openings to Sinuses

Uvula

Nostril

Mouth

Spinal Cord

Tongue

Spinal Column

Trachea (airway)

Esophagus

pockets in the bones; the best that I can figure is that they are designed to make one's face lighter and reduce neck strain.

The nose has two separate channels, separated by a thin structure called the *septum*. The nasal lining is a moist surface called the *mucosa*. It contains many blood vessels just beneath the surface, which supply heat to warm the air, provide moisture, and allow cells of the immune system to rapidly access the nose. The sinuses are connected to the nasal passageways by narrow openings called *ostia*. The sinuses are also lined with mucosa, which contains many microscopic hairs called *cilia*. A thin, clear mucus is secreted in the sinuses, and the cilia beat together like oars on a boat, sweeping this sheet of mucus through the ostia and out through the nose. Any particles, including viruses and bacteria, that enter the sinuses become stuck to this flypaper-like mucus and are carried out by this process. The quality and consistency of the mucus, as well as the openings of the ostia, are crucially important in keeping the sinuses clean and healthy. Sinusitis occurs when this system fails.

This chapter will review those diseases that affect the structure or function of the nose and sinuses: colds, sinusitis, and nosebleeds.

Colds

Colds are minor viral infections of the mucosal lining of the nose and throat. At least eight families of viruses exist that are known to cause colds. One of them, the Rhinovirus family, includes over 100 varieties. With such a large number of viruses causing this condition, a "cure for the common cold" is not expected any time soon.

Colds are the leading reason for office visits to the doctor each year in the United States. When a virus attacks the mucosa, the immune system initiates a reaction that causes most of the symptoms experienced. The blood vessels beneath the surface of the mucosa swell, forcing fluid to leak into the tissue under the mucosa, which causes swelling and a runny nose. Infection-fighting cells release chemicals in the mucosa, causing further tissue swelling and thickening and discoloration of the mucus. Protective reflexes such as sneezing and coughing are triggered. The narrow sinus ostia can become plugged by the swelling, which creates pressure in the sinus cavities and facial pain.

Although over 90 percent of upper respiratory infections seen by doctors are caused by viruses, one-half to two-thirds of patients experiencing these symptoms are treated with antibiotics. Patients have been trained to expect and often demand antibiotic therapy. In a recent survey, 40 percent of educated adults thought antibiotics helped with the common cold. Physicians lack the time to educate patients properly about the cause of their symptoms and the risks of antibiotics. This has led to significant problems with antibiotic resistance and unneeded exposure of patients to the potential side effects of drug therapy.

The average adult has two to six colds a year. Adults with young children, and those who work with children, have more. Prevention includes avoiding close contact with others, washing hands, and keeping your fingers and hands away from your face. Most colds should be treated with time and symptomatic therapy. Adequate hydration is very

> **Did You Know...**
>
> ...that colds cannot be treated with antibiotics? Colds are caused by viruses, which—unlike bacteria—do not respond to antibiotics. (For more information about viruses, bacteria, and antibiotics, see *Chapter 5: Infections and Antibiotics* on page 29.)
>
> The best treatment for a cold? Unfortunately, there is no magic treatment for a cold other than time, relief of symptoms, and vigilance for signs of secondary infections caused by bacteria taking advantage of the moist and congested environment created by the virus.

important. Acetaminophen or ibuprofen can help with fever and discomfort. Decongestants can help reduce swelling and nasal drainage. Topical decongestant nose sprays are useful in the first 48 to 72 hours, although problems with rebound swelling after the medication wears off begin to develop at that point. Antihistamines have only limited use; they tend to thicken the mucus and can further plug up the sinus ostia. Warm saltwater nasal douches are quite beneficial; steam can also help to loosen nasal secretions. If a cold begins to worsen after the first five days, a secondary bacterial sinusitis may be developing that may warrant antibiotic therapy; otherwise, most patients do not need antibiotics.

Many therapies have been adopted over the years to prevent and treat colds, including large doses of vitamin C. Numerous studies show that vitamin C has no effect on catching a cold or the length of the cold, and the use of large amounts of vitamin C is not advised. Conflicting evidence exists about whether zinc lozenges are helpful; they may slightly shorten the length of a cold. Echinacea also appears to shorten a cold's duration when used at the onset of symptoms. It does not help to take this product long-term and, in fact, this may diminish the strength of the immune system. There is no evidence that working or exercise will prolong a cold or worsen the symptoms, though this type of activity may increase the chances of spreading the cold to others.

Sinusitis

Sinusitis means infection of the sinus cavities. Sinus pain does not necessarily mean sinus infection. When mucosal swelling blocks the openings to the sinuses, pressure build-up in the sinuses can cause considerable pain even without infection. Symptoms of sinus infections include facial pressure, postnasal drainage, nasal congestion and obstruction, a change in taste or smell, eye or dental pressure or pain, fever, fatigue, ear pain, and cough. The chemicals in tobacco smoke interfere with the natural cleansing mechanism of the sinuses by thickening the mucus and paralyzing the cilia; therefore, smokers have more frequent sinus infections. A cold that worsens after four or five days can mean that a secondary sinus infection has developed. A doctor's decision to treat a probable sinus infection is often based on a best guess consideration of the available evidence; it is hard to prove or disprove whether a sinus actually is infected during the average office visit.

Sinus infections are classified based on their duration. *Acute sinus infections* last less than 4 weeks. *Recurrent acute infections* mean 4 or more episodes within 12 months, each lasting 7 to 10 days, with at least 8 weeks of no symptoms between infections. Patients with recurrent acute infections usually have some underlying anatomic abnormality or allergy that predisposes them to frequent infections. *Subacute infections*, by definition, last between 4 and 12 weeks. *Chronic infections* are infections lasting longer than 12 weeks. Plain x-rays of the sinuses are of limited value in determining whether a sinus is infected, especially for acute sinusitis; therefore, I rarely order them. CT scans of the sinuses are much more accurate in diagnosing sinusitis, and are used for the evaluation of chronic or recurrent disease.

Medical management includes efforts to drain the sinuses and antibiotics to treat the likely cause of infection. Topical decongestants are effective in shrinking the mucosal lining of the nose and helping to open the ostia so that the sinuses can drain. These can be used safely up to 72 hours, but use beyond this time increases the risk for severe rebound congestion after the spray wears off, which can lead to addiction to the sprays. Systemic decongestants, such as pseudoephedrine, are useful in patients who can tolerate them, as are the anti-inflammatory effects of topical steroid sprays and pills. Antihistamines do not help appreciably with sinus congestion due to infection. They thicken and dry the mucus, which worsens the drainage problem, and are not recommended. Medications such as guaifenesin to thin the mucus are commonly used; although no firm data exists to prove that they work, I use them since they seem to help and have virtually no side effects. Most antibiotics for acute sinusitis are given for 10 to 14 days, and should not be stopped until 7 days after the symptoms have resolved. Longer courses are given to those with recurrent or complicated disease.

No FDA-approved antibiotic therapy exists for chronic sinusitis. This disease requires management by an ear, nose, and throat (ENT) specialist, which may include prolonged antibody therapy or special surgical drainage techniques. Chronic infections are seen in those with anatomic abnormalities that interfere with drainage, allergies, immune reaction to fungal infections, smokers, and those with certain diseases that interfere with sinus or immune function.

Allergic Rhinitis

Allergic rhinitis is a sinus condition that is triggered by an allergic reaction to substances that are inhaled through the nose. I discuss this condition in more detail in *Allergic Rhinitis* on page 23.

Nosebleeds

Since the nose has so many blood vessels just under the surface to help warm and humidify the air, it is not surprising that nosebleeds are common. Nosebleeds usually result from dry or weak nasal membranes, trauma caused by impact or forceful blowing of the nose, or abnormal surface blood vessels. The usual source of a nosebleed is from the rich supply of blood vessels in the septum of the nose. First aid involves putting steady pressure over the bridge of the nose, icing the region, or using topical decongestants (nose drops or sprays), which shrink the blood vessels and help stop bleeding. Petroleum jelly applied inside the tip of the nose is useful in keeping the mucosa moist to reduce cracking and bleeding. Studies show that estrogen cream placed in the nose twice daily for a month will thicken the lining of the nose and reduce bleeding. Patients with recurrent nosebleeds need evaluation by an ENT specialist, who may cauterize the involved blood vessels.

CHAPTER 19

The Throat

The throat serves as a common pathway for both swallowing and breathing. Because of its location at the beginning of both the gastrointestinal tract and respiratory systems, it can affect or be affected by processes that involve either system. It must direct air to the lungs during breathing and protect the lungs from exposure to substances in the mouth that are being swallowed. Given its important location, rich supply of sensory nerves, and constant activity patients are usually acutely aware when the throat is having problems, and throat related concerns prompt a substantial number of visits to the doctor.

This chapter will review those diseases that affect the structure or function of the throat: sore throat and tonsillitis, hoarseness, aphthous ulcers (canker sores), and bad breath.

Sore Throat and Tonsillitis

Sore throats are a common reason for primary care office visits. Everyone worries about Strep throat (an infection caused by the Group-A beta-hemolytic streptococcal bacteria), which accounts for only 10 to 15 percent of sore throats in adults. Other causes of throat discomfort include viral infections, throat dryness (caused by low humidity environments, excessive mouth breathing, dehydration, or medications), smoking and other forms of pollution, vocal abuse (yelling), acid reflux, and cancer.

Viral sore throats are often associated with nasal congestion, discharge, and cough. These symptoms are unusual in Strep throat. Strep throat usually occurs suddenly and is associated with fever greater than 101 degrees Fahrenheit, a white or yellow coating on the throat and tonsils, and swollen lymph nodes in the neck. Unfortunately, none of these signs is specific enough to make a diagnosis. If a patient has a known exposure to Strep throat and compatible symptoms, I usually treat him or her without further testing. Rapid Strep tests in adults are relatively unreliable. They are useful if positive in confirming infection, but negative tests do not mean the absence of infection. Standard throat cultures are more accurate but take up to three days to show a result.

The treatment of Strep throat with antibiotics does not shorten the duration of the sore throat; Strep throat usually resolves itself in 7 to 10 days, whether antibiotics are taken or not. Strep throat is treated to prevent complications such as peritonsillar abscess formation, the spreading of the streptococcal infection, and Rheumatic Fever. In Rheumatic Fever, it is felt that after exposure to the streptococcal organism, the immune system makes antibodies that mistakenly recognize normal parts of the body instead of other streptococci. These erring antibodies then create an immune reaction against normal tissues, leading to Rheumatic Fever, a disease that affects the heart and joints. Rheumatic Fever can be prevented in over 90 percent of patients if antibiotics are started for proven Strep throat within the first week of sore throat symptoms. Penicillin remains the drug of choice in patients who are not allergic to it.

Mononucleosis, an infection caused by the Epstein-Barr virus, is common in teenagers and young adults. Fatigue, weakness, generalized aching, markedly enlarged lymph nodes, hepatitis (with symptoms of nausea and appetite loss), and an enlarged spleen may accompany the sore throat of "Mono." Most patients improve with time and rest, and symptomatic therapy is all that is required. Patients with severe symptoms may benefit from the anti-inflammatory effects of a short course of steroids, though some studies suggest that this carries a risk of prolonging the overall course of the illness.

Sore throats respond to warm saltwater gargles, adequate hydration, and pain control. Acetaminophen and ibuprofen are useful therapies, and lozenges containing local anesthetics may help. Avoid tobacco smoke and other irritants.

Warning signs of serious throat problems include difficulty swallowing or breathing, unusual symptom severity (pain or fever), a sore throat accompanied by a rash, or symptoms that last more than two weeks.

Tonsillitis is an inflammation of the tonsils, which are collections of lymph tissue in the throat. The tonsils can become swollen, bright red, and spotted with pus. Tonsillitis is also usually viral in adults, and simply needs supportive care and time to resolve. Patients who have documented streptococcal pharyngitis 3 times within 12 months should discuss a tonsillectomy with their doctor.

Hoarseness

The vocal cords are thin membranous structures in the larynx that vibrate together and produce sound. *Hoarseness* occurs when these membranes are swollen or otherwise injured and cannot vibrate together normally.

Causes of hoarseness include viral infections, allergy, postnasal drainage, vocal abuse, cigarette smoke and other pollution, gastroesophageal reflux, cancers of the larynx (more common in smokers and those who consume excessive alcohol), vocal cord nodules, and diseases that affect the recurrent laryngeal nerve, which regulates muscular control of vocal cord tension.

Most causes of hoarseness are treated with time and voice rest. Allowing the vocal cords to rest reduces further irritation to them and allows them to heal. Whispering places great tension on the vocal cords and worsens hoarseness. If you must talk, try normal voice volumes and see what comes out—don't whisper. You can also try using a humidifier to add moisture to the air, keeping yourself well hydrated, and treating nasal congestion to reduce mouth breathing. Allowing air to pass through the nose first will warm and humidify it, reducing irritation to the throat.

If hoarseness persists longer than two or three weeks, the vocal cords must be directly examined to show the cause and guide further therapy.

Aphthous Ulcers (Canker Sores)

Aphthous ulcers are small, shallow, painful ulcers that occur in the lining of the mouth. They can occur as individual lesions or in crops and usually involve the linings of the cheeks, tongue, and inside of the lips. They commonly occur after superficial trauma to the mouth (such as a tooth rubbing the cheek or tongue) or along with other medical illnesses. The cause of aphthous ulcers is unknown. The sores usually heal by themselves in 7 to 10 days.

Treatment includes avoiding substances that irritate the ulcers, such as coffee, spicy and salty foods, and citrus fruits. Saltwater rinses or hydrogen peroxide (1 tablespoon in 8 ounces of water) may soothe the lesions. Many over-the-counter remedies are available with variable benefit. For severe or recurrent lesions, prescription oral pastes are available that can speed healing for some.

Rarely, patients can develop debilitating continuous crops of aphthous ulcers. These often defy all currently available treatments; however, some doctors are trying experimental medications that suppress the function of the immune system to help reduce the frequency and severity of aphthous ulcer outbreaks.

Bad Breath

A noticeable odor to the breath is not uncommon. It can occur from local causes in the mouth or upper airway, or from gases expelled as you breathe out—reflecting problems in the lungs or metabolic processes that generate gases with odors. *Halitosis* is the medical name for continuous bad breath.

Local Causes

- Bacteria in the mouth ferment leftover food products. This can occur in crevices in the tonsils or tongue, from plaque build-up or cavities in the teeth, from diseased gums, or from appliances in the mouth (braces or dentures) that aren't properly cleaned.
- A lack of moisture in the mouth leads to a loss of the natural cleansing and infection fighting properties of saliva. This can occur from aging, medications, mouth breathing, smoking, stress, and diseases that affect the salivary glands. Mouthwashes that contain alcohol temporarily help, but the alcohol dries the membranes further and worsens the problem.
- In sinusitis or other upper respiratory infections, chemical processes in infected mucus release odorous compounds.
- Byproducts of tobacco smoke smell by themselves, but also interfere with the natural cleansing mechanisms of the respiratory tract.

General Causes

- Foods may contain odorous substances that evaporate. The foods are digested and absorbed into the bloodstream, the blood passes through the lungs, and the dissolved chemicals in the food diffuse into the air in the lungs and are breathed out. This includes onions, garlic, alcohol, coffee, and less commonly broccoli, cabbage, cauliflower, horseradish, and peppers.
- High-protein, low-carbohydrate diets lead to a metabolic process called *ketosis*. This creates ketones, a volatile gas that is released through the blood to the lungs.
- Poorly controlled diabetes can result in ketoacidosis, in which ketones and acetone are exhaled.
- Renal and liver failure leads to a build-up of waste products in the bloodstream that create volatile odorous gases.

Treatment

You can treat, or at least improve, bad breath as follows:

- **Seek a medical evaluation.** Your doctor will look for an underlying cause.
- **Practice good oral hygiene.** Brush and floss teeth regularly. Brush your tongue, especially if it seems coated or discolored. Visit your dentist for professional cleaning twice yearly or as advised.
- **Keep your mouth well hydrated.** Drink enough fluid (see *Water* on page 11 to help you calculate how much liquid you should drink each day). Discuss with your doctor alternatives to any medications that seem to be drying you out.
- **Eliminate from your diet the foods that are associated with halitosis.** These foods include onions, garlic, alcohol, coffee, broccoli, cabbage, cauliflower, horseradish, and peppers.
- **Stop smoking.**

CHAPTER 20

Glandular and Metabolic Diseases

Glands are organs spread throughout the body that manufacture and release chemicals that can have a variety of effects on the tissues and processes far removed from the gland's location. Glands in the brain regulate hormone production from other organs. The thyroid gland in the neck produces thyroid hormone, which helps regulate the metabolism of the body. Parathyroid glands regulate calcium in the body. The pancreas produces insulin to regulate blood sugar. Diseases that affect glands become evident when the normal functioning of the gland becomes impaired, causing problems in the body that are usually controlled by the gland's actions.

This chapter will review those diseases that affect the structure or function of the glands and metabolism: diabetes mellitus, hypoglycemia, osteoporosis, thyroid conditions (hypothyroidism, hyperthyroidism, thyroiditis, and thyroid nodules), and hemochromatosis.

Diabetes Mellitus

Diabetes mellitus effects 1 in every 17 Americans, half of whom don't know that they have it. The incidence of diabetes has dramatically increased in the past two decades, attributed to increased obesity, decreased physical activity, and the increased consumption of prepared, highly dense foods (fast food). Because symptoms of diabetes usually do not appear until the patient has had the disease over ten years, it is only detected in its early stages by screening laboratory tests.

Normally, the gastrointestinal tract breaks down carbohydrates in foods (grains, fruits, vegetables, dairy products) into glucose, which is transported into the bloodstream. Insulin is a hormone produced by the pancreas that transfers glucose from the bloodstream into cells, where it is either burned up for energy or stored. When food is not available in the gastrointestinal tract for processing, the liver produces glucose through a process called gluconeogenesis. This provides a steady source for the body's energy needs.

In diabetes, insulin doesn't function normally. The muscle and fat cells, among others, appear to be resistant to the effects of insulin. This leads to higher levels of glucose than normal in the bloodstream. The liver cells do not seem to recognize insulin or glucose levels and continue to produce excessive amounts of glucose. The pancreas recognizes the higher sugar levels and pumps out more insulin to try to lower it.

This extra insulin triggers a variety of metabolic problems—it increases the risk for atherosclerosis, elevates triglycerides, lowers healthy HDL cholesterol, increases blood pressure, and increases blood-clotting tendencies. Elevated insulin levels may also fuel tumor growth, possibly accounting for the increased incidence of breast, colon, liver, and prostate cancer seen in diabetics.

Eventually, the pancreas cannot keep up with the need for extra amounts of insulin, sugars continue to rise, and damage occurs to tiny blood vessels. This leads to damage to the structures that these tiny blood vessels supply, affecting nerves, kidneys, the eye, the heart, and the brain and increasing the risk for infection. Diabetes is the leading cause of blindness in the United States, as well as kidney failure (one of every three patients with kidney failure on dialysis is diabetic) and amputations that are not directly due to traumatic injury. Fifty to sixty percent of diabetics have neuropathy (loss of peripheral nerve function), and heart attack and stroke are two to four times more frequent in diabetics than non-diabetics.

Symptoms of advanced diabetes include fatigue, weight loss, frequent urination, excessive thirst or hunger, changes in vision, numbness or burning in the feet, and the slow healing of wounds.

Screening for Diabetes

Screening for diabetes involves checking the glucose level (blood sugar) after an overnight fast. A normal level is less than 110. Doctors compare this normal level with a patient's level to help them diagnose diabetes as follows:

Patients with a fasting blood sugar level of...	Are felt to have...
110–125	Impaired glucose tolerance and are at high risk for progression to diabetes. These patients need to lose weight, exercise, and be monitored for diabetes closely.
Greater than 126 on two occasions	Diabetes
Greater than 200 on one occasion, and symptoms of diabetes	Diabetes

An older test, the glucose tolerance test, involves giving a set amount of sugar in a drink and checking the blood sugar level two hours later. A blood sugar reading above 200 is classified as diabetes. This test is rarely done except to look for gestational diabetes in pregnancy. The hemoglobin A1c test (HgbA1c) provides a measure of the average blood sugar readings over the past three months by measuring changes in hemoglobin caused by elevated blood sugars. This is a useful yardstick to monitor the control of diabetes over time, and can be used as a screening test to detect diabetes.

Suggested screening programs include checking a fasting blood sugar at least every three years after age 45, or more frequently if risks for diabetes are present. Risks include obesity, a relative with diabetes, ethnic risk (African American, Hispanic, American Indian, Asian), previous gestational diabetes or a baby greater than 9 pounds at birth, high blood pressure, or lipid abnormalities (HDL cholesterol less than 35 or triglycerides greater than 250). Men who drink more than two drinks a day are twice as likely to develop diabetes as those who average less. Alcohol affects insulin resistance. It is estimated that alcohol use may account for as much as 25 percent of insulin resistant diabetes.

Treating diabetes by controlling blood sugar improves symptoms such as blurred vision, frequent urination, fatigue, weight gain, vaginal yeast infections, and cholesterol abnormalities. Numerous studies have been conducted to prove that controlling diabetes helps prevent more serious complications. The Diabetes Control and Complications Trial showed a 50 to 75 percent reduction in the development or progression of diabeties-related eye disease, kidney disease, and neurological disease from intense diabetes therapy. The United Kingdom Perspective Diabetes Study showed that for every 1 percent that therapy decreases HgbA1c, there is a 35 percent decrease in the rate of microvascular disease complications. This blood sugar control does not seem to prevent disease related to diabetes in large blood vessels, such as the risk for heart disease and stroke. Therefore, other risk factors for these diseases, such as hypertension and lipid abnormalities, must be treated more aggressively in patients with diabetes. Goals for therapy include a HgbA1c of less than 7 percent, blood sugars of from 80 to 120 before meals, less than 140 two hours after eating, and a bedtime blood sugar of 100 to 140.

Diabetes Management Plan

I regard my patients with diabetes as being in charge of the management of their own disease. They must fully understand their disease and take the principal role in controlling it. I see myself as more of a consultant and resource to them as needed in the management of their disease. The following guidelines are useful in planning the management of diabetes:

- **Stated long-term and short-term goals.** "I will consult a nutritionist and start a diet before our next visit." "I will exercise 30 minutes at least five days weekly." "My blood sugars and HgbA1c will be within goals of therapy in six months."
- **Patient and family education.** I prefer one-on-one counseling by a trained diabetic educator, supplemented by classes at our Diabetes Center, and self-education from books and Internet resources.
- **Individualized nutritional assessment and treatment.** One diet plan does not fit all; developing a diet that you can live with and enjoy is crucial. A few visits with a nutritionist skilled in diabetes education are well worth the effort.
- **Lifestyle changes—exercise, smoking cessation, and weight loss.** A twelve-year study was conducted of men with diabetes, with an average age of 50. After accounting for all other variables, this study found that those men who did not exercise regularly were 170 percent more likely to die over the next twelve years of

the study than men who exercised regularly. Diabetes and smoking together more than quadrupled future risk for heart disease and stroke.

- **Monitoring.** As a diabetic, you should do the following at scheduled intervals:
  - Routinely monitor the blood sugar level at home at a frequency agreed upon with your doctor. Some patients with labile diabetes need blood sugar readings at least four times daily. Most of my patients with stable, non-insulin dependent diabetes on therapy can get by with checking their blood sugar twice daily, three days a week.
  - Obtain HgbA1c exams every three months. If the disease is under control and you do not use insulin, every six months is adequate.
  - Monitor kidney function by receiving annual blood tests of kidney function and urine protein levels.
  - Inspect the feet for blisters, sores, or for other problems daily. Because of circulatory problems and difficulty in fighting infections, diabetics are at high risk for limb loss from minor foot infections. Because of neurological problems, many diabetics cannot feel trauma to the bottom of their feet.
  - Receive annual comprehensive eye examinations. Diabetes can affect the blood vessels that supply the retina. If these changes are caught early, laser treatments are available to treat the vascular changes and preserve vision. Waiting until you notice a change in vision is much too late.
  - Seek regular physician visits and examinations.
- **Medications.** Medications for diabetes act through several different mechanisms: stimulating the pancreas to release more insulin, reducing production of glucose by the liver, increasing insulin sensitivity in the tissues, slowing conversion of starch into glucose in the gastrointestinal tract, and reducing the rate of glucose absorption. Most diabetics should be on multiple medications for best control. A discussion of different diabetes medications is beyond the scope of this book but, in general, medications are selected based on individual patient characteristics and desires, response, and side effects.
- **Aggressive treatment of co-morbid conditions (other medical conditions affecting the same organs that diabetes attacks).**
  - Kidney disease. Diabetes accounts for 42 percent of all new cases of kidney failure. Patients with diabetes survive less well on dialysis than patients with kidney failure from other diseases. The five-year survival on dialysis is only 17 percent, half that of patients with kidney failure from high blood pressure complications. Diabetic kidney disease is detected by monitoring blood tests of kidney function and by looking for excessive amounts of protein in the urine. Microalbumin, a protein in the urine that is a sensitive marker for early kidney disease in diabetics, should be measured annually. Blood pressure medications called ACE inhibitors help reduce protein excretion and preserve kidney function in diabetics. Some evidence exists that ACE inhibitors should be started in all diabetics to prevent kidney and other complications before they develop.

— Hypertension. The goal for blood pressure control in diabetics is a systolic blood pressure below 130 and a diastolic blood pressure below 85. (Traditional blood pressure goals are less than 140/90 in non-diabetics.)

— Heart disease and lipids. The expected life span of a diabetic with no history of heart disease is equal to the life span of a non-diabetic the same age that has already had one heart attack. Thus, goals for lipid therapy in diabetics are the same as for those with heart patients. LDL cholesterol should be less than 100; triglycerides should be less than 150. All diabetics over age 40 should be on daily aspirin therapy if they can tolerate it. One recent study—the HOPE Study—showed that the use of an ACE inhibitor reduced the risk of heart attack, stroke, and death in diabetics; this study provides another argument for placing all diabetics on ACE inhibitors.

• **Routine dental examinations.** Because diabetes affects the small blood vessels that nourish the teeth and gums, diabetics are more likely to experience problems with mouth dryness and dental disease. In addition, the immune systems of diabetics are less able to fight infections. Regular dental evaluations can detect developing problems in the mouth sooner, leading to prevention—or early treatment—of dental disease.

• **Vaccinations.** Diabetic patients should receive the following vaccinations to help maintain overall good health:

— Pneumovax to prevent complications from pneumococcal infections

— Annual influenza vaccine

Hypoglycemia

The syndrome of *hypoglycemia* refers to a symptomatic, often sudden, lowering of the blood sugar. Symptoms include shaking, fast heartbeat, sweating, anxiety, dizziness, hunger, vision loss, extreme weakness, headache, and irritability. Ingesting sugar promptly relieves symptoms. Why patients experience hypoglycemia is frequently unknown; possible contributors include too little food, excessive exercise, over consumption of concentrated sweets, excessive use of diabetic medications, or rarer metabolic problems that affect blood sugar metabolism. Hypoglycemia must be distinguished from anxiety disorders and other medical problems that can mimic its symptoms.

Treatment of hypoglycemia is largely nutritional. Most patients with significant hypoglycemia benefit from a formal nutritional consultation to help outline a proper diet. Principles of dietary therapy include avoiding simple carbohydrates such as sugar, jelly, honey, and candy. The average recommended diet includes 50 percent complex carbohydrates, 20 percent protein, and 30 percent fat. Small, frequent meals are important as well as protein snacks to help provide a more steady level sugar supply.

As diabetic patients age, changes in their liver and kidney function occur that can affect the metabolism (breakdown) of their diabetic medications. This can mean that their medications begin to last longer and have a greater blood sugar lowering effect. If an elderly diabetic begins to experience confusion or other possible symptoms related to low blood sugars, a reduction in the dose of his or her diabetic medication may be required.

Osteoporosis

It is easy to conceive of bones as being made of concrete, hard rigid structures that supply structure and support to the body. Nothing could be further from the truth. The normal wear and tear of human activity causes microscopic cracks in bone. This would ultimately lead to weak and brittle bones if the skeleton were stagnant. In fact, living bone is constantly renewing itself. Bone cells called *osteoclasts* chemically break down bone, developing crevices in existing bone. This activity stimulates other cells, called osteoblasts, to fill cracks with new bone. Every few years, all portions of your skeleton have been replaced with new bone.

Bone mass peaks in the early 30s. After this age, most people lose approximately 1 percent of bone mass a year. As more and more bone is lost, the bone becomes weaker and more brittle, a condition known as *osteoporosis*.

Osteoporosis occurs earlier in women as a consequence of the natural fall in the production of estrogen at menopause. Men can also develop osteoporosis, but typically not until their 70s because they have thicker bones to begin with and lose bone mass at a slower pace than women.

Osteoporosis increases the risk for fracture, mostly of the hip, spine, and wrist. When a person fractures a hip from osteoporosis, statistics show that he or she is two to five times more likely to die in the following year than someone of similar health without a hip fracture. Although the exact reason is unknown, these deaths are thought to be related to complications of bed rest, loss of strength and increased risk of future falls and trauma, depression and its complications, or the possibility that the hip fracture itself represented unseen deterioration in health not picked up in the comparison studies. Of those with hip fractures, 50 percent are never able to walk independently again. Osteoporosis needs to be prevented, detected, and treated before fractures occur.

The major risk factors for osteoporosis include postmenopause without estrogen support, age, white or Asian ancestry, and family history of osteoporosis. Minor risk factors include lack of regular exercise, smoking, excessive alcohol intake, inadequate calcium intake, medication side effects, and low body weight.

It is important to prevent osteoporosis by consuming adequate calcium during childhood and adult years. This is particularly a problem in adolescent girls and young women, who for many reasons reduce their intake of dairy products, the primary source of calcium. This age group also tends to ingest more soft drinks, which contain phosphates that chemically promote further calcium loss from the bones. I recommend an average of 1,200 milligrams (mg) of calcium intake every day for my patients. Give yourself credit for approximately 250 mg of calcium for every average serving size dairy product you consume. Make up the remainder of calcium with calcium supplements, which are best absorbed with food and should be taken at mealtime.

Weight-bearing exercise also helps strengthen the bone density, and is a crucial component of a healthy lifestyle. Eliminate smoking. Postmenopausal women who choose not to take estrogen should consume 1,500 mg of calcium a day, as well as ensure an intake of 400 to 800 units of vitamin D daily.

Screening for Osteoporosis

Effective screening for osteoporosis consists of the use of a bone densitometer. This instrument is used to calculate bone density at two sites—the hip and the spine—and compare the measured bone density to expected bone density. I recommend screening all women at the start of menopause if they choose not to take estrogen supplements and treating them if they are found to have a low bone density. If the bone density is normal, I recommend taking a second bone density two years later to look for any progressive bone loss and then, if necessary, discussing treatment options.

For women who choose to take estrogen supplements during menopause, only 15 percent will go on to develop significant osteoporosis; bone density loss occurs much more slowly than in women who don't take estrogen. Therefore, if a woman decides to take estrogen when menopause begins, I delay the first bone density test for five to ten years unless other risk factors are present. There are no firm guidelines for the detection of osteoporosis in elderly men.

Treatment Options

Extra calcium and vitamin D alone *do not* adequately treat osteoporosis. Other treatments must be used in conjunction with these supplements. Options include:

- **Estrogen.** Estrogen use both prevents the development of osteoporosis and treats it when it occurs. Estrogens are among the most effective medications available. Although plant-derived ("natural") estrogens do not yet have the data to support their use in the prevention or treatment of osteoporosis, other synthetic estrogens have shown a 50 percent reduction in vertebral fractures from osteoporosis. A new class of medications, the "SERMs" (Selective Estrogen Receptor Modifiers, such as raloxifene) have shown a similar reduction in vertebral fracture rates.

- **Bisphosphonates.** Bisphosphonates (Fosamax, Actonel, and others) are medications that interfere with the working of bone-eating osteoclasts. As a consequence, less bone is broken down, leading to an increase in bone density and a reduction in fracture rates. Bisphosphonates require special care in their use. They are poorly absorbed from the stomach and must be taken with a full, eight-ounce glass of water on an empty stomach. No other food, vitamins, or pills should be introduced into the stomach until the medication has had at least 30 minutes to be absorbed. Because bisphosphonates can also be extremely irritating to the lining of the esophagus, the patient is advised to remain fully upright (walking, standing, or sitting) for 30 minutes after swallowing the pill to minimize the risk of esophageal irritation. Fortunately, new formulations of these drugs allow the drug to be taken once a week instead of daily, making the detailed regimen less demanding.

- **Calcitonin.** Calcitonin also inhibits osteoclasts, preventing bone destruction. This medication also helps relieve pain associated with fractures resulting from osteoporosis. It is administered as a nose spray or self-injection.
- **Statins.** Surprising results from treatment of high cholesterol in women with statin drugs show that women on these drugs for at least one year have a 50 percent decrease in the rate of hip fracture. The statin medications seem to increase bone density by stimulating bone growth (osteoblasts), and may prove quite useful in this disease. Research on the use of statins is ongoing.

The Thyroid

The thyroid gland is a butterfly-shaped gland located over the windpipe in the front of the neck. It produces thyroid hormones, which serve to regulate many processes in the body and help set the body's metabolic rate. The production of thyroid hormone is precisely controlled.

Thyroid releasing hormone (TRH) from the hypothalamus stimulates production of thyroid stimulating hormone (TSH), which then stimulates thyroid hormone production and release. The thyroid hormones produced in the gland are categorized into two types: T4 (the majority of hormones produced) and T3. T4 hormones are converted in the tissues to the active hormone, T3. These hormones are carried in the bloodstream on proteins. Many feedback loops between the hypothalamus, pituitary, and thyroid glands help regulate the amount of hormone produced. Significant amounts of thyroid hormone are stored in the thyroid gland prior to their release.

Physicians evaluate the thyroid gland using the following methods:

- **Palpation.** The thyroid gland can easily be felt in most necks. Doctors palpate the thyroid by manipulating it with their fingers to determine its size and detect any irregularities.
- **Blood tests.** The hormones produced in the thyroid, as well as the protein carriers in the bloodstream, can be measured. New ultrasensitive, precise TSH tests have changed the way that thyroid function is monitored. Now, instead of a confusing array of thyroid tests, most physicians simply use the TSH and T4 levels to monitor thyroid function and disease. There is an expected range for TSH; if too much thyroid hormone is present, the pituitary gland stops sending its signal to produce more thyroid hormone and the TSH level falls. If not enough thyroid hormone is present, the pituitary increases its production of TSH to signal the thyroid gland to work harder. Measuring T4 hormone levels can be useful when the TSH levels are borderline.
- **Ultrasound.** This non-invasive test is useful for confirming the size and features of the thyroid gland. In this test, jelly is rubbed on the skin over the thyroid gland to improve the images; then, ultrasound waves are used to look at the size and internal structure of the gland. Lumps in the gland can be checked to see if they are solid or cystic, and appropriate further studies planned.

- **Radioactive iodine scans.** The thyroid gland avidly takes up iodine. Radioactive iodine scans are a safe and important tool to look at precise anatomic and functional information about the thyroid gland.
- **Needle aspiration.** In this procedure performed in the office, experienced physicians use a thin needle to extract tissue samples from the thyroid nodules. By analyzing these tissue samples, the physician can determine whether they might be cancerous.

Hypothyroidism

Hypothyroidism is the under-production of thyroid hormone. Severe hypothyroidism can be life threatening. Symptoms of milder hypothyroidism include fatigue, sluggishness, weight gain, hair loss, skin thickening, enlargement of the thyroid gland, constipation, and depression. Hypothyroidism is treated by providing synthetic thyroid hormone in tablet form; these synthetic thyroid hormone supplements are chemically identical to the hormone naturally produced by the body. After a patient has taken a steady dose of a thyroid supplement for six weeks, the physician can measure the patient's own TSH level to determine whether the dose selected is correct and then adjust the dose upward or downward to bring the TSH level into a normal range.

Some patients have *sub-clinical hypothyroidism.* These patients have no recognized symptoms but a slight elevation in TSH is noted on laboratory testing. The T4 level in these patients is often within normal range. Some evidence exists that even though the patient has no symptoms, this slight elevation in TSH should be treated with extra thyroid hormone. Benefits could include improved memory, an enhanced response to antidepressants if the patient is depressed, better cholesterol profiles, and relief of fatigue. In some cases, a patient with borderline TSH levels is placed on a thyroid hormone supplement for three to six months to see if they feel better. Often the symptoms of hypothyroidism are so subtle that patients don't realize that they had them until they feel better.

Because of the frequency of sub-clinical hypothyroidism, I recommend screening for the disease with TSH testing every five years after age 35 in women. This disease is less common in men, and testing guidelines are not available for them.

Hyperthyroidism

Hyperthyroidism occurs when too much hormone is produced as a result of an irritated thyroid gland that is releasing previously stored hormone or from a thyroid gland that is being excessively stimulated to manufacture and release extra hormone. Symptoms of hyperthyroidism include tremor, sweating, fast heartbeat, diarrhea, anxiety, poor sleeping and concentration abilities, and weight loss. Significant hyperthyroidism can be life threatening.

As in hypothyroidism, some patients have sub-clinical hyperthyroidism. Their laboratory tests show that the TSH level is slightly suppressed, but the thyroid hormone (T4) levels are normal. Sub-clinical hyperthyroidism has been shown to be a risk factor for lower bone density; it also increases the risk for irregular heartbeats, including a three-fold increase in the rate of atrial fibrillation, a chaotic heart rhythm that can be associated with significant medical consequences. Patients with sub-clinical hyperthyroidism can also progress over time to more severe disease. Treatment options for sub-clinical hyperthyroidism should be discussed with your personal physician.

Causes of hyperthyroidism include Grave's disease and thyroiditis. In *Grave's disease*, the body's immune system produces an antibody that stimulates the thyroid gland in the same way that TSH does. This leads to excess production and release of thyroid hormone that is not controlled by the body's usual feedback mechanisms. Grave's disease can be treated with medication, although current drugs have significant side effects and frequent recurrence of the disease after the drugs are stopped. In most patients with Grave's disease, radioactive iodine therapy can be given. This iodine is taken up avidly by the thyroid gland and destroys it. The patient is left dependent on taking supplemental thyroid hormone, but this is relatively easy to do.

Thyroiditis

In *thyroiditis*, usually either the immune system or a viral infection irritates the thyroid gland, causing thyroid hormone that has already been produced to be released in excessive quantities. Hashimoto's thyroiditis is the most common autoimmune form of thyroiditis in which the body develops an autoimmune reaction that destroys the thyroid gland. Initially, stored hormone is released in excessive quantities, resulting in hyperthyroidism. Eventually, as more of the gland is destroyed no more thyroid hormone is left to be released, and hypothyroidism develops.

Thyroid Nodules

Thyroid nodules—lumps and bumps in the thyroid gland—are common. By palpation, nodules can be detected in 4 to 7 percent of the population. Autopsy studies of thyroid glands in people who die for other reasons show nodules in 50 percent of them. Of all thyroid nodules, approximately 5 percent are malignant. Aspiration of the nodule with a fine needle, followed by examination of cells in the laboratory, is the fastest, easiest, and safest way to evaluate thyroid nodules. Results of this test may show that the cells obtained are benign (where the nodule simply needs to be followed over time for changes), malignant or suspicious (where surgery is needed to remove a portion of gland), or "non-diagnostic," which calls for either a second biopsy or surgery, at the discretion of physician and patient.

A *goiter* is an enlarged, lumpy thyroid gland. If the evaluation shows that the goiter is benign and it is not causing symptoms, no treatment is needed unless it is cosmetically desired. Previously, supplemental thyroid hormone therapy was given in an attempt to turn off the TSH signal and shrink the goiter. The benefits of this are controversial; only 25 percent of goiters shrink with this type of therapy and some risks are associated with providing extra hormone. If you are considering this type of therapy, discuss it with your doctor. It may be reasonable to try this suppression therapy in a younger patient to see if there is some improvement; if no significant response is obtained within a year, I would recommend stopping this form of therapy.

Thyroid cancers include *papillary thyroid cancer* (80 percent), *follicular cell cancer* (10 to 15 percent), *medullary cancer* (5 percent, often inherited), and *undifferentiated anaplastic cancer* (5 percent). Papillary and follicular cell cancers are relatively benign, and often surgery can cure them. Since the thyroid tissues absorb iodine so well, at set times after surgery radioactive iodine scanning can be used to detect any residual cancer, and high doses of radioactive iodine can be used to treat any leftover disease.

Hemochromatosis

Iron is essential to health. It is needed to produce hemoglobin, which transports oxygen. Six percent of Americans (15 percent of young women) need extra iron, and it is frequently advised as a supplement. Healthy people absorb about 10 percent of the iron in the foods they eat.

Hemochromatosis is a metabolic disease of iron metabolism in which the intestine absorbs excessive iron. Two genes exist for hemochromatosis. If the patient has one of these genes, his or her body absorbs about 15 percent of the iron in food, rather than the normal 10 percent; if the patient has both genes, the body absorbs up to 20 percent. Throw in a few multivitamins and iron supplements, and significant amounts of iron can be absorbed.

The body lacks the ability to excrete iron through the kidneys as it can for most other substances. Women lose a fair amount of iron through menstrual blood loss. Small amounts of iron are lost in shed skin cells. Despite these small losses of iron, if the body continues to absorb excessive amounts of iron, an overload of iron occurs that is associated with cancers, heart disease, arthritis, chronic fatigue, diabetes, liver damage, and impotence.

Hemochromatosis is one of the most common inherited metabolic diseases. One of every eight people carries a single gene for hemochromatosis; one in every 250 carries both genes. Detection requires measuring iron levels in the bloodstream. If these tests are suspicious for iron overload, a blood test for genetic testing can confirm whether the genes are present. A liver biopsy can also confirm the presence of excessive iron. If a patient is diagnosed with hemochromatosis, all blood relatives should be checked.

Treatment for hemochromatosis is relatively simple when the disease is caught early. The iron excess must be unloaded; this is accomplished by drawing a unit of blood regularly (every one to two weeks) until the patient's iron levels are normal, then periodically (usually four times a year) to maintain a normal iron count.

CHAPTER 21

The Heart and Cardiovascular System

The heart is a two-part muscle that pumps blood throughout the body. The right side of the heart receives used blood from the body and pumps it to the lungs where waste gases are released and the blood is supplied with oxygen. This oxygen-rich blood then returns to the left side of the heart, where it is pumped to the body.

The Heart

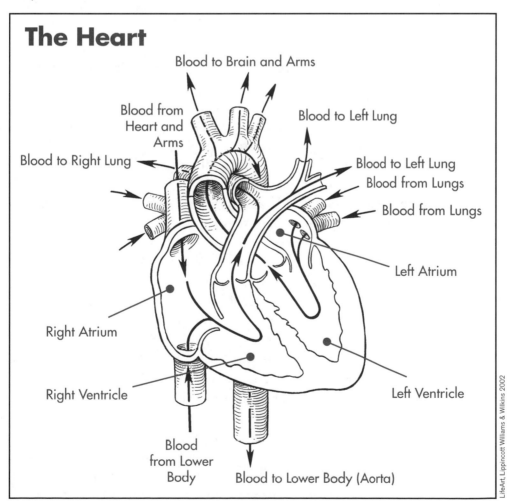

Blood to Brain and Arms

Blood from Heart and Arms

Blood to Left Lung

Blood to Right Lung

Blood to Left Lung
Blood from Lungs

Blood from Lungs

Left Atrium

Right Atrium

Left Ventricle

Right Ventricle

Blood from Lower Body

Blood to Lower Body (Aorta)

LifeArt, Lippincott Williams & Wilkins 2002

Each side of the heart has two chambers. The first chamber, the *atrium*, receives the blood and functions as a primer pump for the second chamber, the *ventricle*. The ventricles are larger, more powerful chambers in that they must pump blood throughout the lungs or body. On each side, a one-way valve to keep blood flowing in the correct direction separates the atrium and ventricle. This valve opens when blood flows from the atria to the ventricles, and closes when the ventricles contract so that blood does not leak backwards into the atria. On the right side of the heart, this is the *tricuspid valve*. On the left side of the heart, it is called the *mitral valve*.

When the ventricles contract, blood must again pass through a one-way valve. The right ventricle pumps blood through the pulmonic valve into the lungs. The left ventricle pumps blood through the aortic valve into the *aorta*, a large blood vessel from which all other arteries branch. The pulmonic and aortic valves prevent blood from leaking back into the ventricles between contractions.

The atria and ventricles contract in a rhythmic, organized fashion. This is accomplished by special bundles of neurological tissue within the heart muscle that initiate a heartbeat and propagate it along predetermined pathways through the heart muscle so that the muscle contracts in a way that optimizes efficient blood flow.

The heart must also supply blood to itself. A rich and constant blood supply is needed since the heart muscle is always working. This blood supply is provided through *coronary arteries*, which begin off of the first part of the aorta and travel along the surface of the heart muscle.

Arteries are blood vessels that carry blood away from the heart to the tissues. When the heart muscle contracts, it generates a pressure that drives blood forward. The arteries can tolerate this pressure because they are thick-walled, muscular vessels that can initially expand to accept blood flow, and then recoil as blood flows from them into the tissues. Arteries divide into smaller and smaller vessels, eventually feeding *capillaries*. Capillaries are the tiniest of blood vessels, with very thin walls so that oxygen and other nutrients can easily pass into the tissues that they supply.

Veins are blood vessels into which used blood from the capillaries flows. These tiny veins merge into larger and larger veins that return blood to the heart. Veins have thinner walls and depend on the contractions of surrounding muscles to squeeze blood back up to the heart. The veins have one-way valves similar to the heart so that blood can only flow in the correct direction. The best example of this process is the rhythmic contraction of leg muscles while walking that push blood uphill to the heart.

This chapter will review those diseases that affect the structure or function of the cardiovascular system: hypertension, varicose veins, valve function (valvular heart disease and mitral valve prolapse), irregular heartbeat (palpitations and atrial fibrillation), high cholesterol, abnormalities of blood vessel walls (atherosclerosis, peripheral vascular disease, and aortic aneurysm), congestive heart failure, chest pain (angina), and blood vessel blockage and clots (myocardial infarction, cerebrovascular disease and stroke, and thromboembolic disease). We will also look at various procedures used to diagnose heart problems and see how to prevent heart disease from happening in the first place.

Hypertension

When the left ventricle contracts, it generates a peak pressure that drives blood forward. This peak pressure is the *systolic blood pressure*. The blood pressure then slowly falls until the next contraction of the ventricle. The lowest blood pressure before this next wave of blood comes is called the *diastolic blood pressure*.

These pressures can be determined with a blood pressure cuff. Most commonly, this cuff is placed over the upper arm. The cuff is pumped up until its pressure exceeds the systolic blood pressure, which causes the large artery in the upper arm to collapse since more pressure is being exerted on the outside of the vessel than from the inside. A stethoscope is applied over this artery; since there is no blood flow, there is no noise. The pressure in the blood pressure cuff is then slowly decreased. When the pressure in the cuff falls below the systolic blood pressure, the artery transiently opens at peak pressure and a noise is heard. This first noise marks the systolic blood pressure. Once the blood pressure in the artery falls below the pressure in the cuff, the artery collapses again and no blood flow is heard. As the pressure in the blood pressure cuff is lowered, the listener will hear intermittent opening of the artery when the pressure in the cuff is somewhere between the systolic and diastolic blood pressures. Once the pressure in the cuff falls below the diastolic blood pressure, the artery stays open all of the time, and the opening and closing noises are no longer heard. When this absence of sound is first detected, the pressure shown on the cuff is recorded as the diastolic blood pressure.

An expected range for normal blood pressure exists. *Hypertension* occurs when blood pressure climbs above this range. *Systolic hypertension* is defined as an upper blood pressure (systolic) measurement of greater than or equal to 140. *Diastolic hypertension* is defined as a lower blood pressure (diastolic) measurement of greater than or equal to 90. This 140/90 number is somewhat arbitrary. Diseases associated with hypertension, such as heart disease and stroke, occur at increasing frequency when the blood pressures are above this range. However, patients with blood pressures significantly lower than 140/90 have even lower rates of these diseases than patients with a "normal" blood pressure of 139/89. Most patients should have a blood pressure less than 130/85 to minimize their risk.

Classification of Blood Pressure

	Systolic	Diastolic
Normal	less than 130	less than 85
High Normal	130–139	85–89
Hypertension		
Stage 1 (mild)	140–159	90–99
Stage 2 (moderate)	160–179	100–109
Stage 3 (severe)	180–209	110–119
Stage 4 (very severe)	greater than 209	greater than 119

Most elevated blood pressure is classified as essential hypertension, which means that there is no identifiable cause. This is felt to be genetically programmed, and often there is a family history of hypertension. Rarely, blood pressure is elevated because of kidney, blood vessel, or hormonal problems. Clues to this would be hypertension at a young age, the sudden development of severe hypertension, or elevated blood pressure that doesn't respond to the usual drug therapy.

Hypertension has no symptoms and is detected by screening blood pressure measurements. Everyone should have his or her blood pressure checked annually. Those with previous readings in the high normal range, or with a family history of hypertension, should be examined more often.

Once an elevated blood pressure is detected, I ask my patients to purchase a blood pressure cuff. They bring it to the office where we determine if it functions correctly and that their technique is acceptable, and then they monitor their blood pressure at home. On subsequent office visits, I can review several blood pressures to make the best decisions regarding their therapy, rather than rely on a spot check that day in the office. Studies show that 20 to 30 percent of those who have high blood pressure in the office are normal outside of the office setting. It is silly to rely only on blood pressure readings inside the doctor's office. Many things, including the stress and anxiety of being in a doctor's office to begin with, can affect blood pressure and result in over-treatment with unneeded costs and medication side effects.

Hypertension increases the risk for coronary heart disease, kidney failure, and stroke. A 20-year Swedish study of 1,000 men age 50 looked at the effect of high blood pressure on cognitive function. At age 70, these men were given tests of attention, calculation, memory, and thinking speed. Men with higher initial blood pressure at 50 achieved lower scores on cognitive testing at 70. These results were explained by *vascular dementia*, or tiny strokes that had occurred in the brains of patients with hypertension.

Therapy for high blood pressure includes weight control, sodium restriction, moderation in alcohol intake (fewer than two drinks a day in men and fewer than one drink a day in women), regular aerobic exercise, and cessation of tobacco smoking. If the hypertension is mild and no other risk factors for heart disease exist, 6 to 12 weeks of effort with these lifestyle changes should be considered before drug therapy.

Drug therapy for hypertension is proven to reduce the risk of heart attack, stroke, and other diseases associated with elevated blood pressure. Many drugs are available for the treatment of hypertension. These drugs affect the speed and force of heart muscle contractions, the muscular tone in the arteries (which affects the resistance to blood flow through them), the volume of blood, and/or chemical and hormonal regulation of blood pressure. Therapy is tailored for each patient based on factors such as age and race, coexisting diseases, and patient sensitivity to side effects. Studies have shown that the older medications in the diuretic and the beta-blocker classes provide the most significant health benefits, along with some remarkable new data about the benefits of newer drugs such as angiotensin converting enzyme inhibitors (ACE inhibitors) and angiotensin receptor blockers (ARBs). A discussion of specific drug therapy is beyond the scope of this book.

Varicose Veins

Varicose veins occur in 10 to 20 percent of the population. Arteries, which carry pressurized blood from the heart to the tissues, are muscular blood vessels with thicker walls. Veins, which carry used blood from the tissues back to the heart, are thin walled. They depend on being squeezed by surrounding muscles to send blood back to the heart and contain one-way valves to prevent the back flow of blood between muscular contractions. The development of varicose veins indicates that this system has been overwhelmed. The veins dilate, the valves fail, and the resulting increase in pressure can create enlarged, twisted veins under the skin of the leg.

Varicose veins follow inherited patterns. They occur more commonly with aging, with women being four times more likely to develop them as men. Tenderness, aching, or a sensation of heaviness may accompany varicose veins. Ankles may swell as fluid leaks into the tissues from the increased pressure in the veins. The skin may become stained with the pigments from blood cells and, in severe cases, skin ulcers may develop.

Patients with varicose veins should avoid activities that further increase the pressure in veins. They should elevate the legs whenever possible, avoid sitting or standing for prolonged periods, and avoid constipation or other activities that would cause straining. Regular exercise such as walking can help.

Treatment options include prescription and over-the-counter compression stockings that help relieve the heaviness and reduce swelling. A procedure called vein sclerotherapy—performed mostly for cosmetic reasons—involves injecting an irritating substance into the vein that causes it to shut down. Surgical procedures range from minor procedures that involve removing small segments of the superficial veins through tiny skin punctures to extensive operations where the entire venous system of the leg is addressed. Since there is no effective therapy for the high venous pressures created once the valves in the deep veins are damaged, most procedures for varicose veins are temporary and new problem areas develop over time. Varicose vein treatment centers have been set up by many different types of physicians with a variety of backgrounds and training. It is best to work with your personal physician for a referral to a reputable center.

Valvular Heart Disease and Mitral Valve Prolapse

The heart valves are structures between the primer pump (atrium) and the main pump (ventricle) on each side of the heart, or between the ventricle and exiting blood vessel (aorta or pulmonary artery). They function to ensure that the squeezing heart chamber pushes blood forward, not backward. *Valvular heart disease* refers to diseases of the heart valves that interfere with blood flow. Valves can have trouble opening or closing, resulting in the following conditions:

- *Valvular stenosis* refers to a valve that does not open all the way as it should, which makes it harder for the blood to flow through it.

- *Valvular regurgitation* refers to a valve that does not close properly, which allows blood to leak backward when the heart contracts.

Depending on which valve is affected and the severity of the dysfunction, valvular heart disease can cause symptoms such as shortness of breath, abnormal heart rhythms, or loss of consciousness. Valvular heart disease is detected by listening to the heart valves with a stethoscope or imaging the heart with ultrasound during echocardiography. Some types of heart valve disease cause turbulent blood flow, which increases the likelihood of a heart valve infection when bacteria get into the bloodstream. Patients with these types of heart valve disease need antibiotics before dental and other procedures that might introduce bacteria into the blood.

Mitral valve prolapse refers to a common abnormality of the mitral valve, which is located between the left atrium and left ventricle. The mitral valve has two leaflets that swing open and closed like a saloon door. On the ventricular side, the leaflets are held by strands of tissue that look like parachute cords. These allow the mitral valve to close properly when the powerful left ventricle is contracting and not swing too far back into the left atrium, which would lead to regurgitation. Mitral valve prolapse occurs when one or both of the leaflets of the mitral valve billow back into the left atrium as the ventricle contracts.

Mitral valve prolapse occurs in 3 to 6 percent of the United States population. Most patients with mitral valve prolapse are without symptoms and never know that they have it. If mitral valve prolapse is not associated with significant regurgitation, antibiotics are not needed and the condition is merely a curious finding on physical examination.

For unknown reasons, some patients with mitral valve prolapse have significant symptoms including unusual patterns of chest pain, anxiety, palpitations, shortness of breath, and fatigue. At times, these symptoms can be severe and incapacitating. Rarely, patients with mitral valve prolapse have sustained episodes of tachycardia (an abnormally fast heart rhythm). Since mitral valve prolapse is so common, this is probably coincidence rather than causally related. Patients with symptomatic mitral valve prolapse need an evaluation and reassurance. Symptoms tend to worsen with dehydration, and can be improved by adequate fluid intake. Occasionally, medications called beta-blockers are needed to control the chest pain and palpitations.

Palpitations and Atrial Fibrillation

The heart has a natural pacemaker called the *sinoatrial node*. This region in the heart initiates the heartbeat 60 to 110 times a minute, on average. The electrical impulses from the sinoatrial node travel down a pathway of specialized conduction tissue and propagate the signal for heart muscle contraction throughout the heart in an organized fashion. Typically, the heart rhythm orchestrated from the sinoatrial node is very regular.

Every cell in the heart has the potential to take over the pacemaking function of the sinoatrial node. Occasionally, one of these cells will get impatient and fire a signal before the sinoatrial node does. This new signal usurps the regular signal and begins the wave of electrical activity that controls the heartbeat. If the new signal occurs close to the time the sinoatrial signal was due, you don't notice anything amiss. If the new signal occurs out of the usual rhythm, you might notice a skip in the heartbeat.

When the sinoatrial node senses a signal from elsewhere in the heart, it pauses, resets, and then begins its usual rhythm again. Blood in motion has inertia and continues to flow into the heart while the rhythm resets. Thus, with the next heartbeat the heart may be fuller with blood than usual, creating the sensation of a forceful heartbeat. Put a few of these forceful extra beats together, and you may sense an irregular heartbeat, or *palpitations*.

Everyone has these extra heartbeats. Some people are exquisitely sensitive to them and feel every one; some feel none. Certain substances and conditions increase the number of extra beats: stimulants such as caffeine or decongestants, inadequate sleep, anxiety or emotional excitement, and mitral valve prolapse are commonly related. Usually these beats are harmless and have no health consequences.

Other disturbances in the heart rhythm can occur, either as spontaneous "short circuits" in the electrical system or as a reflection of underlying heart disease. One of the most common disturbances is *atrial fibrillation*.

In atrial fibrillation, the underlying heart rhythm completely breaks down and the electrical activity in the atria is chaotic. Electrical impulses are intermittently transmitted along the upper portions of the conduction system, resulting in an irregular heartbeat. While the ventricle continues to contract methodically due to the intact lower conducting system, the atria (primer pumps) completely lose organized electrical activity and simply quiver. The efficiency of the heart falls as a result of the primer pump's lack of function and some areas of stagnant blood flow develop in the quivering atria, which can lead to blood clot formation.

Atrial fibrillation occurs in 2 percent of the population and is more common with advancing age. Patients with atrial fibrillation are three to five times more likely to suffer a stroke. They are also more likely to die within 10 years, primarily due to strokes and the fact that atrial fibrillation is a marker for underlying heart disease.

Symptoms

Symptoms of atrial fibrillation include palpitations, episodes of passing out, fatigue, and shortness of breath. Some patients with atrial fibrillation are unaware of this rhythm disturbance, and it is detected only during a routine medical examination or when the patient experiences a complication, such as a stroke or congestive heart failure. Conditions that increase the likelihood of atrial fibrillation include diseases affecting the blood supply or structure of the heart, thyroid disease, chronic obstructive pulmonary disease, severe infection, blood clots to the lung, or trauma.

Treatment

Treatment of atrial fibrillation consists of controlling the heart rate, re-establishing a normal rhythm when possible, and preventing stroke. Many drugs are available to control the heart rate but their administration typically requires a hospital stay until the patient is stabilized.

If a doctor is certain that a patient arrived for evaluation immediately after developing atrial fibrillation, then efforts to restore the heart's normal rhythm can begin right away. Otherwise, patients discovered to be in atrial fibrillation need to be protected from the possibility that a small blood clot has developed in their atrium. If a clot has developed and the patient is converted back into a normal rhythm, the contracting atria can push the clot out where it will travel upstream and potentially cause a stroke. These patients are prescribed anticoagulant medications (blood thinners) for at least three weeks before attempting to restore their normal heart rhythm and then maintained on blood thinners until it is certain that they will remain in normal rhythm.

The longer that atrial fibrillation has been present, the less likely a normal heart rhythm can be restored. Atrial fibrillation seems to cause a remodeling of the heart's electrical system and, after a while, normal rhythms cannot be achieved. Atrial fibrillation also tends to recur. The best available medications only maintain normal heart rhythms for one year in 60 to 70 percent of patients.

This leaves a lot of patients in chronic atrial fibrillation, where they are stuck with this rhythm. The heart rate and most other symptoms can be controlled; however, the quivering atria remain as a potential source of blood clots. Multiple studies show that the use of prescription blood thinners such as warfarin significantly reduces the risk of stroke. Overall, the risk of stroke is reduced from 4.5 percent per year without blood thinners to 1.4 percent with them. The use of blood thinners for certain atrial fibrillation patients with a lower risk for stoke—including patients less than 65 years old without hypertension, history of stroke or transient ischemic attack (see *Cerebrovascular Disease and Stroke* on page 174), congestive heart failure, diabetes, atherosclerotic coronary vascular disease, valvular heart disease, or thyroid disease—should be decided on an individual basis.

High Cholesterol

Cholesterol is manufactured by the body and obtained from foods of animal origin. It is hauled through the bloodstream by lipoproteins. The two principal types of lipoproteins are:

- *LDL (low density lipoprotein)* dumps cholesterol into the arterial wall, contributing to atherosclerosis. LDL is the "bad" cholesterol conductor and is most directly related to the development of heart and blood vessel diseases.
- *HDL (high density lipoprotein)* carries cholesterol out of the arteries into the liver for disposal. HDL is the "good" cholesterol conductor and provides some protection against the development of disease.

In addition to the absolute levels of LDL and HDL cholesterol, the risk of heart disease depends on the ratio of the LDL to HDL cholesterol and the size of the LDL and HDL particles themselves. An ideal LDL/HDL ratio would be less than 2.5. In general, larger sized LDL and HDL particles are healthier than smaller ones. The cholesterol particle size can currently only be measured by a few specialized labs in the United States.

Triglycerides are a second fatty substance that independently increases the risk for heart disease. High triglyceride levels can reduce the HDL (the "good" cholesterol conductor) level. Triglyceride-bearing lipoproteins can dump triglycerides directly into the vessel wall, where the body breaks the triglycerides down into small, dense LDL particles that are considered quite dangerous. In an eight-year study in Denmark, those with the highest triglyceride levels were twice as likely to develop myocardial infarction than their peers. Several studies show higher triglyceride levels in patients who have had strokes.

Cholesterol and triglyceride levels are monitored using a blood test. Before the blood test, you should avoid rigorous exercise for 24 hours and consume nothing but water and any medications you may currently be taking in the 12 hours before the blood is drawn.

What is an Optimal Cholesterol Level?

Cholesterol testing reveals five measurements: a total cholesterol level, which measures the total of all types of cholesterol, a low density lipoprotein (LDL) level, a high density lipoprotein (HDL) level, a ratio of LDL to HDL, and a triglyceride (TG) level. Optimal levels for each of these measurements is as follows:

Your...	Should be...
Cholesterol level	Less than 200
LDL level	Less than 130
HDL level	Greater than 50
LDL/HDL ratio	Less than 2.5
Triglyceride level	Less than 150

When is medical care necessary to reduce cholesterol? Your doctor has access to a statistical model to predict the likelihood that you will have a heart attack within the next 10 years. The Framingham Risk Assessment System uses age, gender, systolic blood pressure, and cholesterol values to calculate this risk. If your risk of a heart attack in the next 10 years is 20 percent or greater, you should be treated as aggressively as someone who has already had a heart attack. New guidelines suggest the need for cholesterol-reducing medication in patients with coronary artery disease or diabetes and LDL levels greater than 100. Medical therapy should also be considered if you have other risk factors for heart disease (hypertension, smoking, a family history of heart disease) and your LDL is greater than 130, or if you are otherwise healthy but your LDL remains greater than 160 despite diet and exercise therapy.

Recent studies have begun to look at the differences in the size of the LDL and HDL cholesterol particles. Patients with small LDL particles are at significantly higher risk for atherosclerotic diseases, even if their overall cholesterol numbers look good. These studies are attempting to determine if medications that induce changes in particle size will help reduce this risk. The outcome of these studies may lead to significant changes in cholesterol management.

Lowering Cholesterol

On average, diet can lower cholesterol by 10 to 15 percent. Here are some guidelines for lowering cholesterol (for more details, see *Chapter 2: Common Sense Nutrition* on page 9.

- Restrict your total fat intake to less than 30 percent of the calories you consume daily.
- Minimize your intake of saturated fat (animal proteins, palm oil, coconut oils).
- Restrict your intake of polyunsaturated fats (sunflower, safflower, corn, soybean oils) to 10 percent of your total fat intake. Monounsaturated fats (olive oil, peanuts, canola and flax seed oils) are healthier oils; try to use them in your cooking, or choose foods that contain them, instead of polyunsaturated fats where you can.
- Avoid the use of partially hydrogenated oils (margarine, shortening, processed foods), which are a source of trans-fatty acids that increase LDL-cholesterol while reducing HDL-cholesterol.

In addition to diet, regular aerobic exercise helps lower total and LDL cholesterol levels and raise HDL cholesterol levels. Obese patients can also raise their HDL levels by losing weight; smokers can raise theirs when they stop smoking.

A proper diet and exercise program are essential to the management of cholesterol. Patients without established cardiovascular disease are typically placed on a three- to six-month trial of diet and exercise therapy before considering cholesterol-lowering medications; for patients with known cardiovascular disease, changes in diet and exercise habits are often accompanied by immediate drug therapy. Even for patients who require medication for cholesterol reduction, diet and exercise therapy play an essential role in maximizing the response to these medications.

Why Reduce Cholesterol?

Multiple medical studies show that if cholesterol is lowered by any means, benefits are noticeable within one to three years for men and women. Cardiac catheterization data, where x-ray pictures are taken of the coronary arteries in patients with established heart disease, do not show any reduction in the size of these cholesterol deposits in patients on cholesterol-lowering therapy. The benefits of drug therapy are felt to be related to more stable plaque deposits and a decreased risk of these deposits rupturing. When studies of interventional angioplasty (using a catheter directed balloon to open up clogged arteries) are compared to cholesterol drug therapy, most patients are found to fare better with drug therapy. In a recently reported West Scotland Study, 6,595 men ages 45 to 64 without a history of heart disease were given a cholesterol lowering medication (pravastatin). Those patients on drug therapy achieved a 30 percent reduction in the rate of heart disease and cardiovascular death. Similar findings of a benefit of cholesterol reducing medications in patients for whom they were not traditionally prescribed was reported in the Heart Protection Study using simvastatin, another agent in this class.

What are "Statin" Drugs?

Pravastatin and simvastatin are examples of drugs in the *statin* class. These drugs block a step in the biochemical manufacturing of cholesterol in the body. They are generally safe and effective, with few significant side effects. Drugs in this class are proven to reduce the risk of future heart attack and death in patients who have documented heart disease or damage and appear effective in preventing the first heart attack in patients with high cholesterol.

Serious but rare side effects include muscle irritation and abnormalities in liver chemistries. The risks and benefits of cholesterol reduction therapy should be discussed with your doctor, who can perform periodic lab work and examinations to monitor for these problems.

No clinical studies confirm that medications to lower moderately elevated triglyceride levels (150 to 400) offer any benefit that outweighs the drug risks. What can you do to sharply reduce triglycerides, then, without taking drugs? You can lose weight, quit smoking, exercise regularly, minimize your sugar, alcohol and fat intake, and eat fatty fish rich in omega-3 fatty acids, such as salmon.

Niacin is a supplement that lowers cholesterol and triglyceride levels while increasing HDL cholesterol levels. Niacin has been shown to favorably increase the size of the LDL and HDL cholesterol subcomponents. It is a difficult supplement to take. Common side effects include stomach irritation and rather uncomfortable skin flushing and itching. Homocysteine, a substance in the blood related to the risk for heart disease, seems to be adversely affected by niacin. The use of niacin in cholesterol therapy is currently being investigated.

Atherosclerosis (Narrowing of the Blood Vessels)

The *vascular endothelium* is the smooth lining on the inside of blood vessels. It is flexible, expanding and contracting with the vessel. This surface promotes smooth blood flow and helps prevent the formation of blood clots. *Atherosclerosis* is a process that occurs in this lining, leading to the deposits of cholesterol and other substances, causing damage to and narrowing of the artery.

Atherosclerosis progresses through several stages. In *pre-atherosclerosis*, no visible changes are seen in the vascular lining but it produces less of the chemical nitric oxide and doesn't relax as well. *Adaptive thickening* occurs as early as age four or five as the lining of the blood vessel begins to thicken at shear points (areas of turbulent blood flow). Later, white blood cells called *macrophages* deposit in the lining of the blood vessel and become filled with fat. These cells are felt to be involved in an inflammatory process within the blood vessel lining that may ultimately weaken the developing cholesterol plaque. Gradually, small pools of lipid (cholesterol, triglycerides, and other fatty substances) begin to form on top of these deposits. A cap called a *fibroadenoma* begins to form over this portion of the vessel; this cap is composed of fibrous (scar-like) tissue and smooth muscle, and is an area of active inflammation and metabolic activity. When this stage is reached, this collective deposit, called *complex plaque*, can crack, ulcerate, rupture, or tear off and expose its internal contents—fats, inflammatory cells, and fibrin—to the bloodstream. The body sees this break in the plaque as a cut or injury and forms a blood clot to patch up the damage. While forming a blood clot may be a good idea for a cut on your finger, a clot on a fractured plaque in a coronary artery leading to your heart may plug up all blood flow through the vessel and lead to a heart attack or death.

Atherosclerosis was thought to develop gradually and to cause problems only when the plaque built up large enough to significantly block the flow of blood through an artery. According to the laws of physics, it takes about a 70 percent blockage of a pipe to significantly affect the flow of fluid similar to blood through it. Thus, it was expected that patients should develop warning symptoms of decreased coronary blood flow once their atherosclerosis was severe enough, or the disease could be discovered by stress testing, before the vessel completely closed and damage was done to the heart muscle.

More recent studies show that this prior understanding of the nature of heart disease is incorrect. Studies show that 90 percent of heart attacks occur in lesions of active plaque that only block 30 to 50 percent of the blood vessel. These lesions are softer, have a thinner cap, are full of fat and inflammatory cells that weaken the cap, and have little smooth muscle in them to provide stability. Lesions that block greater than 70 percent of the blood vessel, and thus would be expected to produce warning symptoms or be discoverable by stress tests, account for less than 14 percent of heart attacks.

Why do these smaller plaques rupture? This is a key question of modern cardiology. Plaque rupture appears related to the amount of lipid in the plaque, the thickness and maturity of the cap covering the plaque, and the amount of inflammation in the plaque. Again relying on physics, Laplace's law tells us the relationship between the circumferential stress on the wall of the vessel and the size of that vessel. Calculations show that the wall stress on a fibroadenoma blocking 50 percent of the vessel is five times greater than that on a 90 percent lesion. This greater stress is speculated to be the cause of the greater numbers of ruptures seen in smaller plaques.

Current research focuses on preventing the development of atheromatous plaques and the rupture of those that have already formed. Anti-inflammatory medications, such as aspirin or ibuprofen, may reduce the inflammation in the plaque and make it more stable. Some of the damage to the plaque occurs from the oxidation of LDL cholesterol; studies are underway to evaluate the use of antioxidant diets and pill supplements to prevent this. Some cholesterol-lowering drugs and blood pressure medications seem to toughen the fibrous cap and may stabilize the plaque. Blood pressure medications such as beta-blockers reduce the sheer force between peak systolic and lowest diastolic blood pressure, reducing the tendency to cause plaques to rupture. Researchers are evaluating therapies to prevent the formation of blood clots on fractured plaques and thus interrupt the final step that leads to blood vessel blockage. Some researchers are also looking into the role certain bacteria may play in plaque development and rupture and whether antibiotic therapy can be of benefit.

Peripheral Vascular Disease

The same process of atherosclerosis described above that occurs in the coronary arteries can involve any artery. *Peripheral vascular disease* refers to disease that occurs in the blood vessels supplying blood to the body. These blood vessels are typically larger; therefore, larger amounts of plaque build-up are required to significantly block them. Although blockages in these blood vessels don't cause strokes or heart attacks, they can lead to pain in the extremities or complications such as poorly healing wounds or limb amputation.

Symptoms

Chronic pain in the legs is a symptom of peripheral vascular disease. With walking, the muscles need more oxygen. If their blood supply is blocked, they can't receive adequate oxygen and, with exercise, develop a painful cramping that eases with rest. Often, patients know just how far they can walk before the pain begins and they adjust their activities accordingly. Other signs of peripheral vascular disease include numbness, tingling in the legs, weakness, a burning or aching pain in the feet at rest, a sore on the leg that won't heal, cold legs or feet, color changes in the feet (red or bluish when hanging down, white or pale when elevated), and loss of skin appendages such as hair and nails. The risk factors for peripheral vascular disease include age over 50, tobacco smoking, diabetes, obesity, hypertension, hypercholesterolemia, and a family history of heart or vascular disease.

Physicians diagnose this disease by taking a careful patient history and comparing blood pressures in the arms and ankles. The blood pressure in the arms should be similar to that found in the ankles; a significant discrepancy means that the blood supply is restricted. To help find the blockage, physicians use the Doppler ultrasound test on the leg vessels to measure the degree of obstruction and other radiological testing such as MRA (magnetic resonance angiography) to provide a precise roadmap of the arterial system.

Treatment

Two important ways a patient can alleviate peripheral vascular disease symptoms are to exercise more and—if a smoker—to stop smoking. Patients with stable peripheral vascular disease on a regular walking program can actually open up new pathways for blood to flow around the obstructions and significantly increase their pain-free walking time. Smoking causes the muscular wall of diseased arteries to spasm and narrow, as well as restrict the amount of oxygen available in the bloodstream. If the patient has other diseases associated with peripheral vascular disease, such as hypertension and diabetes, those diseases should be treated aggressively as well.

Some critical blockages can be opened by procedures such as angioplasty, stent, or bypass. In *angioplasty*, an incision is made under local anesthesia to gain access to a blood vessel and a catheter is passed to the area of blockage where a balloon is inflated to crush the blockage open. Often, a tiny spring called a *stent* is placed at the area of blockage to keep the blood vessel from closing again, and medications are used to keep this area from forming a blood clot until the blood vessel lining grows into the stent. Sometimes the blockages are severe enough to require surgical placement of a new blood vessel (*bypass*) to route blood flow around the area of obstruction. This only works if the blood vessels beyond the area of obstruction are healthy enough to accept the new blood flow.

Aortic Aneurysm

An *aneurysm* is defined as a localized swelling in a blood vessel of greater than 50 percent of its usual diameter. In the aorta, two types of aneurysms are classified based on their location:

- *Thoracic (chest) aorta aneurysms*, where the blood vessels dilate to diameters greater than 3.5 to 4.0 centimeters
- *Abdominal aorta aneurysms*, where the blood vessels dilate to diameters greater than 3.0 centimeters

Abdominal aortic aneurysms occur more often in men than women, with the possibility of experiencing one increasing with advancing age. They occur in 3 percent of the general population and in 9 percent of those with hypertension and coronary artery disease. Of those patients with abdominal aortic aneurysms, greater than 20 percent of their immediate family will also develop this condition as they age. Abdominal aortic aneurysm is the 13th leading cause of death in the United States; thoracic aortic aneurysms are much less common.

Most aneurysms enlarge by 4 millimeters a year. The risk of rupture is related to size, the presence of emphysema, and diastolic blood pressure. Half of all patients with ruptured abdominal aortic aneurysms die; 90 percent of patients with ruptured thoracic aortic aneurysms die. If the aneurysm is identified before it ruptures, in experienced hands surgery to repair the aneurysm can drop the mortality rate to 2 percent and 10 percent, respectively.

If an abdominal aortic aneurysm is smaller than 4 centimeters, it is observed with serial ultrasounds or CT scans every 6 to 12 months. If it is 5 centimeters or greater, surgical repair is advised in a patient in otherwise acceptable condition. Intervention for abdominal aortic aneurysms between 4 and 5 centimeters is considered on an individual basis based on the patient's health and life expectancy. Because of the higher operative risk, thoracic aortic aneurysms are often observed until they reach 6 centimeters before operative repair is considered.

The techniques to surgically repair aneurysms before they rupture have been practiced since the 1950s. Recent efforts have involved techniques to repair the diseased blood vessel by placing a tiny metal tube called a stent in the region of the aneurysm; this technique is called an *endovascular repair*. Candidates for this technique are usually decided by their health and the anatomy of the blood vessel around the aneurysm. Patients with this type of repair avoid a major incision, lose less blood, and are out of the hospital faster; however, there are drawbacks—the operative mortality is the same, endovascular repairs are more expensive, and patients who have received this type of repair are obligated to have CT scans every six months for the rest of their lives to monitor the condition of the graft.

Congestive Heart Failure

Congestive heart failure occurs when the heart is unable to keep up with the workload demanded of it. This typically happens when the left ventricle becomes weaker, dilates like an inflating balloon, and is unable to generate sufficient force to create proper blood flow. Fluid then begins to back up in the lungs and body, causing shortness of breath and swelling in the legs, ankles, and arms. Some patients have a very different cause for congestive heart failure—*diastolic dysfunction*. With this condition, the left ventricle is thick and stiff and does not relax adequately for blood to flow into it, resulting in the same problems of fluid backup and similar symptoms.

Five million people in the United States are diagnosed with congestive heart failure. This includes 1 percent of all adults over age 50 and greater than 10 percent of adults in their eighties. Congestive heart failure is responsible for 250,000 deaths a year; the majority of these occur suddenly. If a patient has no symptoms of congestive heart failure but an echocardiogram shows that the left ventricle is beginning to fail, ejecting less than 40 percent of the blood with each contraction, the five-year survival for this individual is only 50 percent. For patients with severe congestive heart failure, the five-year survival is much less.

Symptoms

Congestive heart failure has nonspecific symptoms, including shortness of breath with exertion and when lying down, sudden episodes of shortness of breath at night, fluid collection in the ankles and limbs, and fatigue. It can be confirmed by findings on physical examination and by testing such as chest x-rays and tests of heart function.

Causes

The causes of congestive heart failure include atherosclerotic ischemic heart disease (disease of the arteries supplying the heart muscle), valvular heart disease (see *Valvular Heart Disease and Mitral Valve Prolapse* on page 157), alcohol excess and other drug abuse, hypertension, viral infections of the heart muscle, thyroid disease, and idiopathic (unknown) causes. Additional risk factors for congestive heart failure include diabetes, age, obesity, and smoking. Sometimes congestive heart failure only becomes evident when the heart is stressed to do more work, such as with fever, anemia, abnormally fast heart rhythms, infections, or salt and fluid overload. Looking for these reversible stressors is important in evaluating and managing heart failure.

The New York Heart Association's classification for congestive heart failure is widely used for prognosis and assessing disability.

This level...	Indicates...
Class 1	No limitation of physical activity; patient has no symptoms during ordinary physical activity
Class 2	Slight limitation of physical activity; comfortable at rest; patient has symptoms during ordinary physical activity (can no longer play that third set of tennis)
Class 3	Marked limitation of physical activity; comfortable at rest; patient has symptoms during less than ordinary activity (difficulty walking to the mailbox)
Class 4	Unable to carry on any physical activity without discomfort; patient has symptoms while resting

---

Treatment

Congestive heart failure is treated as follows:

- Assess the health of the coronary arteries and decrease any risk for new cardiac injury. Treat associated disorders such as hypertension (see *Hypertension* on page 155) and elevated cholesterol (see *High Cholesterol* on page 160).
- Maintain proper fluid balance, restrict salt intake, and control weight. Water intake is generally not the problem; it is salt that holds water within the cardiovascular system, leading to fluid retention and swelling of the limbs.
- Improve physical conditioning. Supervised physical exercise programs in all but the most severe congestive heart failure patients reduce symptoms and improve physical abilities.
- Avoid the use of medications that can worsen congestive heart failure, including calcium antagonist used for blood pressure control and anti-inflammatory medications (NSAIDs) used for arthritis.

Many medications are useful in the treatment of congestive heart failure. Of the ones listed below, only ACE inhibitors and beta-blockers have been shown to decrease mortality.

- **Digoxin.** Digoxin is a medication that can treat the residual symptoms of congestive heart failure after the fluid overload is controlled. Although it has no direct effect on whether a patient survives congestive heart failure, digoxin can increase exercise tolerance and decrease the frequency of hospitalization in patients with congestive heart failure. Digoxin levels must be monitored in the bloodstream; excessively high levels can be lethal.

- **Diuretics.** Diuretics are useful in managing fluid retention. Patients often can monitor their weight at home and adjust their dosages of diuretics as needed. Diuretics relieve symptoms but have not yet proven to prolong survival. Side effects include depletion of potassium and magnesium, which can make heart function worse and promote abnormal heart rhythms. Diuretics can activate a hormonal system called the renin-angiotensin system that can worsen congestive heart failure if it is not carefully monitored and treated.

- **Spironolactone.** Spironolactone is a diuretic that also blocks the effect of the hormone aldosterone, which regulates the balance of salt and water in the body. In a recent study reported in the *New England Journal of Medicine*, 1,663 patients with congestive heart failure and an ejection fraction—a measurement of the percentage of blood ejected from the ventricle with each contraction—of less than 35 percent were treated with a low dose of spironolactone and followed for two years. Patients treated with this drug had a 30 percent decrease in mortality or rehospitalization. The significance of this response is largely unknown, since few of the patients in the study were on the recommended doses of ACE inhibitors and fewer than 10 percent were on beta-blockers (see below).

- **ACE inhibitors.** ACE inhibitors interfere with the metabolic steps in the formation of angiotensin II, an important vasoconstrictor (a chemical that causes arteries to narrow) in patients with congestive heart failure. After one to three months of therapy, the average congestive heart failure patient notes improved symptoms and exercise tolerance. ACE inhibitors slow the progression of heart disease and prolong survival. Patients who use these drugs experience a 20 to 25 percent reduction in mortality rates and a 30 to 35 percent decrease in the combined risk of hospitalization and death. Benefits extend to all age groups and appear to be greatest at higher doses. Side effects of ACE inhibitors include excessively low blood pressure, kidney dysfunction, and cough.

- **Beta-blockers.** Doctors used to avoid prescribing beta-blockers for congestive heart failure patients because these drugs can further depress left ventricular function. It is now understood that many of the forces that drive congestive heart failure involve the sympathetic nervous system, which is blocked by beta-blockers. Several long-term studies show that beta-blockers actually improve heart function and heart failure classification over time, and can decrease mortality by 35 percent in patients with congestive heart failure. Because of their negative effects on heart function, congestive heart failure patients must be started on very low doses of certain beta-blockers and monitored carefully as the dose is slowly increased over time. Physically, patients may feel worse the first six weeks on the beta-blocker therapy, but then should improve.

The progression and treatment of congestive heart failure is still being studied. Based on available data, all patients with congestive heart failure should be taking ACE inhibitors and beta-blockers unless a strong argument exists against their use.

Most of the references about congestive heart failure thus far have referred to patients with systolic dysfunction—when the heart muscle is weak or enlarged and doesn't contract well. Congestive heart failure can also be caused by diastolic dysfunction—when the heart muscle is too thick or stiff and doesn't relax well enough between contractions to allow blood to enter and fill the pumping chambers sufficiently. Patients with diastolic dysfunction are typically older, female, and have a history of hypertension and no evidence of coronary artery disease. Their left ventricular ejection fraction (the percentage of blood ejected from the ventricle with each contraction) is often greater than 50 percent. The stiff left ventricle leads to a backup of fluid in the lungs and legs, creating the classic symptoms of congestive heart failure. Treatment of diastolic dysfunction includes eliminating any significant blockages in the coronary arteries, maintaining a normal sinus rhythm with proper functioning of the primer pump (atrium), and using drug therapy including ACE inhibitors, beta-blockers, another class of medications called calcium channel blockers, and the judicious use of diuretics.

Angina (Chest Pain)

Angina means chest pain, pressure, numbness, or other symptoms caused by a temporary insufficiency of blood flow to the heart. It generally lasts just a few minutes, then resolves. Activities that increase the workload for the heart (for example, exercise or stress) create a need for a greater blood flow to feed the heart muscle. If a coronary artery is diseased and partially blocked, it cannot increase its blood flow rate sufficiently and the heart hurts from the lack of oxygen. Rest reduces demands on the heart and eases angina. *Stable exertional angina* refers to symptoms that are produced each time you attempt to perform at a certain level of exercise. This is generally caused by a fixed blockage that limits flow in a coronary vessel. *Unstable angina* refers to a pattern of increasing chest pain, with subsequent episodes occurring more frequently, with less exertion, lasting longer, or occurring at rest. Unstable angina is often a sign of clot formation on a diseased vessel and needs prompt medical attention.

Myocardial Infarction (Heart Attack)

During a *myocardial infarction* (a heart attack), a coronary artery becomes blocked and, as a result, the heart muscle that depended upon that artery for its blood supply dies. As discussed earlier, this usually occurs when an atheromatous plaque blocks 30 to 60 percent of a blood vessel and ruptures, exposing its contents into the bloodstream and triggering a blood clot that completely shuts off the artery. The amount of muscle damaged correlates with the amount of muscle that depended on the involved coronary artery for its blood supply and whether any other coronary arteries can provide the involved region of heart muscle with an alternative blood supply. Heart muscle that dies cannot grow back.

If you are reading this chapter because you think you are having a heart attack...

STOP!
Put this book down, and
Call 911!

Recognizing the Signs of Heart Attack or Angina:

Sudden onset of chest pain, feeling like a squeezing or pressure sensation that may radiate from the center of the chest to the jaw or arm; chest symptoms usually last from 2 to 20 minutes, or longer if heart damage is occurring. These symptoms are often brought on by physical or emotional stress and are relieved by rest.

Associated symptoms:

- Shortness of breath
- Sweating
- Nausea
- Profound weakness
- Irregular heartbeat
- Loss of consciousness

Be aware of other symptoms: Atypical pain, such as heartburn or pain in the jaw, arm, or back, associated with any of the above symptoms, may represent heart-related pain.

Keep in mind that 30 percent of heart attacks are not associated with any pain sensation at all.

Symptoms

Symptoms of a heart attack include the sudden onset of chest pain, shortness of breath, sweating, nausea, profound weakness, irregular heartbeat, and loss of consciousness. The classic description of chest pain is that of a crushing sensation under the sternum "like an elephant is on my chest," that may radiate to the jaw or left arm. However, many patients experience no pain at all, atypical pain that is misinterpreted as heartburn, or pain that appears in the jaw, arm, or back rather than in the chest. It is estimated that 30 percent of heart attacks are "silent," without chest pain. See your doctor if you experience any unusual symptoms, particularly if you have risk factors for heart disease.

"Time is myocardium!"—that is, that with each passing minute of a heart attack, more heart muscle may be lost. Patients who experience symptoms that suggest a heart attack must be considered to be having a heart attack and be rapidly evaluated until the diagnosis is clear. The doctor will review the patient's history and risk factors and perform a brief examination looking for signs of a failing heart or related conditions. When the heart muscle is injured, the flow of electrical forces through it changes. This can be seen on an electrocardiogram (EKG), which shows deflections in the usual electrical waves that can suggest an acute injury to the heart muscle. When the heart muscle is damaged, chemicals are released into the bloodstream. Measurements of these chemicals, including troponin and CPK isoenzymes, can confirm the presence of heart damage.

Treatment

The goals for therapy of a patient with an acute heart attack are survival, minimization of damage, and reduction in the risk for a second heart attack. If the patient undergoing a heart attack seeks and receives help quickly enough (within the first few hours), the major thrust of effort is to reopen the blocked coronary artery and supply fresh blood to the heart muscle. This can be accomplished in the following ways:

- **Medications that break up and dissolve the clot.** This is referred to as thrombolytic therapy.
- **Urgent cardiac catheterization and balloon angioplasty.** During this procedure, catheters are placed in an artery of the leg or arm and threaded up to the heart. With x-ray assistance, images are created of the heart's blood vessels. Blocked arteries may be opened by passing a balloon through the catheter to the area of blockage and inflating it, crushing the cholesterol and other materials making up the blockage against the walls of the vessel and restoring blood flow.
- **(Occasionally) Emergency coronary artery bypass surgery.** This technique entails surgically placing a new blood vessel to route blood flow around an area of blockage in the original vessel.

The sooner a patient with a suspected heart attack seeks medical assistance, the higher the likelihood of success in re-establishing blood flow.

In the past 30 years, the death rate of patients experiencing acute heart attacks has decreased by 50 percent, thanks to education of the public to seek assistance more quickly for symptoms suggesting a heart attack and an improvement in medical management. The five-year mortality after a heart attack remains high. Women, the elderly, and diabetics are at highest risk of complications after a heart attack.

Numerous drug therapies are available to help improve survival and function after a heart attack.

- **Aspirin.** Aspirin inhibits clot formation by platelets. Studies have shown that the use of aspirin during the heart attack reduced the short-term and two-year death rate by 20 percent. Aspirin is usually given immediately to patients seeking treatment for chest pain, if they are not allergic to it, with doses ranging between 81 and 325 milligrams.
- **Beta-blockers.** These drugs reduce heart rate, lower blood pressure, lower the amount of oxygen the heart's muscle tissue demands, and reduce wall stress in the

heart. Studies of the use of beta-blockers, including over 27,000 patients since the 1970s, show a 14 percent reduction in initial death rates from acute myocardial infarctions associated with these drugs. Patients on long-term beta-blocker therapy are 20 to 25 percent less likely to experience subsequent heart attacks or die. The benefit from beta-blockers is greatest in those with the most extensive heart tissue damage, greatest reduction in left ventricular function, and congestive heart failure (see *Congestive Heart Failure* on page 167).

- **ACE inhibitors.** ACE inhibitors are oral medications usually started within two to three days after a heart attack and continued indefinitely. These drugs lower blood pressure and reduce changes in heart muscle after the heart attack that can lead to congestive heart failure. These drugs also have beneficial effects on blood vessel walls and the cells that make up their lining (endothelial cells). The vessel walls of a patient on an ACE inhibitor seem to grow more flexible, and their cholesterol plaques are not as likely to rupture. A recent study of the use of ACE inhibitors in 9,300 heart patients showed a 25 percent reduction in overall death rate in those patients that took them, even when the traditional indications for the use of these medications (hypertension or congestive heart failure) were absent.

- **Statins.** Statin drugs are cholesterol-lowering medications that can reduce LDL cholesterol by up to 60 percent and are proven to reduce the risk of subsequent attacks in heart patients. Most patients who have experienced a heart attack would benefit from statin drugs, regardless of how low their cholesterol might be. Recent studies suggest a survival advantage when these medications are started immediately after a heart attack.

- **Thrombolytic therapy.** Thrombolytic drugs dissolve blood clots that have occurred on ruptured plaques and in other areas. They restore blood flow similar to that before clotting began. These drugs must be given within a few hours of the onset of a heart attack to be of benefit. These heart-saving medications are not used as often as they could be because many patients arrive for treatment too late to benefit from them. These drugs do increase the risk of bleeding throughout the body, including life-threatening bleeding in the brain, and are therefore given in an intensive care setting under the watchful eye of hospital staff.

- **Heparin and Low Molecular Weight Heparin.** Heparin is a blood thinner that is given following thrombolytic agents to inhibit the formation of new clots. It is administered intravenously or—in the case of the newer version of this drug called Low Molecular Weight Heparin—as twice-daily injections following the heart attack during the course of hospitalization to reduce the likelihood of subsequent attacks.

- **Glycoprotein receptor inhibitors (GPIIb-IIIa inhibitors).** Platelets are present in the bloodstream at all times. When the body forms a blood clot, these platelets become "activated" or turned on, and begin to clump together. The activation of platelets occurs when a signal is received through the stimulation of a certain receptor of the surface of the platelet—the GPIIb-IIIa receptor. Activated platelets become large and sticky and group together to form clots. It is felt that microscopic platelet plugs play a role in reducing flow to areas of injured heart muscle, worsening the damage. In addition, when the coronary arteries are re-opened by angioplasty and stents, platelet clots can form and block the vessel up again. Drugs that are GPIIb-IIIa receptor inhibitors block the GPIIb-IIIa receptors on the platelet surface and keep the platelets from activating. These drugs are dramatically effective in increasing the benefit of thrombolytic drugs and urgent vessel opening procedures.

- **Cardiac rehabilitation.** Cardiac rehabilitation through structured exercise programs after a heart attack has proven to increase the chances of survival.

Strategies for treatment of patients after heart attack are changing. Most patients with heart disease should be taking three or four medications, in addition to a healthy diet, exercise programs, and healthy habits.

Cerebrovascular Disease and Stroke

> **If you think that you or someone that you know is having a stroke, call 911, not the doctor's office. You have less than three hours from the first symptom to receive drug therapy that might reverse the stroke.**
>
> ### Recognizing the Signs of Stroke:
> - Sudden onset of weakness, numbness, or tingling on one side of the body
> - Drooling
> - Difficulty with speech, either forming words or understanding them
> - Difficulty walking
> - Sudden loss of vision, in one eye or one side of the visual field
> - Severe, unexplained dizziness, lack of coordination, or falling
> - Severe, unexplained headache, often with vomiting and loss of consciousness

A brain receives its blood supply from two large vessels in the front of the neck (the right and left carotid arteries) and two smaller vessels in the back of the neck (vertebral arteries). These arteries supply oxygen-rich blood to the brain. These vessels divide into smaller and smaller branches that feed discrete areas of brain. If blood flow is blocked by a blood clot or cholesterol plaque, symptoms may be seen immediately. If a minor blood vessel is involved, the surrounding vessels may take over, supplying blood and resolving the symptoms. If the interruption of blood flow is not restored or bypassed, the brain dies (a condition called an *ischemic stroke*). If the blood vessel is weakened, bursts, and bleeds into the brain, this results in a condition called a *hemorrhagic stroke*.

Strokes can occur from the changes of atherosclerosis in the blood vessels feeding the heart, similar to that described for coronary artery disease. Strokes can also occur from blood clots that develop elsewhere and are carried in the blood vessel to the brain, blocking the blood vessel off once the clot reaches a vessel smaller than itself. These are called *embolic strokes*.

Symptoms

The portion of the brain that is injured dictates what symptoms develop. See the text box on the previous page for signs of stroke.

Not all strokes have symptoms. Some occur in silent areas of the brain. A research study performed 3,415 Magnetic Resonance Imaging (MRI) tests of the brains of people greater than 65 years of age. One-third of these individuals showed changes of a previous stroke while none had recognized symptoms of a stroke. These subjects were put through a variety of cognitive and physical tests. Individuals with previous silent strokes performed measurably worse on these functional tests.

A *transient ischemic attack* is identical to a stroke, but symptoms fully resolve in minutes. The average attack lasts five to seven minutes; if symptoms persist longer than one hour, they will disappear within 24 hours in only 14 percent of patients. Previously, it didn't matter whether a patient was experiencing a transient ischemic attack or a stroke—there was little that doctors could do to sway the outcome. Now there are several medications that can dissolve blood clots within the arteries of the heart or brain. These medications must be administered within three hours of the onset of symptoms of a stroke. Administered after this time frame, these drugs cannot help recover brain function and can even increase the risk of bleeding within the brain and death.

Most major emergency rooms now have procedures to rapidly identify and evaluate patients who are experiencing symptoms suggestive of a stroke, attempting to get the patient evaluated in time to take advantage of these new drugs. Unfortunately, the biggest delay still occurs in the time it takes a patient or those around him to recognize the possibility of a stroke in progress and seek medical attention. Several community-based educational programs are now in place to teach patients how to recognize the symptoms of a stroke quickly, and act promptly to seek medical care.

Risk Factors

Several risk factors for stroke have been identified:
- Previous transient ischemic attack
- Atrial fibrillation (see *Palpitations and Atrial Fibrillation* on page 158)
- Hypertension (see *Hypertension* on page 155)
- Hypercholesterolemia (see *High Cholesterol* on page 160)
- Smoking
- Diabetes (see *Diabetes Mellitus* on page 141)
- Heart disease
- Central obesity (abdominal fat)
- Sleep apnea
- High homocysteine levels
- Chronic stress and anger
- Race (African Americans have a stroke mortality rate twice that of whites)
- Geography (strokes are more common in the South)

These risk factors can be modified as follows:

- If patients with transient ischemic attacks can be identified, physicians may also be able to pinpoint correctable causes for the symptoms and treat the patient with medication or surgical procedures to help prevent a stroke. Patients with transient ischemic attacks have a 4 percent risk of stroke within one month, 13 percent within one year, and 50 percent risk within five years. In addition, 50 percent of patients with transient ischemic attacks develop heart attacks within five years. Unfortunately, many patients who experience these attacks never discuss them with their physicians and lose out on any chance to prevent these devastating subsequent events.
- Atrial fibrillation accounts for one-half of recognized embolic strokes. Use of prescription-strength blood thinners in these patients reduces the stroke risk by greater than 70 percent. In those who cannot take these blood thinners, aspirin reduces the stroke risk by one-third. See *Palpitations and Atrial Fibrillation* on page 158 for more information about this condition.
- Treatment of hypertension reduces stroke risk by 40 percent. See *Hypertension* on page 158 for more information about this condition.
- Three major studies show a 30 percent reduction in strokes in patients taking statin medications for their elevated cholesterol. See *High Cholesterol* on page 155 for more information about these medications.
- Smoking increases the risk for stroke. This risk is proportional to the number of cigarettes smoked per day; for example, smoking two packs of cigarettes a day doubles the stroke risk. Once a smoker stops smoking, it takes two years for their stroke risk to return to that of a similar patient who has never smoked.

Treatment

Patients who have signs of a stroke and seek treatment within three hours of the onset of their symptoms can receive new intravenous medications that help dissolve the blood clot responsible for the stroke. These drugs can only be used for individuals having an ischemic stroke who are certain when their symptoms began (and are within the three-hour window for therapy), whose neurological deficit is measurable (demonstrated weakness or other neurologic changes on examination), and whose head CT scans show no evidence of bleeding in the brain. The use of clot-dissolving drugs can dramatically improve or eliminate all signs of the stroke; however, these drugs are not without risk. The main risk is serious bleeding in the brain, which affects 4 to 6 percent of stroke patients who take these medications. This risk varies based on the size and severity of the stroke. For this reason, clot-dissolving drugs are given only in an emergency room or intensive care setting where patients can be carefully monitored. Patients who do not qualify for clot-dissolving drugs include those who seek treatment too late (unfortunately, a common occurrence), patients with previous stroke or head trauma within three months, major surgery within the previous 14 days, a history of gastrointestinal bleeding within the past three weeks, excessively high blood pressure, a seizure associated with the stroke, or certain laboratory abnormalities.

Patients who have had transient ischemic attacks or abnormal noises in their neck on their physical examination may undergo a carotid ultrasound to look for evidence of atherosclerosis in their neck vessels. Patients whose carotid arteries are blocked more 70 percent may benefit from a surgical procedure called an *endarterectomy* to prevent a stroke. In this procedure, the diseased carotid vessel is cleaned out. Studies have shown that with a good surgeon and proper patient selection, this procedure can reduce the risk of any stroke resulting from vessel blockage of this extent from 26 percent to 9 percent and the risk of a major or fatal stroke from 13.1 percent to 2.5 percent.

Thromboembolic Disease (Blood Clots)

The body must keep the blood fluid so that it can flow through small blood vessels and nourish the tissues. It must also be able to stop bleeding should a cut or other trauma occur. To do this, opposite and competing chemical systems exist that create and break down blood clots. A very delicate balance exists between these two systems; a breakdown in this balance creates bleeding (*hemorrhage*) or clotting (*thrombosis*).

Deep venous thrombosis is a blood clot in the larger veins, particularly the leg. This blood clot interferes with blood draining from the leg, leading to swelling of one leg, warmth, and redness. The leg may be painful or tender to the touch. This condition occurs in up to 1 in 1,000 people each year.

Risk Factors

Risk factors for this condition include:

- Recent orthopedic or abdominal surgery
- Trauma, including fractures of the spine, pelvis, hip, and leg
- Immobilization from illness or prolonged travel (particularly prolonged air travel)
- Cancer
- Pregnancy
- Estrogen use. Oral contraceptive pills increase the risk, particularly in the first six months of their use. A study reported in the January 2000 issue of *Archives of Internal Medicine* followed eight patients who experienced deep venous thrombosis while taking birth control pills. Seven of these patients were found to have inherited defects in the coagulation system. It is felt that birth control pills may primarily be of risk to women who already have coagulation disorders, even though they have never previously experienced problems.
- Dehydration
- Previous clots
- Inherited disorders of the coagulation system

Patients with deep venous thrombosis are identified by their symptoms, physical exam findings, and testing. In the most common test, a Doppler ultrasound looks at images of veins and the blood flow pattern through them. This test detects blood clots and the reduced blood flow associated with them. Doppler ultrasounds are not very good at visualizing the veins in the calf, however, where smaller blood clots can be very difficult to detect.

Treatment

Treatment of deep venous thrombosis involves the use of blood thinners to prevent the development of further clots while the body's own clot-dissolving system slowly removes the original ones. Heparin is a common blood thinner given continuously by vein. It acts immediately and requires an intravenous catheter and blood draws to monitor adjustments in its dose and effect. A newer version of this drug called Low Molecular Weight Heparin is dosed by weight and given as twice-daily injections. It does not require an intravenous catheter or laboratory monitoring. Warfarin (Coumadin) is a pill that works in the liver to block the body's production of blood clotting proteins. It takes several days to take full effect, and the body's response to it is monitored by blood tests. Most patients are initially treated with a rapid-acting form of heparin and then transitioned to warfarin for continued therapy. This initial course of therapy will last from three to six months in uncomplicated cases.

Patients with blood clots that involve only the deep veins of the leg below the knee require thoughtful consideration and close observation over time. The risk of pulmonary embolism in this type of clot is only 5 to 10 percent and usually occurs after the clot has extended up into the thigh. Selected patients with calf-only blood clots may be observed with repeated ultrasounds over a few weeks to monitor for any evidence of clot progression into the thigh. If this does not occur, the clot may dissolve on its own and the risks associated with the use of blood thinners can be avoided.

Patients with blood clots that involve only the small veins directly beneath the skin, a condition called *superficial thrombophlebitis*, are treated with moist heat and anti-inflammatory medications such as ibuprofen. This condition occurs most commonly after trauma to a vein, such as from an intravenous catheter or a mechanical injury (a blow or scraping injury to the skin over the vein). These clots do not break off and travel to other places; therefore, the use of blood thinners is not warranted.

Complications

A blood clot in a deep vein can damage the valves in that vein, leading to increased pressure in them as blood attempts to return to the heart. In the long term, this pressure will distend the veins and can result in dilated superficial veins (*varicose veins*), fluid retention in the legs, discoloration, and skin breakdown. This is called the *post-phlebitic syndrome*.

A blood clot in a deep vein can also break off and travel to the heart and lungs. This is called a *pulmonary embolism*. If the blood clot is large enough, it can create life-threatening complications. Patients with a pulmonary embolism may experience very subtle or very obvious symptoms including shortness of breath, chest pain, and fast heartbeat or cardiac arrhythmias (see *Palpitations and Atrial Fibrillation* on page 158). Patients with massive pulmonary emboli may experience loss of consciousness, cardiac arrest, or shock.

Pulmonary emboli are confirmed by findings on exam, chest x-ray, and blood gases along with specialized testing including scans to compare air and blood flow in regions of the lung. Most pulmonary emboli are treated with support and the same therapy as deep venous thrombosis. Patients who continue to have emboli despite the use of blood thinners, or who cannot take blood thinners because of other medical problems, may have a metallic filter (an "umbrella") placed in the large central vein in the abdomen (the vena cava) to prevent further clots from traveling up the vena cava and reaching the heart.

Treatment for a pulmonary embolism varies depending on the location and severity of the embolism. Patients with life-threatening pulmonary emboli may be treated with thrombolytic therapy in an attempt to dissolve the clot, which, in early studies of its use in intensive care units, has shown a reduction in the death rate from 30 percent to 8 percent. Patients with smaller pulmonary emboli simply need supportive care and blood thinners.

Cardiac Diagnostic Procedures

The most useful cardiac diagnostic procedures occur when your physician's skilled ears and brain are listening to you describe your symptoms. This time-tested technique should not be lost in the ever-advancing technology of modern cardiology.

The Stethoscope

As blood flows through the heart, various noises are created. These occur from the turbulent blood flow through different chambers and vessels, as well as the sounds of blood flowing through valves and the noise made by valves themselves as they open and close. The trained listener can recognize normal and abnormal heart sounds and correlate them with probable changes in the structure or function of the heart.

The Electrocardiogram (EKG)

When the heart muscle contracts, chemical changes in the muscle generate an electrical impulse. The electrocardiogram (EKG) measures these waves of electrical impulses on the surface of the chest. This reading is similar among most individuals. When the heart muscle is injured, diseased, or damaged, the electrical impulses that are generated change. This creates deflections in the resulting electrical field on the chest and causes characteristic changes in the pattern seen on the EKG. The trained observer can recognize a normal heart, a diseased conduction system, a heart undergoing damage (heart attack), or a heart that has already been damaged by the precise patterns seen on the surface EKG.

The Treadmill Stress Test

In the treadmill stress test, a surface EKG recording is made continuously before, during, and after a set exercise program. This continuous recording tracks the heart rate response to exercise, any problems in heart rhythm, and any changes in the electrical fields that occur during exercise. How long it takes for the heart to speed up to certain levels, what level of exercise is tolerated, and what symptoms develop during exercise provide a measure of the physical condition of the test subject. The blood pressure response to exercise is also measured and provides clues to the health of the heart. If an area of heart muscle is being fed by a coronary artery with a significant blockage (70 percent or greater), that area may not receive adequate blood flow during exercise to meet its energy needs. This creates an injury current, which shows up as characteristic deflections in the electrical field measured by the surface EKG.

Some patients, particularly women and patients with conduction abnormalities on their EKGs, have changes in their EKGs during exercise that cannot be interpreted. In these patients, additional measurements during the stress test can help increase its usefulness.

A stress echocardiogram compares ultrasound images of the heart immediately before and after exercise. This looks for the presence or absence of expected changes in heart muscle motion with exercise (with exercise, healthy heart muscle will increase the speed and vigor of its contractions) and detects abnormalities in heart muscle or valvular function that occur under the stress of exercise. (See *The Echocardiogram* on page 180 for more information about this test.)

A nuclear medicine stress test uses one of several chemicals during the exercise test, and then looks at special x-ray results that show how that chemical is distributed through the heart muscle during exercise. For example, thallium is a radioactive chemical taken up by healthy heart cells. At peak exercise, an injection of thallium is given. The heart is then x-rayed to see how the thallium is distributed through the heart. Bright spots on the imaging screen indicate that healthy muscle cells are taking up the thallium and are therefore receiving the blood flow they need during exercise, while the cells receiving inadequate flow will not take up the thallium and appear darker on the scan. A few hours later, another x-ray is taken to see whether any dark areas from the previous scan are brighter, indicating that some heart muscle cells receive inadequate flow during exercise but are still alive and take up the thallium when given enough time to do so. Dark areas that remain dark on the second scan indicate dead muscle areas.

Some patients are unable to participate in the treadmill test because of underlying lung disease or orthopedic problems. These patients can be given chemicals to mimic the effects of exercise on the heart and the stress test can proceed as above.

The Echocardiogram

This noninvasive (that is, no needles or tubes) test uses ultrasound to look at the size of the heart's chambers, the motion of heart muscle, and the structure and function of heart valves. Doppler techniques measure the speed of blood flow across valves, which can be used to calculate their function.

The Cardiac Catheterization

The cardiac catheterization is a common procedure that is performed in a hospital to investigate symptoms or test results that suggest heart disease, to diagnose heart problems, and to guide therapy.

In this procedure, under local anesthesia, an incision is made over a large artery in the groin or arm. A long, flexible tube called a catheter is inserted into the blood vessel and steered upstream under x-ray guidance to the heart. Once in place, this catheter can be used to measure pressures in the heart and major blood vessels and to inject x-ray fluid to investigate the structure of the heart and coronary arteries. The test checks for clogged arteries, the pumping ability of the heart, the function of heart valves, and overall heart structure.

A film of the x-ray images obtained during this procedure is made and later reviewed by a team of cardiologists and cardiovascular surgeons. The details of anatomy, heart muscle movement, and blood flow are used to pinpoint problems and to guide the selection of appropriate therapy.

Angioplasty uses the catheter to open clogged arteries by expanding a balloon several times within an area of plaque and crushing it against the side of the vessel wall. When this heals, the artery should remain open for blood flow. A small percentage of the time, attempts to perform an angioplasty will result in damage to the blood vessel. Occasionally, this damage will require immediate open heart surgery to repair it and save the heart muscle supplied by that artery. For this reason, angioplasties can't always be done at the time of the initial diagnostic cardiac catheterization. Arrangements must be made to have a surgical team immediately available to assist with any complications that may arise.

Atherectomy employs a roto-router type device that chews up and removes plaque. Some procedures utilize a laser to assist in this process.

Stents are metal spring-like devices that are placed in arteries after the above procedures to help hold them open.

In general, a cardiac catheterization is a serious procedure but is relatively safe in skilled hands. The major risks of the procedure include bleeding or clotting, rupture of the heart muscle or a blood vessel, allergic reaction to x-ray fluids, heart attack, stroke, and death. If your doctor recommends a cardiac catheterization, he or she feels that the possible risks of your heart disease and the benefits of the information gained or therapy provided to you during the procedure outweigh the theoretical risks.

It is hoped that one day noninvasive techniques, such as MRA (magnetic resonance angiography), will replace the diagnostic portions of the cardiac catheterization.

The Electrophysiology Study (EPS)

An electrophysiology study (EPS) is performed on patients to investigate abnormal rhythm disturbances (arrhythmias) in the heart. This procedure is performed similarly to a cardiac catheterization, except that the catheters placed in the heart are special catheters to stimulate and record electrical activity. A map of how electrical activity flows through the heart is created, and attempts are made to reproduce the patient's arrhythmia while they are in the lab. If this can be accomplished, medications can be tried in the lab to prevent the arrhythmia, or additional catheters can be used to electrically zap the conducting system so that the arrhythmia can no longer occur. This procedure carries the same risks as a cardiac catheterization.

CT Scans and Heart Disease

Calcium is related to the presence of atherosclerosis. Rapid Computerized Tomography scan (CT scan) techniques are able to detect the presence of calcium in coronary blood vessels, leading the media and various medical professionals to conclude and publicize that these tests are useful in screening for heart disease. Unfortunately, this test produces inconsistent results and therefore does not yet appear to be a clinically useful technique.

In a study of 632 patients who received rapid CT scans and then were followed over 32 months, 4 percent of these patients experienced a heart attack or died during the study period. When the calcium scores obtained on the original CT scans for these patients were reviewed, the vast majority of these patients had only mild or moderate elevations in their calcium scores. This is consistent with the pathophysiology of heart attacks discussed at the beginning of this chapter—heart attacks occur when a soft, partially obstructing plaque ruptures, not when an old calcified plaque finally chokes off the blood flow. I think that the proponents of rapid CT scans for the detection of heart disease are looking for the wrong thing. A second study in which subjects obtained two CT scans from the same scanner, on different days, produced measurements that varied considerably.

Until the technique is better refined, it should be limited to research settings. Currently, CT scanning to screen for heart disease is not covered by insurance and is springing up as a lucrative cash-only business in a variety of settings. Be wary.

Coronary Artery Bypass Surgery

Coronary artery bypass surgery is performed in patients where angioplasty or atherectomy cannot be performed, such as when the area of blockage is too long, is unapproachable for the catheter, or occurs at a branch of a vessel where correcting the blockage would cause a second blockage elsewhere. Other situations in which bypass surgery might be performed instead of other techniques include blockage of the left main artery, blockage of all three vessels with weak heart function, or blockage of two vessels—one of which is the left anterior descending artery supplying the main pumping section of the heart—with diabetes or weak heart function. All of these examples are conditions where a failed attempt to perform angioplasty or atherectomy could be lethal for the patient, without adequate time to make it from the catheterization lab to the surgical suite to fix the problem.

The bypass surgery is performed under general anesthesia. In the standard technique the breastbone is separated, the ribs are spread, and blood is rerouted from the heart through a heart-lung machine. Heart contractions are stopped, the blocked vessels are bypassed with arteries or veins taken from elsewhere in the body, blood is returned from the heart-lung machine, and the heart is restarted. The chest wall is then closed. Most patients are hospitalized after surgery for five to seven days and take three months to return to full activities. During bypass surgery, 1 to 3 percent of patients die; 15 percent experience serious complications, including heart attack, stroke, infection, and kidney problems.

A newer technique for bypass surgery in selected patients involves what is known as a "mini-thoracotomy," where a small opening is made between the ribs through which the heart is repaired. This technique requires a skilled surgical team and can only be used in patients whose blockages are in locations that can be accessed by the instruments used in the technique. Other techniques include performing bypass of limited areas without ever stopping the heart or using the heart–lung bypass machine. This may be required when the aorta is too diseased to clamp it off in order to hook up the heart–lung bypass.

Preventing Heart Disease

So far, we have talked about heart diseases, their symptoms, and their treatment. More important than their treatment, though, is their prevention. Preventing heart disease involves identifying the risk factors associated with the development of heart disease and modifying or eliminating them. Risk factors include:

- **Cholesterol.** Patients should have fasting lipid profiles at least every five years, beginning by age 18. Patients with existing heart disease should be aggressively treated for cholesterol disorders, including drug therapy.
- **Tobacco.** Tobacco smoking narrows and injures arteries, reduces the amount of oxygen in the bloodstream, chemically stimulates the process of blood clotting, and lowers HDL cholesterol. Smoking only one to four cigarettes a day doubles the risk of heart disease. Prevention of smoking in adolescents and young adults, as well as cessation of smoking in all adults, should be a high-priority national health goal. See *Chapter 7: Smoking* for more information.
- **Diabetes.** Patients with diabetes face the same future risk of heart attack as heart patients who have already had one. Most diabetics have diabetes at least ten years before the disease is discovered. Diabetes needs to be detected earlier; aggressive blood sugar control in diabetics may help reduce the development of blood vessel diseases. Other risk factors in diabetics, such as high cholesterol, should be treated as aggressively as possible. See *Diabetes Mellitus* on page 141 for more information.
- **Hypertension.** Elevated blood pressure is a major risk factor for heart disease. Not only are people with severely high blood pressure at risk; two-thirds of patients who have experienced heart attacks have only mild or high normal blood

pressure readings. Control of blood pressure in studies has shown a 40 percent reduction in the risk of stroke and a 20 percent reduction in the risk of heart attack.

- **Family history.** Patients whose immediate family members have heart disease are at a high risk of developing this disease themselves. Other risk factors for heart disease should be treated aggressively in these patients, and they should be appropriately monitored for the development of heart problems.

- **Exercise habits.** Several studies of men and women who exercise regularly over many years show that this relates to a reduced risk for cardiovascular disease and death. Aerobic exercise and strength training reduce blood pressure, raise HDL cholesterol, improve circulation to the heart, induce chemical changes that inhibit clot formation, and increase the activity of the parasympathetic nervous system on the heart, which reduces the risk for some heart rhythm disturbances. See *Chapter 1: Physical Fitness* for more information about beginning an exercise program.

- **Blood clotting tendencies.** Aspirin therapy reduces the ability of platelets to form blood clots, theoretically decreasing the risk of clot formation on irritated cholesterol plaques in arteries. In addition, aspirin has anti-inflammatory properties, which may help reduce the amount of inflammation in atheromatous plaques and make them less likely to rupture. Long-term studies of men (Physicians Health Study) and women (Israeli BIP trial) show a reduction in heart-related events in patients who regularly take aspirin. I advise a dose of 81 milligrams daily in patients who are able to tolerate aspirin therapy.

- **Prevention of oxidation.** The role of antioxidant supplements in the prevention or treatment of heart disease is controversial. A 1993 nurses and physicians health study showed a 40 percent reduction in risk for heart disease in patients who took high levels of vitamin E. Some well-designed studies since that time have failed to reproduce this benefit. Recent studies suggest that supplemental vitamin E may diminish the beneficial HDL raising effects of some cholesterol medications. I advise my patients to consume a diet high in antioxidants, but I no longer advise pills as a reliable source of them.

- **High homocysteine levels.** *Homocysteine* is an amino acid (protein building block) produced in the body. High levels of homocysteine oxidize LDL cholesterol and increase blood clotting. A rare inherited disease with extremely high homocysteine levels is associated with a high risk for cardiovascular disease at a very early age. Normal homocysteine levels are from 5 to 15, with optimal levels below 10. Consuming folate (400 micrograms), Vitamin B_6 (50 milligrams), and Vitamin B_{12} (50 micrograms) daily reduces the levels of homocysteine. Most individuals can meet these needs by eating cereal and grains (since the FDA requires supplements in these products) and leafy green vegetables. Extra vitamin B_{12} may be needed after age 50 since the body becomes less efficient in absorbing it with age. Patients with premature cardiovascular disease should have their homocysteine levels evaluated. I fudge on the science a bit, and ask all of my patients with risk factors for heart disease to take a B-complex multivitamin with folate.

- **Estrogen.** Estrogen affects lipids, coagulation, platelets, and the function of blood vessel lining. When taken in pill form, it decreases LDL and increases HDL. Over 20 studies of estrogen replacement therapy after menopause suggest an average 40 percent reduction in the relative risk of heart disease for those women who took it. Thus, estrogen has been traditionally advised as a means to reduce the risk for heart disease for postmenopausal women. The data to support this was all from observational studies, in which large populations of women were surveyed and their habits and traits were examined in comparison to the type of medical problems that they experienced. More recent studies, with a more precise scientific design, have created significant confusion. The Heart and Estrogen/Progestin Replacement Study (HERS) followed 2,700 women with known heart disease; in this study, estrogen was given to half of the women and a placebo pill was given to the other half. After 4.1 years of follow-up, no overall benefit was seen from estrogen use. In the first year of the HERS trial, a 50 percent increase in cardiovascular events was noted in the group taking estrogens. The second and third years of the study showed no difference in the two groups. Toward the end of the study, the opposite trend was seen—cardiovascular events that would appear to have reached statistical significance if the study had been continued were reduced. Estrogen increases blood clotting but also leads to an improvement in the lipid profile. It is felt that the early years of the study showed the effect of blood clotting in women with known heart disease, and that the later years of the study were beginning to show the benefits of estrogen on lipids and other issues. Future studies hope to pinpoint which women are more likely to benefit from estrogen replacement therapy. For now, much is left to judgment and personal preference. See *Chapter 26: Women's Health* for more information about estrogen therapy.
- **Elevated C-reactive protein.** High sensitivity C-reactive protein is a marker for inflammation, and recent studies show that high C-reactive protein levels correlate with the risk of cardiovascular disease. The use of this test is an evolving issue; it is unknown whether therapies given in an attempt to improve test results have any benefit on cardiovascular disease.
- **Chlamydia.** Chlamydia is an infectious agent that is frequently found in atheromatous plaques. It is uncertain whether these organisms play a role in the development or maturation of atheromatous plaques or whether they are innocent bystanders in this disease. Further studies about the role of these organisms and any response to antibiotic therapy are ongoing.
- **Stress.** Stress and hostility appear to play a role in the development of heart disease. Emotional stress speeds up the heart rate, elevates blood pressure, stimulates chemicals that form clots and inhibits their breakdown, narrows coronary arteries, and alters heart rhythms. In addition to these physiological changes, hostile individuals alienate others and thus have a lack of social support and more unhealthy habits. In the Multiple Risk Factor Intervention Trial (MRFIT) study of risk factors in heart disease, hostile people were 50 percent more likely to develop coronary disease or have a heart attack. In a study of men at Harvard, the angriest/grumpicst men experienced three times the risk for heart attack than the mellowest.

CHAPTER 22

The Respiratory System

The main function of the lungs is to obtain oxygen for the body and eliminate waste gases (carbon dioxide). Air flows from the mouth and nose to the windpipe, or *trachea*. The trachea divides into branches called *bronchi*, which lead to the right and left lung. These airways then divide again and again until the tiniest of airways called the *terminal bronchioles* are reached, which are capped with several tiny air

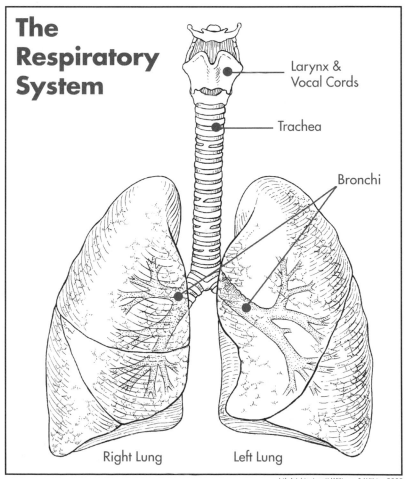

The Respiratory System

Larynx & Vocal Cords

Trachea

Bronchi

Right Lung   Left Lung

LifeArt, Lippincott Williams & Wilkins 2002

sacs called *alveoli*. These end structures look like very small bunches of grapes. All the airways except the tiniest ones are lined with a blood vessel-rich membrane that contains glands, smooth muscle fibers, and tiny hairs called *cilia*. The glands secrete a thin layer of mucus which helps keep the airways moist and acts as flypaper in catching dust and other particles. The cilia beat rhythmically together so that this layer of mucus is slowly swept up the airways and out the trachea, constantly cleansing the lungs, along a passageway called the *mucociliary elevator*. Paralleling these divisions of the airways are divisions of blood vessels. *Pulmonary arteries* take used oxygen-poor blood from the right side of the heart to the lungs; *pulmonary veins* return blood freshly supplied with oxygen from the lungs to the left side of the heart, where it is pumped to the rest of the body.

The thin-walled alveoli form a membrane between the air in the lungs and the blood in the blood vessels. Only two cells thick, this membrane allows gases to easily diffuse across it to supply the blood with oxygen and relieve it of carbon dioxide. If the surface area of the alveoli were spread out flat, the size of the membrane would approach that of a football field.

Air is moved into the lungs primarily by the diaphragm, a dome-shaped muscle at the base of the lungs that separates the chest cavity from the abdomen. When the diaphragm contracts, it pulls down and creates a negative pressure inside the chest cavity, causing air to flow into the lungs. When the diaphragm relaxes, the chest wall and lungs recoil, exerting pressure and pushing the air out. When the body is breathing hard, other muscles are involved.

Examining Lung Function

Your physician can use several different means to assess the function of your lungs, including:

- **Asking you directly.** Speaking with you about the symptoms and signs you may have noticed provides the bulk of needed information. You may be asked about your breathing, cough pattern, and sputum production. Are you short of breath at rest? What level of physical activity can you perform before getting winded? Does position influence your breathing? Do you feel smothered when you lie down? Does sitting up help? Do you ever wheeze (hear high-pitched musical noises while breathing, indicating that your airway is narrowed)? Your tobacco smoke and environmental toxin exposure are crucially important, as well as allergies or other upper respiratory conditions that might affect your breathing.

- **Examination.** Examining the lungs includes observing the chest cage shape and movement. Do the ribs expand normally? Does the chest cage have normal dimensions? Are extra muscles in the neck and abdomen being used because of labored breathing? Does the body exhibit other signs of an inadequate oxygen supply? Listening to the lungs during breathing checks for normal air movement and detects areas where extra sounds are present (caused by excessive mucus, inflammation, or narrowing of the airways), or where expected sounds are absent (such as the absence of adequate air flow caused by fluid, obstruction, or infected lung tissue).

- **Chest x-rays.** X-rays of the chest provide information about the physical state of the lungs. X-rays are partially blocked by solid tissue, such as bones, the heart, blood-filled vessels, or collections of fluid. These areas show up as white on an x-ray film. X-rays pass through air, such as in the lungs, and these areas appear darker on the film. Diseases such as pneumonia cause mucus and other debris to collect in the lung tissue, creating a whiter area on the film. Likewise, tumors or collections of fluid show up as white areas. An experienced x-ray reader knows what a normal x-ray should look like; changes in the expected pattern provide clues to the disease process in the lungs. Other methods of looking at lung structure include CT scans—a three-dimensional form of x-ray—and bronchoscopy, in which a pulmonary physician uses a lighted fiber-optic scope in a sedated patient to directly examine the airways for disease.

- **Pulmonary function tests.** Pulmonary function tests look at the volumes of air in the lung, the speed at which air can move through the airway during breathing, and the efficiency of the lung at exchanging gases. The *arterial blood gas* test uses a sample of blood drawn from an artery to measure lung function by seeing how much oxygen and carbon dioxide exists in blood that has recently passed through the lung. *Spirometry* involves breathing forcefully into a device that measures airflow and comparing the airflow to known normal rates. Diseases that inflame and narrow the airways (like asthma) reduce maximum airflow rates. *Lung volume measurements* examine the total amount of air contained in the lungs, as well as the amount of air that can be moved out of the lungs with effort. In diseases like emphysema, the lungs may contain more than the normal amount of air; however, because the lung tissue is diseased, it cannot move all of the air effectively and "air trapping" occurs, resulting in a lesser amount of usable air exchange with each breath.

This chapter will discuss common ways that lung structure and function are challenged: cough, infection (bronchitis and pneumonia), inflammation (asthma), breakdown in structure (chronic obstructive pulmonary disease and emphysema), and abnormalities in the control of airflow (sleep apnea).

Cough

Cough is one of the body's important defense mechanisms. Several times a day, the lungs will forcefully contract, producing airflow rates as high as 500 miles per hour. This serves to expel irritants, such as dust or heavy secretions, from the airway. Although coughing is normal, the frequency of coughing can increase and become bothersome, for several reasons:

- **The common cold.** Excessive secretions that drip into the airway trigger cough.
- **Allergies.** Allergic reactions may produce inflammation of the airways and excessive secretions.

- **Respiratory tract infections**. Infections of the respiratory tract, including influenza, bronchitis, and pneumonia, also cause excessive cough.
- **Smoking.** Tobacco smoke damages the mucociliary elevator resulting in thickened and stagnant secretions, depositing irritating debris in the lungs.
- **Drug side effects.** ACE inhibitors, used for the treatment of hypertension and heart disease, or drugs that dry secretions, can cause persistent coughing.
- **Heart causes.** Congestive heart failure causes fluid build-up in the lungs, triggering a cough that increases with exertion or gets worse when lying down.
- **Gastroesophageal reflux.** Backwash of stomach acid into the esophagus can trigger a neurological reflex that causes coughing.

Cough therapies include expectorants, which help thin the mucus so that it is more easily expelled with each cough, and cough suppressants (both over-the-counter and prescription drugs including codeine derivatives) and lozenges and other topical anesthetics, which suppress the cough reflex. While these therapies are somewhat beneficial, it is important to treat the cause of the cough, not just cover it up.

Bronchitis

Bronchitis is an infection of the large- and medium-sized airways. Acute infectious bronchitis in patients without underlying lung disease is almost always caused by a virus. These infections are highly contagious, being easily passed from person to person in the droplets of respiratory secretions produced by a sneeze or cough. Bronchitis is characterized by a sudden illness with a cough that usually produces only scanty amounts of phlegm. Other symptoms include nasal discharge, sore throat, a burning sensation in the windpipe, malaise, and low-grade fevers or chills. The symptoms are worse in the first few days but should significantly improve or resolve, without treatment, within a week.

If symptoms worsen after the first five days, a secondary bacterial infection may have occurred. This means that some bacteria have taken advantage of the chaos of inflammation and secretions in the lung caused by the virus, causing a second infection in the same area. This second infection may require the use of antibiotics. Bacterial bronchitis can also follow excessive tobacco use, thickening of respiratory secretions (from dehydration, medication side effects, or underlying lung disease), excessive alcohol intake, or general anesthesia. Symptoms include a more frequent and severe cough, production of pus-filled phlegm, chest congestion and discomfort, wheezing, and shortness of breath.

Because acute bronchitis spreads quickly through workplaces, schools, and communities, it is a frequent cause for office visits in primary care. It is best treated with time and therapy for symptoms, including rest and adequate fluid intake to avoid dehydration and keep secretions thin, acetaminophen or ibuprofen to help with fever and discomfort, and medications to assist with coughing.

Why not just treat everyone with antibiotics? Antibiotics treat bacterial infections, not viral infections. Since acute infectious bronchitis is caused by a virus, antibiotics will not be effective and may even do more harm than good (see *Chapter 5: Infections and*

Antibiotics for more information). However, they can be prescribed if the acute bronchitis develops into the secondary bacterial infection we mentioned earlier.

Patients with underlying lung disease, such as asthma or emphysema, are at higher risk from upper respiratory infections since their lungs don't work as well to clear them and because their lung function isn't strong enough to make up for the stress of infection. They are typically treated more aggressively for bronchitis and similar infections, including the earlier use of antibiotic therapy.

Pneumonia

Pneumonia is an infection of the lungs, including the small airways and alveoli. It is a serious disease. One out of eight people who are hospitalized with pneumonia dies, despite aggressive therapy. While clinical studies have identified the most common bacterial types of pneumonia, the exact cause of an individual pneumonia is rarely known; in fact, fewer than 40 percent of the cultures taken from hospitalized patients—and even fewer cultures of patients who are evaluated and treated in a doctor's office—reveal the identity of the specific organism responsible for the infection. Patients are promptly treated with drugs to cover the most likely causes based on the characteristics of the infection and the pattern of disease present in the community.

Symptoms

Symptoms of pneumonia include fever and chills, an increase in respiratory rate, cough, sputum production that may be bloody and full of pus, shortness of breath, malaise and fatigue, and chest pain. If the pneumonia irritates the lining of the lung, a particular pattern of sharp, localized, and severe chest pain called *pleurisy* is produced with each breath that is often worsened or improved by certain positions. Some types of pneumonia are associated with more widespread symptoms: headache, muscle aches, confusion, nausea, or rashes. Pneumonias are much more serious in elderly patients in that they are associated with fewer symptoms and an elderly patient can become quite ill before a problem is obvious.

Physicians diagnose pneumonia by symptoms, findings on physical examination (extra noises in the chest or the lack of usual sounds, dullness to tapping on the chest wall), and x-ray abnormalities. Patients with upper respiratory infections, such as bronchitis, that seem to worsen after the first four or five days should be reexamined for this complication.

Treatment

Pneumonia requires a complete course of antibiotics and follow-up assessment by your physician to ensure that the infection is responding and eventually resolves with treatment. While the infection may respond to 10 to 14 days of antibiotics, it is often several weeks until patients feel normal. Activities and responsibilities during this recovery time should be adjusted to allow for more rapid and complete recovery.

Some patients require hospitalization for treatment of their pneumonia, although with the latest generations of oral antibiotics this is becoming less common. Guidelines for consideration of hospitalization include patients older than 60, those with coexisting illness (chronic obstructive pulmonary disease, diabetes, renal failure, congestive heart failure, chronic alcohol abuse, previous loss of spleen), and those with signs of significant pneumonia, such as a respiratory rate greater than 30, low blood pressure, fever greater than 101 degrees Fahrenheit, or confusion.

Asthma

Asthma is a chronic, inflammatory disease of the small airways (bronchioles). White blood cells called *eosinophils* and numerous other cells and chemicals in the immune system are involved in the inflammatory reactions of asthma. This disease is characterized by swelling of the lining of these small airways, mucus production, and spasm of the smooth muscle in the airway wall that further narrows the airway. Asthma affects 14 million Americans, one-third of whom are children. Eighty percent of patients with asthma develop it in childhood before age ten.

Symptoms

Symptoms of asthma include recurrent wheezing, shortness of breath, a feeling of tightness in the chest, or a cough that lasts for more than a week. Physicians diagnose it by reviewing symptoms and measuring episodic changes in lung function. If these changes in lung function are reversible and other causes are excluded, asthma is diagnosed.

This chronic inflammation of the airways causes them to narrow as the muscles around them spasm and contract. It also makes the airways excessively sensitive to substances in the air. In these swollen, spasmodic airways, plugs of mucus can trap air within the lungs and interfere with the expulsion of used air and the intake of fresh air.

The cause of asthma is unknown, although the disease tends to be inherited. Children whose father, mother, or sibling has asthma are three times more likely to develop asthma. Environment also plays a role. When cotton fabrics were introduced to an isolated population in New Guinea, a 50-fold increase in the incidence of asthma was seen. This was felt to be related to creating favorable indoor conditions for dust mites.

Triggers of an asthma response include those related to allergy (for example, molds, animal dander, dust mites, cockroach debris, food additives and medications) and others not related to allergy (for example, chemical fumes, perfumes, smoke, infections, exercise, cold air and gastroesophageal reflux). Because these triggers can often be tracked through a person's history, keeping a diary of asthma activity can help identify them. Asthma that worsens in certain seasons may be associated with other allergy symptoms from pollens and molds; allergy testing and shots may help. Asthma flaring after making the bed or vacuuming may relate to dust mites. Asthma responses around pets may relate to animal dander; responses in barns, basements, or bathrooms may relate to mold. Chronic sinus infections are common causes of respiratory problems in asthmatics; the sinus symptoms themselves may be very subtle and not noticed in the midst of all the asthma activity.

Avoiding asthma triggers is crucial. Dust mites are microscopic creatures in all homes; they live off of shed human skin and, due to changes in heat and humidity, are more prevalent from July to December. Dust mite exposure can be minimized by changes in the home environment. For example, remove bedroom carpets and damp mop the floor weekly. Minimize the use of heavy drapes and fabric-covered furniture. Launder curtains every other month. Cover bedding and pillows in special allergy-reducing fabrics or vinyl. Use a dehumidifier to lower indoor humidity. Dust mites live in blankets and stuffed animals; to kill them in these items, place the items in the freezer overnight or wash them in 130-degree water weekly. In research studies where these changes were made, the severity of asthma significantly improved.

Cat dander is problematic for allergy and asthma sufferers. The particle size of cat dander is so small and light that it doesn't fall out of the air from gravity, but remains suspended. It coats clothing and is easily transported. Air quality studies in classrooms show a higher cat dander concentration in the air of schoolrooms that contain children with cats at home.

Nighttime asthma is particularly a problem and—because more than 65 percent of asthma deaths occur at night—should be treated aggressively. A major change in lung mechanics occurs when you lie down. Gravity no longer assists the efforts of the diaphragm, which results in shallower breath and lower lung volumes. Lower lung volumes lead to smaller airways and an increased resistance to airflow. In a body, extra fluid exists between the cells. During the day when a person is upright, gravity gradually causes this extra fluid to trickle down to the legs. At night while supine, gravity is no longer pulling free fluid down to the legs and more fluid collects in the lungs. Studies in asthmatics show that their airways become more inflamed and the muscles in the airways become more "twitchy" or reactive at night. In addition, a variety of nocturnal changes occur in the nerves and hormones that regulate lung function. This is associated with an increase in the numbers of eosinophils in the lining of the airway in the early morning hours.

Management

At our present state of knowledge, asthma cannot be cured. The current goal is to manage the asthmatic's condition to minimize the effects of the disease and its complications. The following are tips for managing asthma:

Know how your asthma is doing—use a peak flow meter.

Several studies show that patients and physicians alike cannot accurately assess the severity of asthma without obtaining objective measurements of airflow. In asthmatic patients whose pulmonary function measurements showed dangerous levels of asthma activity, 61 percent felt that their asthma was doing "ok." It is felt that chronic asthma creates an altered sense of shortness of breath, and patients can't tell when they are in trouble until very late.

Peak flow devices are simple airflow measuring devices that are used as indicators of airway activity in asthmatics. All asthmatics should have one and use it regularly. Since

---

Using a Peak Flow Meter

Here's how to use a peak flow meter:

1. Empty your mouth.
2. Set the peak flow meter back to zero.
3. Stand up straight and take a deep breath.
4. Close your lips around the mouthpiece. Don't block the hole with your tongue.
5. Blow as fast and as hard as you can.
6. Record the best score out of three trials.

---

peak flow readings vary by time of day, baseline readings should be taken the same time every day.

Peak flow results are compared to your best results measured when asthma was inactive, using the following guide:

This zone...	Indicates...
Green	80 to 100 percent of predicted air flow. This is where you should be every day.
Yellow	50 to 80 percent of predicted. Symptoms may include cough, wheezing, shortness of breath, and chest tightness. Sleep or certain activities may be difficult.
Red	Less than 50 percent of predicted. Symptoms may include cough, extreme shortness of breath, difficulty talking or during physical exertion. Wheezing may actually lessen because there is not enough air moving to make noise.

Patients with asthma and their physicians prearrange "action plans," which provide written instructions on what to do with regular and emergency medications and guidelines for when to seek medical help based on the peak flow reading results. Peak flow meters should be regarded as early warning devices—thermometers for asthmatic activity.

Seek aggressive asthma therapy, early.

Seek aggressive asthma therapy early in the course of the disease. Asthma creates permanent changes in the architecture of the lungs, a condition referred to as "airway remodeling." Airway remodeling includes lung tissue scarring, increased numbers of cells in lung tissue, extra fluid in the airway lining, increased smooth muscle mass, and disruption of the structural support of the lung. These changes are felt to occur early in the course of the disease and are permanent. Early, aggressive intervention in asthma appears to prevent or minimize these changes. This is not a disease to ignore and hope that it will go away.

Routinely use controller medication.

Routinely use controller medications—medications that are used regularly to keep asthma under control—such as:

- **Inhaled anti-inflammatories (corticosteroids, cromolyn, and nedocromil sodium).** These prevent airway inflammation, reduce inflammation already present, and make the airways less sensitive to irritants. They must be taken for four to six weeks before maximum benefits are seen.
- **Leukotriene modifiers (montelukast, zafirlukast).** These are pills that block the effects of potent messengers of inflammation, the leukotrienes, preventing inflammation and making the airways less sensitive to irritants.
- **Long-acting bronchodilators (salmeterol and oral forms of albuterol).** These drugs relax the muscles around the airways and reverse and prevent airway narrowing.
- **Oral corticosteroids (prednisone).** These drugs reverse and prevent airway inflammation and reduce mucus in the lung. Unfortunately, potential steroid side effects (such as diabetes, elevated blood pressure, osteoporosis, fluid retention, cataracts, and weakening of the immune system) on the rest of the body limit their use to those with severe asthmatic activity.
- **Combination products.** A currently available product mixes the anti-inflammatory properties of corticosteroids with the long-acting bronchodilating effects of salmeterol to achieve a result superior to either approach alone. This product is administered in a simple-to-use, breath-activated device.

Use reliever medications appropriately.

Reliever medications are medications such as short-acting *beta-agonist inhalers* (albuterol). These drugs relax the muscles around the airways, reducing spasm and opening the airway. They take effect in about five minutes and often last for three to four hours. Used to reverse symptoms that have developed, these drugs are also administered before exercise to prevent anticipated attacks, such as in patients with exercise-induced asthma. A measure of how well controlled a patient's asthma is can be obtained by how infrequently he or she needs the reliever medications. A well-controlled asthmatic should use only one or two cans of albuterol a year.

Patients with more severe asthma do better with multiple medications. Although all of the medications mentioned have risks and side effects that should be discussed with your doctor, the biggest risk by far lies in inadequately treated asthma.

The device in which many asthma medications are delivered is called a *metered dose inhaler* (MDI). Asthma patients should be trained and observed in the proper use of MDIs to make sure they are using them correctly and getting the full benefit of their medications. A spacer is a special chamber attached to the MDI that increases the amount of medication that actually gets to the lung, rather than being sprayed on the mouth and tongue and swallowed. I prefer that all of my patients use spacers whenever possible.

Using a Metered Dose Inhaler

Here's how to use a metered dose inhaler:

1. Remove the cap and shake the inhaler. Check that the opening is free of debris.
2. Attach the spacer.
3. Stand up or sit up straight, tilting the head back slightly.
4. Breathe out as much as comfortable.
5. Hold the canister upright like a pipe, seal lips around the spacer opening (if you are not using a spacer, aim the inhaler from one to two inches to a widely opened mouth).
6. Activate the canister at the beginning—or just before—a breath (if you are not using a spacer, activate at the start of a breath).
7. Continue a slow, deep breath until your lungs are completely full.
8. Hold your breath for 5 to 10 seconds.
9. Exhale slowly.
10. Take one puff at a time and wait 20 seconds or more before the next puff.

Sound complicated? It is. Most patients do not use their MDIs correctly. Have your doctor watch you use your inhaler to ensure that your technique is adequate. Fortunately, technological advances in the delivery of medication to the lungs may help with this problem. Some delivery devices are now activated by the patient's own effort to breathe in, negating the need to try to coordinate activation of the device with your breathing.

Chronic Obstructive Pulmonary Disease

Chronic obstructive pulmonary disease (COPD) is a combination of two diseases: chronic bronchitis and emphysema. Chronic bronchitis is defined by the signs and symptoms that a patient has; it means cough and sputum production for at least three consecutive months, for more than two consecutive years. Emphysema is defined by the physical changes that occur in the lung; it means that the alveoli at the end of the terminal bronchioles have distended and the fine membranes separating them have broken down so that the air sacs are larger (like several small soap bubbles combining to perform bigger bubbles). Chronic bronchitis and emphysema frequently coexist in the same lung. They are difficult diagnoses to separate in any single patient, and are therefore lumped together and classified as COPD.

In COPD, the lining of the small airways is swollen and inflamed, and these airways contain more mucus than lung tissue. Over time, the airways begin to scar, which further narrows them. As the air sacs (alveoli) in emphysema melt together and become larger, the diffusion of oxygen and waste gases through them becomes less efficient. The gases must travel across larger amounts of empty space in the alveoli to reach the membrane where they exchange with gases in the blood. Other structural changes also occur in the lung of a patient with COPD. In the normal lung, the many small alveoli act as a framework of structural support for the small airways, holding them open. When the alveolar walls break down, the small airways are not held open as well and tend to collapse during the pressure of breathing out, trapping gas within the lung. In these areas of trapped gas, oxygen and carbon dioxide cannot be exchanged. This lack of oxygen has secondary effects on the blood flow through the lungs and can cause the blood pressure in the pulmonary circulation to rise. This ultimately can result in heart failure.

Symptoms

When the airways are small and inflamed and tend to collapse under the pressure of breathing out, the lung has difficulty moving air in and out. When the airflow rates fall to 50 percent of normal, patients become short of breath with exertion. When the airflow rates fall to less than 25 percent of normal, shortness of breath is felt even at rest. Unfortunately, once the physiology of COPD is established, it progresses with a slow and relentless loss of further lung function over time.

By far the leading cause of COPD is cigarette smoking. Other contributing causes include pollution, certain occupational exposures, infections, and inherited metabolic defects (alpha-1 antitrypsin deficiency) that affect lung structure. COPD is a leading cause of disability and death in the United States.

Treatment

Treatment of COPD involves first and foremost eliminating further exposure to and damage from tobacco. **It is never too late to stop smoking**. Those with less advanced disease stand to benefit the most, but even those with advanced disease will see an improvement in lung function and oxygenation. A graded physical exercise program can also improve lung function and the body's adaptation to it. Drugs described in (See *Asthma* on page 192 have been used in COPD, with variable benefit. It is essential to control infections in patients with COPD so that the remaining lung function isn't compromised; therefore, antibiotics are used much more freely. Supplemental oxygen can improve symptoms and quality of life.

Sleep Apnea

In *sleep apnea*, the patient stops breathing periodically during sleep. This occurs multiple times throughout the night. More than 90 percent of sleep apnea is obstructive, which means that something is blocking the passage of air into the windpipe. Rarely, sleep apnea has a central cause in which the muscles used in breathing do not get the go-ahead signal to breathe.

Obstructive sleep apnea occurs in 2 percent of women and in 4 percent of men of working age. It occurs more frequently in the elderly, obese, or patients who snore on a daily basis. The overwhelming majority of patients with moderate to severe sleep apnea have not been diagnosed with this condition, are unaware that they have it, and remain untreated.

In this condition, collapse of the upper airway relates to anatomy, size of the airway, shape, and muscle tone. Obesity with enlargement of the soft tissue of the airways is a major mechanism. In some patients, a weight gain of only 5 to 10 pounds can have a dramatic affect on airway diameter, leading to snoring and sleep apnea. In the daytime, neurological signals keep a higher resting muscle tone in the airway, keeping it open. At night, this resting tone is lost and the airway relaxes and closes.

When the airway collapses, fresh air with oxygen is no longer able to reach the lungs and waste gases with carbon dioxide are no longer expelled. The heart rate begins to slow through an effect from the parasympathetic nervous system. The blood pressure falls, and then slowly rises. Oxygen levels fall, which causes the smooth muscle in the walls of the pulmonary arteries to spasm, and carbon dioxide levels increase. After a certain severity is reached, the body declares an emergency and the brain arouses. The patient partially wakes up, often thrashes about a bit, and gasps as airflow is reestablished. The heart rate and blood pressure sharply rise, breathing restarts, and the oxygen levels recover. Once the emergency is over, arousal ends, sleep restarts, and the cycle repeats itself.

Symptoms

The symptoms of sleep apnea include excessive daytime sleepiness, loud intermittent snoring, abnormal physical activity in sleep, psychological problems such as depression, early morning headaches (10 to 20 percent), bed wetting at night, impotence, short-term memory loss, inability to pay attention, chronic fatigue, and concentration problems.

Numerous other medical problems are associated with sleep apnea:

- **Hypertension.** The blood pressure rises in cycles with the apnea at night. Greater than 50 percent of patients with sleep apnea have hypertension during the daytime. It is uncertain whether sleep apnea causes this hypertension or whether both conditions occur in the same patient due to shared risk factors. Most studies of sleep apnea treatment show that the elevation in daytime blood pressure does not improve with sleep apnea therapy.

- **Pulmonary hypertension.** Abnormal elevations in blood vessel pressures in the lungs occur in greater than 15 percent of patients with obstructive sleep apnea. This can lead to significant and irreversible dysfunction of the heart and lungs over time.

- **Cardiac arrhythmias.** Irregular heartbeats occur frequently in patients with sleep apnea. Life-threatening rhythm disturbances can occur when oxygen levels drop severely during apneas.

- **Atherosclerotic cardiovascular disease.** Patients with sleep apnea are more likely to develop atherosclerotic cardiovascular disease (cholesterol deposits and narrowing in the arteries that supply the heart muscle). Again, it is uncertain as to whether sleep apnea causes heart disease or whether both conditions simply occur in the same patient due to shared risk factors.

• **Trauma.** Patients with sleep apnea are seven times more likely to be at fault in motor vehicle accident than those without sleep apnea.

The five-year mortality of patients with obstructive sleep apnea in the moderate to severe range is the same as patients without sleep apnea who have significant heart disease.

Treatment

Medical treatment for sleep apnea is quite limited. Numerous studies show that weight loss can be a significant benefit in decreasing the number of sleep apnea events, improving oxygen saturation, decreasing the upper airway collapsibility, and increasing upper airway size. Significant improvement can be seen with loss of as little as 5 to 10 percent of body weight. Medical evaluation should look for diseases associated with sleep apnea, such as thyroid disease. Changes in posture can be tried. Some patients have less airway obstruction on their side than on their back and benefit from sewing a tennis ball in the back of their nightshirt to encourage them to sleep more often on their side. Treatment of allergies or other causes of nasal obstruction can also help open the airway.

Devices are available that increase the positive pressure in the airway and act as a pneumatic splint in holding the airway open. Continuous positive airway pressure (CPAP) devices have long been the most effective therapies available for sleep apnea. In CPAP therapy, the patient is fitted with a mask or other device that forms a good seal to the nose or nose and mouth. This mask is hooked up to an air pump that forces air down into a patient's airways, increasing the pressure in the airways and holding them open. These devices can be lifesaving, but take significant patient education in the rationale for their use, training in proper use, and management of side effects. Most motivated patients can learn to tolerate these devices and see such a drastic improvement in the quality of their sleep and daytime wakefulness that they are willing to put up with the hassles of their use. Some patients respond to simpler devices in the mouth that extend the jaw forward and help open the airway.

Surgical procedures are sometimes performed on carefully selected patients with sleep apnea whose sleep studies and physical examinations suggest that their sleep apnea is due to physical obstruction of the upper airway from anatomic features that are correctable by surgery. Operations remove some of the redundant soft tissue in the airways, open the passages, and make obstruction of the airway at night less likely. These procedures have a reasonable success rate and require the skill of an ear, nose, and throat (ENT) physician with training and experience in sleep apnea patients. In the most common procedure, the tonsils, uvula, and portion of the back sides of the throat and soft palette are removed; this procedure can cure about 50 percent of patients with sleep apnea and provide marked improvement for another 25 percent of patients.

The Gastrointestinal System

T he gastrointestinal tract serves as a processing plant to extract nutrients from food consumed and to package waste. The teeth tear and grind food. Salivary glands add extra moisture and chemicals that begin to break down food structure. The tongue moves food around in the mouth for more effective chewing and

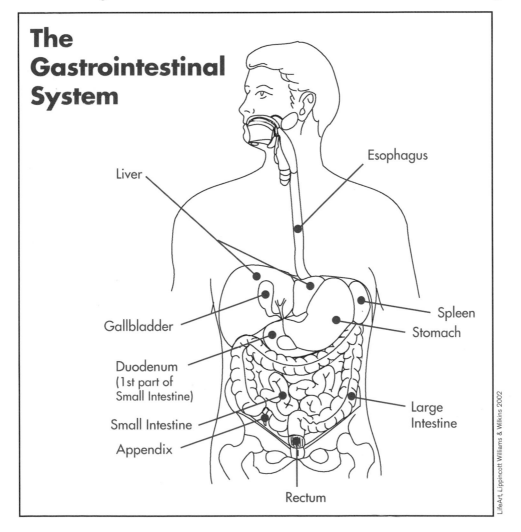

The Gastrointestinal System

- Liver
- Esophagus
- Gallbladder
- Spleen
- Stomach
- Duodenum (1st part of Small Intestine)
- Small Intestine
- Large Intestine
- Appendix
- Rectum

LifeArt, Lippincott Williams & Wilkins 2002

201

forms it into small, soft packets in the back of the mouth for swallowing. The esophagus is the long, muscular tube that transports a food packet from the mouth to the stomach through a series of coordinated muscle contractions that push contents along. This process is effective enough to allow us to swallow water standing on our heads. The esophagus has sphincter muscles at its upper and lower ends, which either relax or tighten to allow food to pass or keep substances from going the wrong way.

The stomach is a strong muscular chamber that adds acids and continues to mix and break down food. In the first part of the small intestines, juices are added from the liver (bile acids) and pancreas (enzymes) to further the digestion process. Most nutrients are absorbed in the small intestines, either by diffusing across the intestinal wall into the bloodstream or by being carried across the lining by special proteins. The large bowel absorbs moisture and stores and packages solid waste for elimination. Bacteria live in the bowel and manufacture important vitamins, which are absorbed by the body. The rectum and anus provide a structure to allow voluntary control over bowel movements.

This chapter will review those diseases that affect the structure or function of the gastrointestinal system: difficulty swallowing (dysphagia), excess acid entering the esophagus (gastroesophageal reflux disease), breakdown in the stomach lining (peptic ulcer disease), growth of crystals in the gallbladder (gallstones), inflammation of the liver (hepatitis), abnormal bowel movements (constipation and diarrhea), bowel disorders (diverticulosis, diverticulitis, irritable bowel syndrome, and inflammatory bowel disease), weakness in veins or muscles surrounding digestive organs (hemorrhoids and hernia), and colon cancer.

Dysphagia (Difficulty Swallowing)

Dysphagia, or difficulty swallowing, has several possible causes. It is best to evaluate this problem by breaking down swallowing into stages. *Transfer dysphagia* refers to problems in the mouth and throat in getting a food packet prepared and to the esophagus. *Transport dysphagia* refers to swallowing problems in the esophagus itself. Difficulty swallowing solids but not liquids usually means a mechanical blockage in the esophagus; difficulty swallowing both solids and liquids usually means a problem in esophageal muscle function or coordination.

In transfer dysphagia, patients have trouble beginning to swallow, for various reasons: the food was not properly chewed, the food goes the wrong way, the upper throat forces are weak, or the upper esophageal sphincter does not relax properly with swallowing. These reasons are typically neurological in origin (for example, stroke) or related to abnormal anatomy in this region. The esophagus may have a herniated pouch (Zenker's diverticulum) that fills with food and gets in the way of swallowing, or the upper esophageal sphincter's muscular tone may be too high. These conditions are detected using a test called a *modified barium swallow*, in which the patient is given a variety of substances to swallow. These substances show up on a detailed x-ray that records the act of swallowing. Treatment of identified swallowing disorders may include training in effective swallowing techniques by a speech pathologist, changes in the consistency of the food consumed, or surgical procedures to relieve blockages or disorders of muscular function.

The difficulty swallowing solid foods found in transport dysphagia can occur intermittently or continuously. Intermittent causes are sometimes related to a *hiatal hernia*. Usually, the transition between the esophagus and the stomach occurs at the level of the diaphragm muscle (which separates the chest and abdominal cavities). In a hiatal hernia, a portion of the stomach protrudes (herniates) up through the diaphragm into the chest cavity. This pushes the bottom of the esophagus away from the diaphragm into the chest cavity, where it functions less efficiently and can produce intermittent problems in swallowing and reflux (washing of stomach contents up into the esophagus). Constant dysphagia implies a fixed mechanical blockage in the esophagus; this most commonly occurs from acid reflux from the stomach, which burns and scars the lining of the esophagus, or from esophageal cancer.

The difficulty in swallowing both solids and liquids found in transport dysphagia occurs from processes that affect the muscle function of the esophagus. Related diseases include:

- Diffuse esophageal spasm, where the muscle contractions are uncoordinated
- Scleroderma, a rheumatological disease where internal scarring of the esophagus stops the contraction of muscles that carry food to the stomach and interferes with the function of the lower esophageal sphincter
- Achalasia, where the lower esophageal sphincter fails to relax with swallowing, and the esophagus above this muscle balloons out and loses its ability to contract

Most swallowing disorders are evaluated initially with a barium swallow. In this test, the patient drinks a glass of barium, a substance that coats the lining of the upper gastrointestinal tract and is seen on x-ray. The physician watches how this barium progresses down the esophagus as it is swallowed to see any abnormalities in structure and function of the upper gastrointestinal tract. Upper endoscopy, in which a gastroenterologist passes a lighted fiber-optic scope through the mouth and stomach of a sedated patient, allows the physician to look directly at structures in the upper gastrointestinal tract, take biopsies of suspicious areas, or use inflatable balloons or other instruments to open narrowed areas.

A third condition that causes a sensation of fullness in the throat—but does not interfere with swallowing—is called *globus*. The cause of this sensation is unknown and often difficult to treat.

Gastroesophageal Reflux Disease

The stomach has a lining of thick mucus that protects it from its own acid. The esophagus has no such protection. A ring-like muscle, the lower esophageal sphincter, exists between the esophagus and stomach to close the lower esophagus and prevent backup of acid. In *gastroesophageal reflux disease* (GERD), this muscle either relaxes at the wrong times or doesn't close completely.

Symptoms

Symptoms of GERD include heartburn, chest pain, asthma, cough, and laryngitis. Often symptoms occur after a large meal, when the excessive pressure in the stomach promotes reflux, or with the ingestion of certain foods that irritate the esophagus or worsen reflux. Upright posture helps keep acid in the stomach; lying down promotes reflux and worsens symptoms. Complications of gastroesophageal reflux disease include ulceration and scar formation in the esophagus that can eventually block swallowing, as well as pre-malignant changes in the cells of the lining of the esophagus called Barrett's esophagus.

Physicians assist patients who experience the classical symptoms of this disease by listening to the patient's description of symptoms and initiating therapy with medications that either reduce the acid content in the stomach or stimulate muscular contractions that promote emptying of the stomach or retard tendencies for substances to wash back into the esophagus. If the patient fails to respond to therapy, or if symptoms continue, the physician then performs an *upper endoscopy* using a lighted fiber-optic scope to look directly into the esophagus. If the patient has difficulty swallowing, the physician often precedes the endoscopy with a barium swallow study to obtain more information about the anatomy and muscular function of the esophagus. If these tests do not pinpoint a cause, the physician may perform other testing such as esophageal manometry, where a tube containing pressure gauges along its surface is placed in the esophagus to determine how well the esophagus contracts to push food to the stomach, and a 24-hour pH probe, in which a thin, acid-sensitive catheter is hooked up to a recorder and passed through the nose into the esophagus to measure acid levels over the course of a day.

Relieving Symptoms

Lifestyle changes to relieve gastroesophageal reflux disease are an important component of any therapy for it. These changes work sufficiently to relieve symptoms in 20 to 25 percent of patients, eliminating the need for additional medication.

- **Elevate the head of the bed by six inches.** Elevating your head while sleeping allows gravity to help keep acid down in the stomach. The most effective way to do this is to place blocks under the bed frame at the head of the bed to give the entire bed a gentle slope. Simply using extra pillows to elevate the head may not be enough because it causes a bend at the waistline, producing more pressure on the stomach and increasing reflux.
- **Sleep on your left side.** This position anatomically places the stomach below the esophagus, reducing reflux.
- **Decrease the size of meals.** A stomach that is less full generates lower pressure, reducing reflux.
- **Avoid foods that make the condition worse.** Citrus juices, tomato products, coffee, and alcohol directly irritate the esophagus. Chocolate, peppermint, alcohol, onions, garlic, and fat cause the lower esophageal sphincter to relax. Fat slows

the emptying of the stomach, creating a longer time for stomach contents to reflux. Carbonated beverages bloat the stomach, increasing pressure and reflux.

- **Avoid lying down until two or three hours after meals.** After this amount of time, food has left the stomach and been passed further along the small intestines. An empty stomach doesn't stimulate acid production, and has limited material within it to reflux.
- **Stop smoking.** Nicotine relaxes the lower esophageal sphincter and increases acid production from the stomach.
- **Lose excess weight.** Reducing the body weight in the abdominal area also reduces pressure on the stomach.
- **Avoid tight belts and garments.** Again, additional pressure on the stomach increases the likelihood of reflux.
- **Avoid potentially harmful medications.** Many drugs lower the tone of the lower esophageal sphincter, including calcium channel blockers (blood pressure medications) and theophylline (a drug for lung disease). Some drugs directly irritate the lining of the esophagus, including arthritis medications and some drugs for osteoporosis.

Treatment

In addition to lifestyle changes, many treatment options are available for gastroesophageal reflux disease. If the patient only experiences occasional heartburn, therapy is needed only when symptoms occur or in circumstances expected to create symptoms. These therapies include antacids and over-the-counter medications that block the production of acid in the stomach. More persistent symptoms require further testing and/or ongoing therapy.

What Medications are Used to Treat GERD?

The two most common classes of medications to reduce stomach acid are H2 blockers and proton pump inhibitors (PPIs).

H2 blockers have been around longer and are available over the counter, in reduced dosage formulations. They begin to work more quickly and are less expensive than PPIs, but aren't quite as effective at suppressing the total level of acid. H2 blockers are particularly effective in suppressing the type of acid secretion that occurs while fasting overnight.

PPIs are currently only available by prescription in the United States. They are more effective at total acid production and healing of acid-related problems in the lining of the upper gastrointestinal tract, but take a few days to achieve their maximum benefit and are much more expensive.

Chronic acid exposure in the esophagus can cause changes in the lining of the esophagus (referred to as Barrett's esophagus), which is a risk for esophageal cancer. The risk of having Barrett's esophagus correlates with the length of time a patient has experienced reflux and the severity of his or her symptoms. Current guidelines recommend an upper endoscopy to screen for the changes of Barrett's esophagus in patients who have had daily heartburn despite one month of treatment, who have had heartburn at least twice weekly for a year, or who have had heartburn at least once a week, every week for five years. White males with symptoms of nighttime acid reflux are especially at risk for Barrett's esophagus.

Patients with chronic gastroesophageal reflux disease symptoms, or whose gastroesophageal reflux disease episodes have actually injured the esophagus (*erosive esophagitis*), are prescribed a maintenance therapy to suppress acid production. The PPI drugs work better for this condition. In patients with erosive esophagus, the use of PPIs heals 91 percent of patients after eight weeks of therapy and, if the PPIs are continued, 80 percent of patients remain healed at one year. If H2 blockers at high doses are used instead, only 50 percent of patients remain healed at one year. Although PPI drugs were initially only approved in the United States for short-term therapy, this restriction is no longer present. Studies in the European literature show that PPI drugs have been used safely in patients for more than 12 years. Several brands of PPIs exist, and the newer drugs in this class seem somewhat better in their degree of acid suppression and symptom relief.

Peptic Ulcer Disease

The stomach is well protected from its own acid. A thick layer of goop made up of mucus coats the stomach. This goop contains high levels of bicarbonate, which buffers the acid. *Ulcers* are sores or craters in the lining of the stomach. A *perforated ulcer* is an ulcer that was deep enough to puncture completely through the stomach wall. In the last ten years, our understanding of ulcer disease has changed dramatically. It used to be felt that ulcers were due to excessive acid secretion; it is now apparent that the overwhelming majority of ulcers are caused by breakdowns in the protective lining of the stomach created by infection with the Helicobacter pylori organism, injury from nonsteroidal anti-inflammatory drugs (NSAIDs), or the effects of tobacco smoke and alcohol use.

Five to ten percent of the U.S. population will experience peptic ulcer disease sometime in their lifetime. Men are twice as likely to get an ulcer as women. Eighty percent of ulcers occur in the first part of the small intestine (duodenum), and most frequently occur between the ages of 45 and 54. Ulcers that occur in the stomach typically occur in patients about 10 years older, and are more likely to be associated with cancer of the lining of the stomach.

Symptoms

Patients with ulcers may experience abdominal pain between the rib cage and the navel or have gastrointestinal bleeding. Whereas food worsens gastroesophageal reflux disease symptoms, food initially buffers the acid in the stomach and may relieve peptic ulcer disease symptoms. Ulcer pain often increases between meals or may awaken the patient at night. If the ulcer causes enough surrounding swelling, it may obstruct the outflow of the stomach, leading to nausea and vomiting. Signs of bleeding may be as obvious as vomiting blood or as subtle as passing sticky, black, tarry stools. When blood passes through the colon, the bacteria in the colon oxidize the iron in blood, turning it from red to black. Black stools may represent a medical emergency, even in the absence of other symptoms, and should be reported to your doctor promptly.

Treatment

Treatment of peptic ulcer disease includes prescribing medication to suppress the production of stomach acid and testing for the H. pylori infection. This testing includes direct examination of samples obtained from the ulcer during endoscopy or blood testing for antibodies indicating infection with H pylori. Successful treatment of this organism using a variety of medications dramatically reduces the risk of future ulcers. A patient who has been treated for ulcer may be advised to have a confirmatory test to prove that the ulcer has completely healed.

Gallstones

The gallbladder is a small sac-like organ at the base of the liver. It stores bile made in the liver and, when stimulated by a fatty meal, contracts to squirt bile into the small intestine to help in the process of digestion. Bile acids contain high concentrations of cholesterol; when this concentration of cholesterol becomes supersaturated in the gallbladder, small crystals begin to form, which can grow into stones called *gallstones*.

The risk for gallstones increases with age, obesity, rapid weight loss, pregnancy, female sex, and family history. Two-thirds of all stones are silent and never cause trouble; these silent stones are incidentally found during testing for other conditions and have a low risk for serious complications. No evidence exists that removing them offers any health benefit when they haven't caused any symptoms.

Symptoms

Some stones block the drainage duct system of the gallbladder. This obstruction produces sudden pain below the right side of the rib cage that typically—though pain patterns vary widely—radiates to the back and shoulder blade. This pain progresses rapidly to its peak intensity, is steady, lasts fewer than three hours, and is often accompanied by nausea. Once one episode of gallbladder pain has occurred, the risk of repeat attacks is significant; 50 percent of patients will have another attack within 12 months.

Cholecystitis occurs when the wall of the gallbladder becomes inflamed. This commonly occurs when a stone obstructs the gallbladder, though 5 to 10 percent of cases occur without stones. In addition to the usual signs of a stone, patients with cholecystitis look sicker, have more tenderness in the right upper quadrant of the abdomen, and may have fever. The pain lasts longer than three hours. Prompt treatment is needed.

Gallbladder disease is primarily diagnosed by the symptoms a patient reports, as well as physical examination and laboratory tests. The gallbladder shares its drainage system with the pancreas; occasionally, gallstones will block the pancreatic drainage route and create *pancreatitis*, which is detectable by history, examination, and additional laboratory tests. (See *Chapter 20: Glandular and Metabolic Diseases* for more information about the pancreas and its function.) Ultrasound is an excellent technique to see the gallbladder; it is more than 95 percent accurate for diagnosis of stones larger than two millimeters. Because stones are easier to see in a distended gallbladder, patients are asked to fast for a gallbladder tests to allow the gallbladder to fill with bile. Another gallbladder test is the hepatobiliary scan, in which the patient fasts and is given an intravenous injection of a radioactive imaging chemical that is excreted into the bile ducts. It is normal to see images of the bile ducts, gallbladder, and small bowel within 30 to 45 minutes. If the gallbladder cannot be seen, it suggests that the duct to it is blocked.

Treatment

Treatment of gallbladder disease is primarily surgical. Laparoscopic surgical techniques have greatly speeded the healing process and reduced complications of gallbladder surgery, and are generally used whenever the anatomy and disease process will allow them. In laparoscopic gallbladder surgery, small incisions are made in the abdominal wall through which the laparoscope (a fiber-optic viewing device) and various instruments are passed. The surgeon operates by manipulating these instruments as the gallbladder and its contents are removed.

Hepatitis

Hepatitis is an inflammation of the liver. *Viral hepatitis* is hepatitis caused by an infectious virus. In most cases, viral hepatitis produces non-specific, flu-like symptoms and goes away on its own without therapy. After exposure to the virus, an incubation period of two weeks to six months may pass before symptoms develop. Symptoms include malaise, loss of appetite, nausea, changes in the senses of taste or smell, low-grade fever, abdominal discomfort, and fatigue. Within six to eight weeks, most patients are well on their way to recovery. Some patients experience a more severe illness, with severe hepatitis and liver failure. Other patients progress to chronic hepatitis, with low-grade ongoing inflammation that can ultimately lead to *cirrhosis* (scarring of the liver) and liver failure.

Hepatitis is classified into types. In this chapter, we will look at three types: hepatitis A, hepatitis B, and hepatitis C.

Hepatitis A

Hepatitis A is transmitted from person to person by ingestion of contaminated foods or secretions. The infection spreads in poor sanitary conditions and where crowding exists. Often, contamination of the water supply by human waste leads to illness in travelers to third-world countries. It takes an average of 30 days to begin experiencing symptoms from the time a patient is first exposed. Hepatitis A can be prevented by vaccination.

Hepatitis B

Hepatitis B is transmitted from person to person by blood or body fluids, including sexual transmission (responsible for at least 50 percent of cases), shared infected needles (drug addiction, tattooing, or body piercing without proper sterilization of equipment), or infected blood. Unlike hepatitis A, the time from exposure to hepatitis B to the onset of symptoms varies; the incubation period averages twelve weeks but can range from four weeks to six months. Persistent infections can develop in 5 to 10 percent of cases. Long-term effects of chronic infection include cirrhosis and liver cancer. Hepatitis B can be prevented by vaccination.

Hepatitis C

Hepatitis C is transferred primarily through blood-to-blood contact. People at risk include those who received blood transfusions before July 1992 (blood has been screened since then) and those sharing drug paraphernalia or other poorly sterilized contaminated devices. Five percent of infected pregnant women can transfer the infection to their babies during birth; less than 1.5 percent of infected men and women infect their sex partners. The incubation period averages seven weeks. Patients are more likely to develop chronic infection and associated illnesses with hepatitis C than with other forms of hepatitis. There is no vaccination for hepatitis C at this time.

Out of 100 people infected with hepatitis C, 85 will develop a chronic infection; within 20 to 30 years, 17 of these people will go on to develop cirrhosis. Four of these people will die from liver failure and two will develop liver cancer. Hepatitis C disease progresses slowly; the time from the original infection to the development of cirrhosis takes 20 to 30 years. We currently are experiencing a silent epidemic of hepatitis C. In a recent blood survey, 8.6 percent of patients hospitalized for other reasons had antibodies in their bloodstream showing previous infection with hepatitis C. Hepatitis C is the leading reason for liver transplantation. Hepatitis C patients who drink alcohol excessively, are older than 40, or who have a second infection with hepatitis A, hepatitis B, or the HIV virus tend to have more severe problems during the course of their illness.

Patients with hepatitis C should be vaccinated against hepatitis A and B, counseled to abstain from alcohol, and educated in preventing the spread of the virus to others. Their liver chemistries and the concentration of the virus in their bloodstream should also be periodically monitored.

For more information about hepatitis vaccinations, see *Chapter 10: Vaccinations and Associated Diseases*.

Treatment

Newer treatment options can lead to a cure for hepatitis C in up to 41 percent of patients. Treatment is currently offered to patients with persistently elevated liver enzymes three times above the normal range, high levels of virus in the bloodstream, and liver biopsies showing early changes of cirrhosis. Given the slow progression of this disease and the rapidly expanding treatment options, patients with hepatitis C who don't meet obvious criteria for treatment should discuss with their doctors whether to take currently available therapy or wait to see if better therapies are developed in the next few years.

Constipation and Diarrhea

Normal bowel movements vary, depending on personal habits and diet, from as often as three times daily to once every three days. As muscle contractions push the contents of the colon toward the anus, the colon absorbs water and salts, forming solid waste. If too much water is absorbed, dry, hard stool results in *constipation*. If too little fluid is absorbed, or if the bowel wall is irritated and secreting fluid, *diarrhea* results. Fiber is crucial in this process; its bulk and texture retain moisture in the stool and help regulate the consistency of the stool.

Constipation

Constipation—the passage of dry, hard bowel movements—usually reduces bowel movements to fewer than three times a week. It is associated with a sensation of abdominal bloating, discomfort, and generalized sluggishness. Causes include a poor diet (that is, the inadequate consumption of fiber), lack of physical exercise, inadequate fluid intake, medications (narcotics, antacids, iron, antidepressants), irritable bowel syndrome, pregnancy, advanced age, travel, long-term abuse of laxatives, a history of ignoring the urge to defecate, thyroid disease, and some neurological diseases.

If an underlying disease is not found, constipation is usually treated through changes in the diet and fiber supplements. Eating beans, whole-grain or bran cereals, and fresh fruits and vegetables may help, as well as limiting meats, cheeses, and highly processed foods. It is important to drink plenty of liquids and exercise daily to help speed the passage of material through the colon. If laxatives are used, bulk-forming agents (laxatives containing substances such as bran that add bulk to the stool) are the safest. Stool softeners help, and lubricants such as glycerin suppositories inserted into the rectum can ease the passage of hard stool. Laxatives that contain stimulants, which cause an artificial contraction of the large intestine in order to move the stool, must be used carefully; long-term use of this type of laxative can damage the neurological net of the colon and cause further malfunction of the colon's muscular contractions.

Diarrhea

Diarrhea refers to the frequent passage of poorly formed stools. Due to the increased muscular activity of the colon, abdominal cramps may accompany diarrhea. Diarrhea is the body's protective way of pushing irritants through the colon quickly, and is a helpful response for some viral and bacterial infections. Although most diarrheas are caused by a virus, diarrhea can also occur as a result of toxins or bacterial contamination of foods, as side effects of antibiotics and other drugs, as part of a stress response, and in relation to intolerance of certain foods. Parasitic infections with Giardia result from drinking contaminated untreated water, such as drinking from streams while hiking or camping. Chronic (greater than two weeks in duration) and recurrent diarrheas can be signs of underlying bowel disease, diabetes, thyroid disease, and other medical conditions.

To treat diarrhea, first stop further stimulation to the gastrointestinal tract by not ingesting food and by drinking small, frequent sips of water to stay hydrated. Don't begin to take drugs to stop diarrhea until six hours after symptoms begin in order to give the colon a chance to clear toxins. Avoid milk and other dairy products during this time; diarrhea flushes the enzyme that helps digest the lactose sugar in dairy products from the lining of the intestine and therefore prevents the stomach from absorbing the lactose, often perpetuating the diarrhea. Fatty and fried foods also seem to perpetuate diarrhea. It is best to stick with easily digested, high-carbohydrate foods such as bananas, rice, baked potato, and applesauce until bowel movements are back to normal.

Medical attention is needed if the stools are black or bloody, if abdominal pain is severe and unrelieved, if you are unable to drink adequate fluids to avoid dehydration, or if the diarrhea is accompanied by fever of 101 degrees Fahrenheit or higher, severe chills, persistent vomiting, or fainting. Medical evaluation is advised if severe diarrhea (that is, a large volume of stool every couple of hours) lasts longer than 24 hours or if mild diarrhea lasts longer than two weeks. If these more severe symptoms are not present, most diarrheas, including those caused by bacteria, will resolve themselves without therapy.

Diverticulosis and Diverticulitis

The colon wall is lined by layers of muscle that help propel stool through it. These layers of muscle reinforce the wall of the colon like a steel-belted tire. Diverticula—small pockets of the colon that push through the muscular layer and resemble sacs protruding from the colon—are formed in weak points of the muscular wall.

When diverticula are present, the condition is known as *diverticulosis*. This condition is normal for patients over age 40. Diverticulosis usually does not cause symptoms and is detected when the colon is examined for other reasons, such as screening for colon cancer. Sometimes, complications can occur, including infection (a condition called *diverticulitis*) and bleeding.

Diverticulitis occurs when the opening between the diverticular pouch and the colon becomes blocked, either by particulate matter in the stool (an undigested seed or nut fragment) or by inflammation and swelling at the mouth of the diverticulum. This leaves some stool walled off within the diverticular pouch. Stool contains bacteria, which begin to thrive and multiply in this confined space, resulting in infection. Pressure builds in the diverticulum, its walls become inflamed, and this inflammation can spread to surrounding tissues resulting in pain. Infected diverticula can rupture, spilling their contents into the abdominal cavity creating an abscess.

As stool passes through the colon, water is absorbed and the stool solidifies. Higher pressures must be generated within the colon to propel the solidifying stool along than are needed to move liquid stool. It is in these zones of higher pressure (the end of the bowel, or sigmoid colon) that most diverticula occur.

Symptoms

Symptoms of diverticulitis include pain and tenderness in the lower left quadrant of the abdomen, fever, and changes in bowel frequency (constipation or diarrhea). Your physician often diagnoses diverticulitis solely on the basis of your symptoms and findings on physical examination. The white blood cell count is often elevated. An abdominal CT scan may show findings that suggest inflammation in the colon wall, but CT scan results can also be entirely normal in early phases of diverticulitis. Endoscopic studies, such as colonoscopy, are usually avoided in patients with acute diverticulitis in fear that the added pressure in the colon created during the examination may cause the infected diverticulum to rupture.

Treatment

Treatment of diverticulitis includes bowel rest, appropriate antibiotics to treat the types of bacteria found in stool, and careful monitoring of the patient. Mild cases are usually treated at home. Bowel rest consists of switching to a diet that is easily digested and doesn't create much fecal matter, such as liquids, thin soups, and carbohydrates. Pain medication is provided, and patients are seen back in the office frequently until they are clearly improving. Some patients are sick enough to require intravenous fluids to allow for complete bowel rest, intravenous antibiotics, and close monitoring in the hospital. The majority of patients will recover without deficits. A few will require surgery to drain an area of abscess or to remove a portion of the colon.

Prevention of diverticulitis involves following the same healthy fiber-rich diet that is recommended for most people. Fiber-rich foods include whole-grain cereals and breads, fruits, and vegetables. Many commercial fiber supplements are also available. The regular intake of fiber and adequate water leads to softer, bulkier stools that are easier for the colon to transport, thus requiring lower pressures to be generated in the end of the colon and less trouble with diverticula. Patients with recurrent bouts of diverticulitis are usually advised to avoid foods that create small, undigested particles in the stool, such as seeds, nuts, and popcorn.

Irritable Bowel Syndrome

Irritable bowel syndrome is classified as a functional bowel disorder. Functional means that there is no discernible abnormality in the structure of the bowel; it just doesn't work properly. This disorder occurs in 15 to 20 percent of adults, women more than men.

Symptoms

Irritable bowel syndrome is characterized by crampy abdominal pain and is associated with alternating painful episodes of diarrhea and constipation, often accompanied by bloating. Bleeding, fever, and weight loss are not symptoms of this syndrome. Episodes may be triggered by eating (eating causes reflex contractions of the bowel, which are heightened by meals with high calories and fat content) and stress (which interacts with the nervous net controlling gut movement).

A formal diagnosis of irritable bowel syndrome requires three months of continuous or recurrent symptoms of abdominal pain that are relieved by defecation, associated with a change in stool consistency or frequency. Two of the following symptoms must also occur:

- Altered stool frequency (greater than three times a day or less than three times a week)
- Altered stool form
- Altered stool passage (straining, urgency, incomplete evacuation)
- Passage of mucus
- Abdominal bloating

The symptoms of irritable bowel syndrome are associated with gastrointestinal motility, the normal muscular contractions in the intestinal wall. It is felt that patients with irritable bowel syndrome abnormally sense and perceive as painful normal activity in the gut. Recent research is studying this abnormal processing of signals from the gut, focusing on 5-hydroxytryptamine receptors that regulate the gastrointestinal tract's muscular contractions and activation of glands. This research is also targeting newer medical therapies to interact in this area.

Treatment

Traditional therapy of irritable bowel syndrome consists of increasing the fiber content of the diet, reducing the fat content of meals, decreasing the consumption of concentrated calories, and eliminating cigarette smoking. These measures reliably quiet some of the most bothersome symptoms of this syndrome. Fiber keeps the bowel distended and helps prevent spasms. The use of low-dose amitriptyline, an older antidepressant medication, helps regulate bowel activity in some patients. Some of the newer antidepressant medications that target the chemical serotonin also seem to help relieve irritable bowel symptoms even in those patients who are not depressed. We are just beginning to understand the complex neurological, hormonal, and chemical control of bowel function and how the system malfunctions in disease.

Inflammatory Bowel Disease

Inflammatory bowel diseases, including *ulcerative colitis* and *Crohn's disease*, are chronic, relapsing disorders characterized by inflammation of the gastrointestinal wall. The causes of these diseases are unknown, but factors in the environment (such as infectious organisms) and genetic predispositions seem to play a role.

In ulcerative colitis, shallow areas of inflammation in the bowel wall begin in the rectum and lower colon and may spread progressively upward. Tiny open sores develop in the colon lining and mucus, pus, and blood are found in the stool. Ulcerative colitis typically develops in younger patients, ages 15 to 40. Symptoms include abdominal pain, bloody diarrhea, fever, fatigue, loss of appetite, weight loss, and dehydration. Occasionally, other organ systems are involved—most likely through the immune system—in ulcerative colitis patients, including the skin, joints, eye, and liver. The disease can vary from mild to severe. Patients with long-term ulcerative colitis are at increased risk for colon cancer.

In Crohn's disease, the entire gastrointestinal tract from mouth to anus may be involved. The disease can skip around, leaving areas of unaffected intestine between areas of activity. Symptoms include abdominal pain, persistent diarrhea, and low-grade fever, occasionally resulting in rectal bleeding and weight loss. Whereas ulcerative colitis is a superficial inflammatory disease, the inflammation in Crohn's disease goes deep and can involve the full thickness of the lining of the gastrointestinal tract. This leads to a higher rate of complications around the colon, including abscesses and fistulas (channels between the bowel and other organs or to the skin) or blockage of the intestines. Other organ systems—including the joints, skin, eyes, and kidneys—may also be affected.

Diagnosis

Inflammatory bowel disease takes some time to diagnose. Blood test results are not specific for these diseases, so sometimes physicians can only go by the suspicious and persistent symptoms their patients experience and their response to therapy over time. To help identify and assess inflammatory bowel disease, physicians sometimes take stool samples to rule out infections in the colon that can masquerade as inflammatory bowel disease or examine the lining of the colon through x-rays or endoscopes.

Treatment

Treatment options for inflammatory bowel disease vary. No specific diet exists for inflammatory bowel disease patients, although some find that certain foods—such as dairy products or raw fruits or vegetables—aggravate their symptoms. Depending on the section of the gastrointestinal tract involved, the body may be unable to absorb certain vitamins well and these must be supplemented. However, mega doses of vitamins have not proven helpful and may cause harm. Medical therapies include drugs that treat pain and diarrhea symptoms, reduce inflammation, or suppress the reactions of the immune system. About 70 percent of patients with Crohn's disease eventually require surgery for complications such as abscesses, perforation, or obstruction, whereas 20 to 25 percent of patients with ulcerative colitis require removal of the colon to control bleeding or treat other complications.

Hemorrhoids

The entire gastrointestinal tract is lined with a rich supply of blood vessels. *Hemorrhoids* are veins at the end of the colon that have become distended and swollen, caused at least in part by excessive pressure on these veins. This can occur as a result of constipation, pregnancy, prolonged sitting or standing, or obesity. Straining to hurry bowel movements can also contribute to hemorrhoids. Hemorrhoids can be internal (still within the anal canal) or external (protruding from the anus).

Symptoms

Irritated hemorrhoids can cause itching, pain, and discomfort. Complications of hemorrhoids include rectal bleeding and thrombosis, in which a blood clot forms within the hemorrhoid. Bleeding from the hemorrhoid usually appears as bright red blood from the rectum, noticed on the toilet paper or on the surface of the stool. Blood from higher up in the colon usually turns dark maroon or black before it is passed, resulting from the colon bacteria's oxidization of iron in the blood. A thrombosed hemorrhoid appears as a firm mass at the anus, which can become exquisitely tender as a result of inflammation in the vein.

Treatment

Treatment of hemorrhoids begins with attempts not to further aggravate them and to relieve the symptoms they cause. Hard, dry stools that accompany constipation irritate the hemorrhoids. To both heal and prevent hemorrhoids, the stools must be moister and soft. This can be accomplished by adding fiber to the diet to create a fiber meshwork in the stool. Fiber can be obtained from fruits, vegetables, and grains or by the use of commercially prepared fiber supplements. Adequate fluid must be taken with the fiber. Stool softeners or lubricants (mineral oil or glycerin suppositories) help the stools to pass without straining. Ice packs to the rectum can help relieve swelling. Sitting in eight or ten inches of warm water is soothing. A variety of over-the-counter medications can provide topical relief. Beware of those that contain an anesthetic such as lidocaine, as contact allergies to these substances can develop. Your doctor can provide steroid creams and suppositories to help relieve inflammation when needed. Occasionally, surgical procedures are required to drain thrombosed hemorrhoids or to remove problematic ones.

Hernia

The lining of the abdominal cavity is reinforced with layers of muscle and connective tissue, like a steel belted tire. When a defect occurs in the structure of the abdominal wall that enables the contents of the abdominal cavity (fat, fluid, intestines, etc.) to bulge through, a *hernia* is created. A *ventral hernia* occurs in the midline of the abdomen between two muscles that run from the chest to the pelvis. An *umbilical hernia* occurs at the belly button. An *inguinal hernia* occurs just to the side of the genitals at the base of the abdomen. In men, an inguinal hernia follows the canal that originally allowed the testicles (which develop in the abdomen) to descend into the scrotum before birth. A *femoral hernia* occurs through the canal where the major blood vessels and nerves pass from the abdomen into the leg.

Symptoms

Hernias can appear as a localized bulge or pain or simply be detected during a routine examination. They are usually more noticeable under circumstances that increase local pressure, such as upright posture or straining. They may disappear entirely when the pressure is relieved, such as by lying down. The major complication of a hernia is called an *incarceration*. This occurs when tissue, such as a loop of intestine, slips through the hernia and becomes stuck. This can result in swelling or twisting sufficient to cut off the blood supply to the herniated tissue, resulting in a medical emergency.

Treatment

Most hernias enlarge with time and are more easily repaired when small. The decision to repair a hernia is based on its location, size, symptoms, and the general health of the patient.

Colon Cancer

Colon cancer is the fourth most common cancer diagnosis and the second leading cause of cancer death in the United States. The odds of developing colon cancer steadily rise with age, continuing to increase even after age 80. The lifetime risk of developing colon cancer is 6 percent. The risk doubles if a family member has had colon cancer; if that family member had cancer before the age of 50, the risk is 20 percent or greater. Survival depends on detecting colon cancer early. Of patients discovered with an early, localized form of the disease and treated, 92 percent were still alive five years later. If the disease has spread to lymph nodes within the immediate vicinity of the colon, the survival rate drops to 62 percent. Only 7 percent of patients are alive at five years if their cancer had spread outside of the abdomen at the time of diagnosis.

The colon (the large intestine) is a long muscular tube that is lined by a rich membrane of tissue called the *mucosa*. Sometimes, growths called *polyps* develop on the mucosal surface, similar to moles on the skin. *Hyperplastic polyps* are small and seem meaningless. *Adenomatous polyps* can progress over a period of time, undergoing changes that lead to colon cancer. It is felt that adenomatous polyps take 10 to 15 years to develop and transition into cancer. The goal of colon cancer prevention is to detect and remove these adenomatous polyps before cancer develops or spreads.

Symptoms

Colon cancer has few symptoms until its later stages. One sign is bloody stool, although not all cancers bleed. Other signs include a persistent change in bowel habits, diarrhea, constipation, a change in stool size or consistency, abdominal pain, loss of appetite, weakness or fatigue, anemia, or an urge to defecate that is not relieved by a bowel movement.

Risks for colon cancer include a previous colon cancer or adenomatous polyp, disease of the bowel such as inflammatory bowel disease or familial polyposis—an inherited disease in which patients form a large number of polyps at an early age—a family history of colon cancer, age, and, in Western civilizations, a meat-based diet. Irritable bowel syndrome is not a risk for colon cancer. However, 95 percent of colon cancer patients have no identified risk.

Reducing the Risk

Several suggestions have been made to reduce the risk for colon cancer. Little hard science exists behind many of these suggestions; they are often based on simple observation of large groups of people with and without colon cancer and are subject to all the bias that affects that type of study.

- **Improve your diet.** Eat a lower fat diet with less red meat. Consider a high-fiber diet supplemented with antioxidants such as folic acid, calcium, and vitamins C, E, and B.
- **Drink less alcohol.** In a Harvard study, men who drank two or more drinks a day doubled their rate of colon cancer.
- **Take aspirin or anti-inflammatory medications daily.** Aspirin or anti-inflammatory drugs block the actions of chemicals called prostaglandins, which may have a role in transitioning adenomatous polyps to cancer.
- **Take estrogens after menopause.** Observational studies show a 30 to 50 percent reduction in colon cancer in postmenopausal women who use estrogens. Better recent scientific studies confirm this benefit.
- **Be physically active.** Regular exercise speeds the passage of waste through the colon, possibly resulting in less time for contact between cancer-causing substances and the colon lining. Studies of the most active exercisers show a 50 percent reduction in the age expected incidence of colon cancer.
- **Don't smoke.** Carcinogens in tobacco smoke reach the colon via the bloodstream, and studies suggest a higher colon cancer rate in smokers.

These prevention hints may be helpful, but preventing colon cancer deaths requires regular and systematic screening for the disease. Since screening involves the detection and removal of intestinal polyps that may have otherwise grown into cancer, colon cancer is one of the few diseases where screening can both detect and prevent cancer. Most patients who get screened and follow through on the results of screening essentially eliminate their chance of dying from this disease.

Screening Tests

- **The digital rectal exam.** In this test, performed during a prostate exam or pelvic exam, the doctor uses a gloved finger to feel for abnormalities in the anus and rectum and to obtain a stool sample for testing. Masses or abnormalities within reach of the finger, such as anorectal cancers, can be identified by touch.

- **Fecal occult blood test (Guaiac test).** Some colon cancers and polyps bleed, resulting in small amounts of blood in the stool that can't be seen with the eye but can be chemically detected. This test involves the collection of small samples of stool from three bowel movements by the patient, which are tested chemically in the doctor's office for blood. The test is relatively cheap and simple to perform and should be done annually after age 50. Some substances can cause false results: Vitamin C in excess of 250 milligrams a day interferes with the chemistry of the test, and blood can be missed. Certain substances may appear as blood falsely in the chemical test. Sufficient quantities of ingested red meat, turnips, radishes, horseradish, or melons can turn the test positive. Blood from other sources, such as menstrual blood, may contaminate the specimen. To maximize the test's effectiveness, follow the instructions for collecting the samples carefully. Use of the stool tests alone, with no other screening, results in a 33 to 40 percent reduction in mortality from colorectal cancer.

- **Flexible sigmoidoscopy examination.** This procedure, performed by many primary care physicians, uses a flexible fiber-optic scope in the office to examine the rectum and most of the left side of the colon for polyps or other abnormalities. Flexible sigmoidoscopes only reach about one third of the colon, penetrating further into the colon usually requires sedation of the patient to control pain. If abnormalities are seen on this limited examination, the doctor can either obtain a biopsy or refer the patient for a complete colonoscopy and biopsies. Preparation for flexible sigmoidoscopy is simple; a light dinner the night before and self-administered enemas the morning of the exam are usually sufficient. No sedation is needed. In my experience, most patients note only minor discomfort or bloating during the procedure, and wonder afterwards what all the fuss was about. A recent study from the Veteran's Administration medical centers showed that combining a fecal occult blood test with a sigmoidoscopy identified 76 percent of the colon cancers discovered on a simultaneous colonoscopy.

- **The colonoscopy.** In essence, the colonoscopy is a larger, more complex sigmoidoscope that is of sufficient length to examine the entire colon. It is also equipped with the tools needed to remove larger polyps. This exam is performed by a physician with special training (usually a gastroenterologist or surgeon) and enables a more thorough examination of the colon. For anatomic reasons, the colonoscope cannot always be passed through the entire colon; Harvard studies show that technical limitations in viewing all portions of the colon during the exam cause small polyps (less than one centimeter) to be missed about 15 percent of the time. Colonoscopy also requires more preparation—usually a day of strong laxatives to clean all contents from the colon. Because of the discomfort of this deep procedure, it requires intravenous sedation and pain medication for the patient and must be done in the hospital or a special center. The risk of complications from the procedure is higher: The rate of perforation of the colon is 1 to 8 per thousand for colonoscopy, increasing to 10 to 20 per thousand if a polyp is removed. (The risk is about one per 10,000 for sigmoidoscopy). In our area, colonoscopy is about ten times the cost of a sigmoidoscopy, not including the additional time lost in preparing for the exam or recovering from the anesthesia.

Other, less common, tests include:

- **Barium enema.** In this x-ray test, laxatives are used to entirely cleanse the colon of stool. Liquid barium is forced into the colon through the rectum as an enema, and the colon is inflated with air. Pictures are taken of the pattern of barium coating on the colon wall. In a study reported in the *New England Journal of Medicine* in June 2000, barium enemas failed to detect 50 percent of polyps one centimeter in size or smaller. Barium enemas have limited use in colorectal cancer screening. The preparation is the same as colonoscopy, and some discomfort is associated with the procedure. Barium enemas are sometimes helpful in examining those portions of the colon that could not be reached in patients who have already had a sigmoid exam.

- **Virtual colonoscopy."** My patients are understandably always asking about colon cancer screening techniques that do not require endoscopy. These techniques currently are research tools only and not ready for prime time. The most common techniques use a CT scanner. The colon must first be entirely cleaned with laxatives. Medication is then given to temporarily paralyze the colon, stopping contractions. The colon is then filled with air. A fast helical CT scanner with a special computer software package then takes x-rays of the colon; the computer program uses these x-rays to reconstruct a three-dimensional image of the colon. Unfortunately, the resolution of the currently available programs is little better than a barium enema, and lesions one centimeter in size or smaller are frequently missed. Abnormal areas detected require a colonoscopy for further evaluation.

My patients are increasingly likely to ask for the more thorough colonoscopy instead of the flexible sigmoidoscopy. Which test do I recommend? I follow the current screening options as outlined by the American Cancer Society, American Gastroenterology Society, and the United States Preventive Services Task Force:

- Annual digital rectal examination, plus one of the following:
  — Annual fecal occult blood test plus flexible sigmoidoscopy every five years, or
  — Complete colonoscopy at age 50, then every ten years if normal

- Patients at high risk of cancer due to a family history or a personal history of previous polyps require special consideration in screening and should discuss this with their doctor. Patients with a family history should begin screening at least ten years before the age of the youngest family member who was diagnosed with colorectal cancer.

(The recommendations for colorectal cancer screening from the U.S. Preventive Services Task Force were published in the July 2002 issue of the *Annals of Internal Medicine*. These recommendations provided addition validation that either the flexible sigmoidoscopy and stool occult blood testing approach or the colonoscopy approach to colorectal cancer screening is acceptable. In the summary of recommendations, the authors stated, "It is unclear whether the increased accuracy of colonoscopy compared with alternative screening methods… offsets the procedure's additional complications, inconvenience, and cost.")

CHAPTER 24

The Urinary System

I n short, the urinary tract serves to clear the blood of waste products, storing and reprocessing those waste products until it is convenient for the body to expel them.

The kidneys are a pair of filters high in the back part of the abdomen. They receive a continuous flow of blood from branches off the aorta, the major artery from the heart. This blood is squeezed through tiny filtering units called *glomeruli*, which separate the blood cells and larger blood components—such as proteins—from the liquid part of the

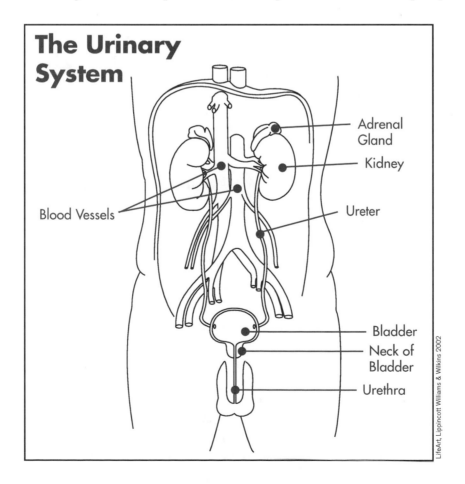

The Urinary System

Adrenal Gland

Kidney

Blood Vessels

Ureter

Bladder

Neck of Bladder

Urethra

LifeArt, Lippincott Williams & Wilkins 2002

blood, the plasma. Initially, this filtered fluid contains both components that the body desires and waste products that it does not. This filtered fluid then passes through a long tube, which is lined with specialized structures that further process the fluid by transferring desired substances—such as certain salts, sugars, and water—back into the body and secreting additional waste products into the filtered fluid. The result is urine.

Once the kidneys have processed the urine, it is passed through two long tubes called *ureters* to the *bladder*, a muscular tank that holds urine until it can be eliminated. The muscles of the bladder stretch as the bladder fills and contract to generate a force to eliminate it.

The bladder neck is a special area at the base of the bladder surrounding the *urethra*, the exiting channel. Muscles that surround the bladder neck can contract, sealing off the bladder and keeping it from leaking, or relax to allow urination. The muscles of the bladder and bladder neck must be closely coordinated to allow for proper bladder function. To urinate, the bladder muscles must contract while the bladder neck muscles relax. To remain continent, the bladder muscles must relax while the bladder neck muscles contract.

The urethra, the tube that exits the bladder and carries urine to be expelled from the body, passes through the pelvic floor muscles. These muscles are under voluntary control and can pinch off the urethra, acting as a stopcock enabling you to make it to the bathroom when you get that intense urge to urinate.

In women, the urethra is a relatively short tube that passes from the bladder to the vagina. It is dependent on the health of the surrounding estrogen-dependent tissues to maintain its support. In men, the urethra passes through the center of the prostate gland as it exits the bladder and is then joined by tubes from the testicles. The urethra then proceeds through the pelvic floor muscles to the penis.

This chapter will discuss common ways that the structure and function of the urinary system are challenged: urinary tract infection, interstitial cystitis, inability to hold urine (incontinence), kidney stones, and sexually transmitted diseases and infections related to the genital/urinary organs (herpes, vaginitis, urethritis, genital warts, chlamydia, and pelvic inflammatory disease).

Urinary Tract Infections

Urinary tract infections occur when bacteria are introduced into the usually sterile urine through the opening of the urethra. This occurs more often in women than in men because of a woman's shorter urethra. The risk for urinary tract infection correlates with several factors. Local factors determine how many bacteria are introduced into the urethra. In the healthy female, the vaginal lining is thick and moist and is colonized by helpful bacteria called *lactobacilli*. These bacteria produce substances that drop the pH of the vagina, which inhibits the growth of other, more harmful bacteria. This natural protection is interrupted by excessive use of antibiotics (which kill the lactobacilli), the loss of estrogen support at menopause (leading to a thinner, dryer vaginal lining), local trauma to the urethra (sexual activity or diaphragms), chemicals (douches and spermicides), other causes of local inflammation (vaginal infections and sexually transmitted diseases), or excessive numbers of bacteria (fecal soiling from incontinence or wiping "back to front").

Bladder function also determines the risk for infection. Bacteria are commonly introduced into the bladder. If the bladder is able to drain rapidly and completely, bacteria that are present are washed out before they can multiply and set up an infection. Bladder drainage may be interrupted if the urethra is narrowed or if the bladder is functioning improperly. The urethra can be narrowed at birth (a cause of bladder infections in children) or scarred by previous infections or procedures. The prostate gland can grow enough to pinch off the urethra as it passes through it, restricting flow and increasing infection risk. In some instances, the bladder itself doesn't function properly. The bladder may lose muscle tone or coordination and not completely empty itself with each contraction. This leaves a leftover pool of stagnant urine in the bladder, giving any bacteria that may be present a chance to multiply and cause an infection. Frequently ignoring the urge to urinate can also lead to bladder malfunctions and infections. I see this frequently in elementary school teachers who cannot easily leave their classrooms.

Some bacteria are more aggressive in causing bladder infections. They have special characteristics that enable them to adhere to the lining of the urethra and bladder and are not washed out as easily during urination.

Symptoms

Symptoms of urinary tract infections include:

- An increase in frequency of urination, including nighttime urination
- Urinary urgency ("I've got to go right now!")
- Pain with urination, both burning at the urethral opening and lower abdominal cramping from bladder spasm
- Incontinence
- Changes in urine smell
- Cloudy or discolored urine
- Fever, chills, and signs of generalized illness
- Low back and side pain with kidney infections

Not all bladder infections are associated with symptoms. Infections without symptoms may be discovered during a routine urinalysis. Most studies suggest that these asymptomatic bladder infections are not associated with adverse health outcomes and do not need to be treated. Exceptions include pregnant women, in whom about 25 percent of bladder infections will proceed upward to kidney infections, patients about to undergo a surgical procedure involving the urinary tract, and some patients with impaired immune defenses.

Treatment Decisions

A decision to treat a patient for a bladder infection is usually based primarily on suggestive symptoms and the results of a dipstick urinalysis in the office. In this procedure, a strip of paper coated with stripes of chemicals is dipped into a urine sample. Within minutes, color changes occur in the various chemical stripes when they detect abnormalities in the urine, such as protein, white blood cells, or red blood cells, which may indicate an infection. In addition to the chemical testing, a urine sample can be spun down in a centrifuge to concentrate the cells in it, which the physician or technician can directly examine under a microscope for signs of infection. Many antibiotics reach high concentrations in the bladder; most uncomplicated infections can be treated with three to five days of antibiotic therapy. A urine culture, in which the urine is sent to a microbiology lab to see if bacteria can be grown from it, is not usually required for proper treatment of this common infection.

Exceptions to this simple treatment approach are multiple. More detailed evaluation and longer courses of therapy are often needed for the following people:

- People with abnormal structure or function of the urinary tract
- People troubled by recurrent infections
- People who experience fever, chills, and side pain—indicating that the upper urinary tract is involved
- People who have recently taken an antibiotic and may have altered their normal flora of bacteria
- All men with infections (because of differences in anatomy)
- Patients who fail to respond to the initial simple approach

If a woman has more than three bladder infections within a twelve-month period, or a man more than one, an evaluation is warranted to look for an underlying reason. Your physician will initiate this evaluation with a thorough history and examination and may refer you to a urologist to evaluate the anatomy and function of your urinary tract. Options for treatment vary depending on the underlying problems discovered. Common techniques to help those with frequent infections include the use of a single dose of antibiotics after sexual activity, daily antibiotics for prevention, or the use of self-start therapy—an open prescription for antibiotics to be self-initiated by a well-educated patient under his or her physician's supervision.

Prevention

The prevention of urinary tract infections includes reducing the numbers of bacteria introduced into the urinary tract and improving urine flow and flushing out bacteria that are present. Avoiding the unnecessary use of antibiotics helps maintain the normal vaginal lactobacillus population, limiting the presence of less desirable bacteria. Women can maintain vaginal health by properly using estrogens after menopause, avoiding chemicals such as douches and spermicides, and wiping from front to back after toileting to reduce the number of fecal bacteria in the vagina. Women can also reduce trauma to the urethra by adequately lubricating the vagina during intercourse. Men and women alike can promote a healthy urine flow by drinking plenty of fluids and promptly voiding when the urge occurs.

Interstitial Cystitis

The symptoms of recurrent bladder infections can be confused with a less common condition called *interstitial cystitis*, a chronic inflammatory disorder of the bladder. Symptoms of interstitial cystitis include recurring pain in the bladder or surrounding areas that can vary from mild to incapacitating, urinary urgency, and a need to frequently urinate. Ninety percent of patients with this disease are women. Despite their symptoms, repeated medical testing shows no evidence of bladder infections in patients with interstitial cystitis, and they do not respond to antibiotic therapy.

Diagnosis

Basic testing for patients suspected of having interstitial cystitis include examination of urine samples, urine cultures, and cystoscopy. In cystoscopy, the physician inserts a flexible tube about the diameter of a pencil into the bladder of the anesthetized patient. The cystoscope is equipped with a light and lenses so that the physician can examine the inside of the bladder, instruments to obtain biopsies of the bladder wall, and a channel to instill fluid into the bladder to stretch it and determine its capacity.

The diagnosis of interstitial cystitis requires:

- Recurrent symptoms of urinary urgency, frequency, and bladder pain
- Cystoscopic evidence of inflammation of the bladder wall
- The absence of infection of other diseases to account for the symptoms

Treatment for interstitial cystitis is hampered by a lack of knowledge about its cause. Most researchers believe that what is diagnosed as interstitial cystitis at this time is not one disease but several diseases with similar features. This may account for the tremendous variability seen in how patients respond to different treatment options.

Treatment Options

Treatment options for interstitial cystitis include:

- **Bladder distention.** Many patients improve after their initial diagnostic evaluation when the bladder is stretched during cystoscopy. Periodic stretching of the bladder under anesthesia may help some patients.
- **Bladder instillation.** Chemicals can be periodically washed into the bladder to relieve symptoms. The most common approach instills DMSO (dimethyl sulfoxide) through a catheter into the bladder weekly for six to eight weeks.
- **Oral medication.** In 1996, the FDA approved one drug for oral use in interstitial cystitis. This drug, pentosan polysulfate sodium, is taken three times a day. The response rate to this medication is 38 percent, but it may take up to six months for maximum benefit to be achieved.
- **Pain medications.** Pain medications, including aspirin, ibuprofen, and prescription pain medications help some patients. Antidepressant medications, which seem

to interfere with the transmission of pain signals in small nerve fibers, help some patients.

- **Diet.** Some patients report benefits from dietary changes that eliminate certain substances, most commonly alcohol, spices, chocolate and other sources of caffeine, acidic foods including tomatoes and citrus fruits, and artificial sweeteners. Elimination of tobacco smoke frequently helps.

- **Surgery.** When all else fails, a variety of surgical techniques have been tried to relieve pain in interstitial cystitis patients. The results are often unpredictable.

Incontinence

Urinary incontinence is defined as an involuntary loss of urine that is sufficient enough to be a problem for the patient. Eighty-five percent of incontinence occurs in women because of the shorter female urethra, the pelvic trauma of childbirth, and the loss of vaginal support that can occur after menopause. Incontinence can be embarrassing, interfering with sleep, travel, desired physical activities, and the willingness to participate in social functions. It can significantly interfere with aspects of functioning that add quality to life. There are also medical aspects to the problems of incontinence—urine is acidic and very caustic to the skin.

Symptoms

Three basic types of incontinence exist, though most patients have a mix of all three:

- *Urge incontinence* is characterized by a sudden urge to void due to overactivity or spasm of the bladder muscles. Patients suffer incontinence if they can't get to the bathroom quickly. They typically go frequently day and night at the most unexpected and inconvenient times. The bladder is excessively sensitive to chemical stimulation; caffeinated beverages create a need to void out of proportion to the amount of liquid consumed.

- *Stress incontinence* refers to involuntary leakage from the bladder as a reaction to the physical pressure of a cough, sneeze, or strain. Patients may experience incontinence when first getting up from bed or a chair if the bladder is full, or when attempting to exercise. They must void frequently to avoid accidents. Stress incontinence is usually the result of weak pelvic floor muscles that provide little support.

- *Overflow incontinence* occurs when the bladder becomes too full. This can be the result of neurological problems that inhibit voiding, weak and over-distended bladder muscles, or an obstruction to bladder outflow such as an enlarged prostate or an abnormal narrowing of the urethra. Patients typically have a slow urinary stream and take a long time to urinate. The bladder dribbles in small amounts, never feels empty, and urges are felt with no results. Patients typically feel the need to urinate often during the night.

Many factors can increase the risk of incontinence. Physical impairment in the elderly and disabled can interfere with the ability to respond quickly to bladder urges. Pregnancy, delivery trauma, and lack of vaginal support create special problems for women. Dementia and other cognitive factors may decrease the awareness of a need to void. Smoking, diabetes, hypertension, cholesterol disorders, and neurological diseases may affect the small nerves that control bladder muscle function.

Treatment

The treatment of incontinence includes both behavioral and medical therapy.

- **Limit fluid intake.** A common recommendation to manage incontinence is to limit the amount of liquid consumed—the "less in, less out" theory. While this is an effective technique, many patients with incontinence are older and already at risk for dehydration. Except for special social occasions, I am very reluctant to ask my patients to limit their fluid intake.
- **Avoid dietary items that tend to stimulate bladder function.** Avoid caffeinated or carbonated beverages, alcohol, citrus fruits and juices, spicy foods, and artificial sweeteners.
- **Void at routine intervals.** Don't wait for the bladder signal to urinate.
- **Lose weight.** Excessive abdominal fat places more external pressure on the bladder, increasing the likelihood of leakage.
- **Replenish the vagina through systemic or topical estrogen replacement therapy.** With the loss of estrogen production at menopause, the estrogen-dependent tissue at the base of the bladder will shrink by one-third or more. Topical estrogen therapy in the vagina at the base of the bladder can be effective for post-menopausal women with thin vaginal linings, but usually takes months to show an improvement in bladder control.
- Strengthen the pelvic muscles. An exercise to strengthen the pelvic floor muscles (called the Kegel exercise) is effective in controlling stress urinary incontinence. Studies show that 80 percent of patients with stress urinary incontinence improve with an eight-week trial of this behavioral therapy. This exercise consists of the following:

What is the Kegel Exercise and How Do I Do It?

The Kegel exercise is a technique used to strengthen the muscles that support the pelvis. Strong pelvic floor muscles help control stress urinary incontinence. Do this exercise as follows:

1. Identify the proper muscles:
   a. Sit on the toilet and start to urinate.
   b. Try to stop the flow of urine midstream by contracting the pelvic floor muscles (pretty much the same ones you use when you don't want to pass gas in public).
2. Once you have identified the right muscles, practice contracting them when you are not urinating. Sustain the contraction for 10 seconds.
3. Repeat this several times, learning to contract these muscles without tensing your abdominal wall.

Perform these exercises three times a day, with 15 contractions each time, in different positions (standing, sitting, or lying down).

- **For those with urge incontinence, practice controlling the reflex.** Urge sensation response training employs a similar method for those with urge incontinence. When the urge to void is first felt, the patient practices controlling the reflex by pausing, relaxing, sitting if possible, and then performing the pelvic floor exercises described in "What is the Kegel Exercise and How Do I Do It?" before walking to the bathroom. Physiologically, if the voluntary muscles of the pelvic floor are contracted at the first sign of bladder urgency, local neurological loops can inhibit the contraction of the smooth muscle of the bladder and temporarily halt the urge to urinate.

- **Take medications to control contractions.** Medications are available to control the contractions of the bladder and the bladder neck. Different receptors on these areas of muscle are usually stimulated by chemical packages released from local nerve endings, leading either to muscular contraction or relaxation. Medications can also stimulate these receptors. Unfortunately, these receptors are present in other areas of the body, and medications that affect them in the bladder also stimulate them elsewhere, leading to side effects in some patients such as dry mouth, constipation, blurring of vision, dry eyes, and confusion. Newer drugs are becoming more selective for the specific receptors in the bladder and promise fewer side effects.

  An extreme technique is to use medication in an attempt to stop all urine flow from the bladder, thus making the patient continent but requiring them to insert a catheter several times daily to drain the bladder. Medication side effects often limit the application of this type of approach.

- **Consider surgery.** Surgical techniques, including collagen injections and repair of the tissue that supports the bladder, are effective for some patients.

Kidney Stones

Kidney stones, the formation of excess calcium and other minerals in the kidneys, occur in about 3 percent of the U.S. population at some point in their lives. About 1 in 1,000 people must seek medical care each year for the management of a kidney stone. Once a patient passes a stone, there is a 15 percent risk that a second stone will be passed within one year, 35 percent within five years, and over 50 percent within ten years.

Symptoms

Kidney stone pain is not subtle. It usually occurs as a sudden, very severe pain on one side of the abdomen. Pain occurs as the stone, which has been formed in the larger fluid spaces of the kidney, tries to pass down the smaller ureter to the bladder. The location of the pain correlates with where the stone gets stuck. If this occurs higher up near the kidney, the pain is in the side. If the stone has migrated down closer to the bladder prior to getting stuck, the pain is in the lower abdomen or groin and may be confused with other types of abdominal pain such as appendicitis. This severe pain is often associated with nausea, vomiting, and sweating. Patients with symptomatic kidney stones usually must seek immediate medical attention due to the severity of their symptoms.

Treatment

The primary focus of medical therapy is to make the proper diagnosis and to provide prompt and effective pain relief. The diagnosis of a kidney stone is usually made by the history provided by the patient and the detection of blood in the urine. In addition to examining the urine, an x-ray of the abdomen may show the location and size of the stone. In 70 to 90 percent of patients (particularly those with stones 5 millimeters or smaller), the kidney stone will pass on its own and medical therapy is primarily support-ive, to control the pain and nausea.

Additional tests include the *intravenous pyelogram* (IVP) and the *spiral CT scan*. The IVP uses a contrast material that is injected in a vein and then filtered by the kidney. X-rays are then taken which detect the contrast material as it forms a silhouette of the kidney and its urine collecting system, often showing the level of obstruction by the stone (no further contrast is seen in the ureter beyond the obstructing stone). A spiral CT scan uses a very fast CT scanner to take a series of cross-sectional x-rays of the abdomen, allowing the radiologist to follow the ureters down from the kidneys to see if they are dilated or blocked.

Since the majority of stones pass spontaneously, most patients are managed without the need for hospitalization. Narcotics to relieve pain, drugs to relieve nausea, and in-structions to maintain a high fluid intake are given. The patient is given a strainer to urinate through so that if passed, the stone can be captured and analyzed. Patients who experience severe pain or nausea that is not responsive to therapy, or have evidence of an obstructing stone complicated by a urinary tract infection, are admitted to the hospital. If the urine is infected and unable to drain, the kidney can become infected and rapidly destroyed or the infection can spread through the bloodstream (this is called *sepsis*).

Several options for therapy exist for patients who are unable to pass their stones. *Lithotripsy* uses ultrasonic shock waves to shatter larger stones into smaller pieces that can be passed more easily. Urologists perform *cystoscopy*, an operative procedure in an anesthetized patient in which a flexible fiber-optic tube is inserted through the urethra into the bladder. Special devices, including baskets and probes, can be inserted through the cystoscope into the ureter to break up, collect, and remove the stones. Tiny metal tubes called *stents* can also be placed in this manner across the blockage, allowing urine flow to protect the kidney and gain time to address the stone.

Why Do Stones Form?

Several theories exist as to why kidney stones form. Urine contains high concentra-tions of certain chemicals, such as calcium oxalate and uric acid. Just as in the childhood science experiment when you kept adding sugar to water until it became supersaturated and formed crystals, crystals can form in the urine when these chemicals concentrate. Once the crystals begin, their surface attracts more of the chemical, which also crystallizes, eventually forming that most painful of rocks, the kidney stone. The theory is that due to inadequate fluid intake, dietary factors, or inherited changes in how the kidney handles these substances, their concentration grows to exceed the amount that can be kept in solution, and crystallization begins.

The urine also contains substances that inhibit the formation of stones, such as magnesium, citrate, and certain proteins. Some patients who form stones may do so because of an inadequate amount of these substances. In addition, the ability of a chemical to stay in solution depends on the pH (acid-base state) of that solution. Patients with abnormal urine pH levels, either due to kidney defects, urinary tract infections, or medication effects, may be more likely to develop certain kinds of stones.

Risk Factors

The risks for stone formation include:
- A previous history of kidney stones
- A family history of kidney stones
- A diet high in animal proteins
- A diet high in sodium
- Inadequate fluid intake, resulting in less than two to three liters of urine a day
- A diet low in calcium. No, this is not a mistake. Since most stones are made of calcium compounds, it would seem to reason that patients with diets high in calcium, or those who take calcium supplements, would have more kidney stones. In fact, studies show that just the opposite is true. It appears that when a diet is low in calcium, the intestine absorbs more oxalate instead. Oxalate in the urine binds with calcium and forms stones.
- Crohn's disease, and other diseases of the small intestine, in which more oxalate is absorbed
- Certain endocrine diseases, such as gout (uric acid stones causing severe pain in the joints) and hyperparathyroidism (excess secretion of parathyroid hormone contributing to calcium stones)

Reducing the Risk

To reduce the risk of future stones:
- Increase fluid consumption so that you produce at least $2\frac{1}{2}$ liters of urine a day. I tell my patients with a history of kidney stones that if they aren't getting up at least once a night to go to the bathroom, they are not drinking enough.
- Decrease animal protein in the diet.
- Decrease sodium in the diet.
- Include an adequate amount of calcium (1,200 to 1,500 milligrams a day, for most people) in your diet.
- Decrease oxalate consumption, including teas, dark colas, and some dark green leafy vegetables.

• Consider the following medications: Thiazide diuretics (HCTZ) to reduce urinary calcium levels, allopurinol for gout to reduce urinary uric acid, and other drugs that alter the urine pH and retard stone development.

Sexually Transmitted Diseases and Genitourinary Infections

Herpes

Herpes simplex is caused by a DNA virus with a genetic structure similar to that in our own cells. The virus is acquired through direct exposure to an infected person and enters the body through abraded skin or through mucus membranes. In most patients, two to twelve days after initial exposure, the patient develops the initial symptoms of itching, burning, and redness at the site of infection. As the epithelial cells die from the infection, they release clear fluid into the skin that classically appears as groups of small blisters on a red base. These blisters are filled with infectious herpes viruses. Flu-like symptoms may develop, lymph nodes in the region of the infection enlarge, and over two to three weeks the initial outbreak crusts over and heals.

The herpes viruses, unfortunately, do not remain just in the skin. They are transported up the nerve roots to the nucleus of the nerves in the sensory ganglia, where they are incorporated into the cell's own DNA structure. Once there, the infection cannot be eliminated and will be present life-long.

Usually, herpes is held in check by the immune system. Over the years, infected people tend to have fewer outbreaks that are less severe. It may not reappear for weeks, months, or even decades. Often, the primary infection is forgotten or may not initially have been recognized. However, if the immune system fails in its surveillance function, the herpes virus can reactivate, travel back down the nerve roots, and cause a new, painful eruption at the same exact spot as previous outbreaks. Triggers of an outbreak can include anything that alters immune function: exposure to ultraviolet light, extremes of temperature, fever, the menstrual cycle, local trauma (including cosmetic surgeries), stress and sleep deprivation, or other illness. The recurrence of herpes can be most distressing, especially when it first occurs decades after the primary infection. About twice a year, I have to carefully explain to a couple that even though they have been married, monogamous, and unaffected for decades, a herpes outbreak in one partner does not prove recent infidelity.

In the United States, one in six adults have genital herpes, and 40 to 60 percent of adults have herpes of the lips (cold sores). These two common locations of herpes are generally associated with different strains of the virus; however, cross contamination can occur. For example, a person with an active herpes sore on the lip can infect his or her partner's genitals during oral sex.

Antiviral therapy is available to suppress reproduction of the herpes virus. Therapy begun soon after an outbreak is apparent can shorten the duration of virus production and shedding, speed healing, and limit the severity of an outbreak. For patients with six or more outbreaks a year, or patients with severe physical or psychological symptoms related to outbreaks, the antiviral medications are prescribed on a daily basis. This practice of suppressive therapy reduces the frequency of viral outbreaks about 80 percent and, although expensive, is usually well tolerated. In intermittent therapy, drugs are taken at the first sign of an outbreak (tingling) or prior to an event expected to cause an outbreak (a trip to the beech or ski slopes) for a limited period of time.

Vaginitis

Vulvovaginitis means inflammation of the female genitalia. Common causes include bacterial vaginosis, candidiasis (yeast infections), trichomoniasis (a parasite), and atrophic vaginitis (from a lack of estrogen support). Vaginal pain or irritation, itching, burning, abnormal discharge, and/or odor often characterize these conditions. While trichomoniasis is sexually transmitted, the causes of other types of vaginal infections are not completely clear. Anything that affects the normal bacterial flora of the vagina can contribute, including antibiotic use, chemicals in the vagina (douching, spermicides, perfumes), and exposure to multiple sexual partners. Vaginitis requires a physical examination of the vaginal mucus to categorize it.

Bacterial vaginosis is the most common vaginal infection. It is associated with an odorous, nonirritating discharge. Itching is not a prominent feature of bacterial vaginosis. In the normal vagina, the lactobacillus bacteria predominate. These bacteria create an acidic environment that keeps down the numbers of other, more aggressive, organisms. In bacterial vaginosis, this population of helpful bacteria is lost and other types of bacteria predominate, which can create irritation, a discharge, and odor. The cause of this condition is not understood. For women with symptoms, this condition can be treated either by oral or intravaginal antibiotics. Oral therapy is less messy and more convenient, but has significantly more side effects. In about a third of women, the infection will recur after therapy.

Candidiasis refers to a yeast infection of the vagina. This infection is characterized by intense itching with little discharge. Burning may occur when urine comes into contact with the inflamed vagina. Candida infections frequently flare just before menstruation when the pH of the vagina drops. These yeast are present in the vagina of normal, healthy women. Their numbers increase under certain conditions, including shifts in vaginal flora after antibiotic use, the use of birth control pills, diabetes, and pregnancy. Although many therapies exist for this condition, none seem superior in their results but some are more convenient to use than others. Recurrence of this infection is common.

Trichomoniasis is a sexually transmitted disease caused by a protozoan parasite. It typically causes intense itching and an irritating discharge that typically worsens after menstruation. This infection requires treatment of both the patient and her sexual partner to ensure a cure.

Atrophic vaginitis is not an infection. It occurs in postmenopausal women from a lack of estrogen support to the estrogen-dependent tissues of the vagina. This leads to a thinning and dryness of the vaginal lining, with resulting burning, soreness, itching, and sensitivity of the vagina. Atrophic vaginitis is frequently associated with incontinence as the tissues supporting the bladder and urethra shrink. The additional moisture and acidic urine lead to further tissue irritation, discomfort, and infections.

Urethritis

Urethritis is an infection of the urethra (the tube draining urine from the bladder). It is characterized by pain with urination and a discharge. Urethritis is divided into that caused by a gonococcal infection (gonorrhea causes 50 percent of cases in a sexually transmitted disease clinic but only 10 percent of cases in an average doctor's office due to the different populations and sexual practices of patients seen in these settings), or other causes (nongonococcal urethritis, from chlamydia and others). Most cases of gonococcal urethritis create abrupt symptoms within four days of exposure, with painful urination and a pussy discharge. Due to the severity of symptoms, most patients seek medical attention within a few days. In contrast, nongonococcal urethritis begins gradually, with intermittent symptoms beginning several days after exposure. The discharge is milkier and patients may delay seeking assistance. The type of urethritis is diagnosed by testing samples of the discharge either by culture or DNA testing. Patients should not urinate within an hour prior to culturing for urethritis to increase the sensitivity of the testing. Urethritis readily responds to antibiotic therapy, but due to the emergence of resistant infections, follow-up testing is needed to ensure successful treatment.

Genital Warts

Genital warts are caused by a viral infection with the human papilloma virus (HPV). They appear as small growths or bumps on the genitals and surrounding areas. They are acquired by direct sexual contact with an infected person, but may not be apparent until months later. HPV lives inside infected cells; treatment involves destroying infected cells and is difficult to accomplish. Warts can return months or years after treatment. Treatment options include topical chemical compounds, some applied only by the physician, others carefully self applied by a trained patient. Laser therapy and surgical approaches are also available.

Chlamydia

Chlamydia is the most common sexually transmitted disease in the United States and other developed countries. It can infect the urethra in men and the cervix, urethra, and the upper genital tract (see *Pelvic Inflammatory Disease*, on the next page) in women. Because up to 80 percent of women and 50 percent of men do not experience any symptoms and therefore do not know they have the disease, they are more likely to infect others and spread the disease. In addition, the lack of symptoms places women at risk of upper genital tract infections as unrecognized lower tract infections progress. Those who do have symptoms report nonspecific vaginal discharges, bleeding in between periods, urethral discharge, and pain with urination. In women under 25 with more than one sexual partner, infection rates of greater than 9 percent have been found in some studies.

This has led to the recommendation for routine testing for chlamydia at the time of the Pap smear in at risk women. This disease can be effectively treated with a single dose of the antibiotic azithromycin, but follow-up testing to ensure clearance of the infection is recommended.

Pelvic Inflammatory Disease

Pelvic inflammatory disease refers to infection of the upper genital tract in women, involving the fallopian tubes, ovaries, and surrounding tissues. This disease results from an untreated infection of the lower genital tract (cervix) that migrates upwards. Gonorrhea and chlamydia are the most recognized types of infections, but the majority of pelvic inflammatory disease cases involve other and often multiple infectious organisms. Symptoms are nonspecific and include generalized abdominal pain, tenderness, and fever. Treatment requires hospitalization and intravenous antibiotics.

One-fourth of all women who have pelvic inflammatory disease will experience long-term consequences. Infertility occurs in 20 percent of women with a history of this disease. Ectopic pregnancies due to scarring in the fallopian tubes are six to ten times more common in women with a history of pelvic inflammatory disease.

CHAPTER 25

The Musculoskeletal System

T he musculoskeletal system provides the framework for support and move-ment of the body. *Bones* provide structural support. *Joints* are where two bones come together and allow for movement. Joints are designed to allow for the necessary movement at a site, while maintaining as much strength and stability as possible. Contrast the simple hinge joint movement of a finger, with limited movement

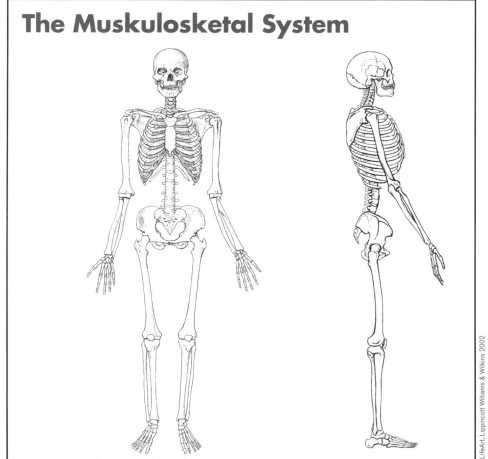

The Muskulosketal System

LifeArt, Lippincott Williams & Wilkins 2002

but great strength and stability, with the freedom of movement allowed by the ball and socket joint of the shoulder, at the price of greater instability and risk of injury. *Ligaments* are tough, fibrous bands that help hold bones together. *Tendons* are similar structures that connect muscle to bone. *Bursas* are fluid-filled sacs that are strategically positioned to allow one structure to glide smoothly over another.

Where two bones meet at a joint, the connecting surfaces of the bones are lined by *cartilage*. This is a tough but slippery substance that reduces friction during movement at the joint, easing movement and keeping the ends of the opposing bones from grinding each other down. A synovial capsule encompasses the joint space, secreting *synovial fluid* to nourish and lubricate the cartilage surface.

Exercise is crucial in maintaining the health of a joint. When the muscles and supporting structures are strong, they absorb the shock of most activity, limiting the forces at the joint surface. When muscles are weak, most of the force is transmitted directly to the joint surface, and this greater force leads to damage.

With such a variety of structures making up the musculoskeletal system, many things can go wrong. Trauma or disease can affect the bone, cartilage, ligaments, tendons, bursas, synovial apparatus, or other supporting structures. In general, those regions of the skeleton that allow for greater movement are more prone to problems. For instance, the neck and lower back are common sites of injury, while it is unusual to have trouble with the less mobile spine in the middle.

This chapter will first focus on general problems that affect the musculoskeletal system and are not restricted to a particular region of the body (arthritis, rheumatoid arthritis, gout, and fibromyalgia), then review more common problems based on body region: foot and ankle (plantar fasciitis and heel spur, bunions, and ankle sprain), knee (arthritis, irregularities in structure, tears in cartilage, ligament injuries, and bursitis), hip (bursitis and arthritis), hand and wrist (ganglion cyst, carpal tunnel syndrome, DeQuervain's tenosynovitis, and arthritis), elbow (tennis elbow, ulnar nerve entrapment, and olecranon bursitis), shoulder (fractures, dislocation, impingement syndrome, subacromial bursitis, frozen shoulder, rotator cuff tendonitis and tears, and arthritis), and spine (neck strain and arthritis, disc ruptures, lower back pain, sciatica, and costochondritis).

Comments about therapy are intentionally limited in this chapter. Most conditions need hands-on evaluation before detailed care instructions can be provided.

Generalized Problems

This section describes musculoskeletal system problems that are not specific to a particular body region.

Arthritis

Osteoarthritis develops when a healthy joint breaks down. The protective pad of cartilage degenerates, the space between the two bones of the joint narrows, microscopic cracks develop on the cartilage and bone surfaces, and irregular new bone growth may occur. This all leads to inflammation and pain within the joint. It is uncertain exactly why this happens, or how to prevent it.

Factors in the development of arthritis include both mechanical and biochemical forces involved in the destruction of cartilage. Arthritis will develop when the rate of cartilage destruction exceeds the rate at which it is rebuilt. Risk factors for the development of arthritis include previous injury, overuse, muscle weakness, and obesity. Genetics, diet, estrogen and other hormone levels, and bone density may play contributing roles.

SYMPTOMS

Arthritis most commonly occurs in the knee, hip, hand (particularly the base of the thumb), and spine. Pain occurs in and around the involved joint, or may be referred to other locations. Patients with hip arthritis (or even hip fracture) may complain primarily of knee pain, when the knee itself is fine. In addition to pain, patients may experience joint stiffness after periods of inactivity, such as after sleeping; with osteoarthritis, this stiffness should resolve in less than 30 minutes of normal morning activity. Joint instability may occur; people with knee or hip problems may experience a sensation of sudden "give-way" weakness while standing. The joints may visibly enlarge, and the range of motion of the joint decreases.

TREATMENT

The goal for therapy of osteoarthritis is to control pain and preserve or improve function while avoiding side effects from medication and other therapies. Several therapeutic options are available:

- **Vitamin D.** Vitamin D is involved in bone metabolism. Studies show that patients with lower vitamin D levels have higher rates of osteoarthritis. Studies are currently in progress to see if supplementing vitamin D will affect the future development or progression of arthritis. But be wary—excessive vitamin D intake (more than 1,000 units a day) can cause serious medical problems.
- **Vitamin C.** Vitamin C is a part of the chemical pathway for the manufacturing of collagen, an important component of cartilage. Animal studies using high-dose vitamin C supplements show reduced arthritis-related joint damage. Observational studies in humans show that individuals with the highest blood levels of vitamin C had the slowest rates of progression in their arthritis. These possible benefits must be balanced by recent studies that suggest that the routine use of greater than 500 milligrams of vitamin C daily may be associated with an increased rate of heart and other vascular disease. I advise obtaining large amounts vitamin C from fruits and vegetables and limiting supplements to no more than 500 milligrams each day.
- **Glucosamine and chondroitin sulfate.** These substances have been available since the 1960s and are a standard of care for veterinary medicine. Their use in humans for the treatment and prevention of osteoarthritis has gained recent popularity. Laboratory studies, sponsored by the manufacturers of these

products, have shown that the use of these supplements increases the production of components of cartilage and decreases the rate of breakdown of cartilage. In clinical practice, glucosamine and chondroitin do seem to reduce arthritis-related pain in some patients. Except for the suggestive results of a few preliminary studies, proof does not yet exist that these supplements prevent or decrease the rate of progression of arthritis. A large study sponsored by the National Institutes of Health is addressing this issue; results will be available in 2004. As with most supplements, the quality of glucosamine and chondroitin available to consumers is quite variable, and they are expensive agents for long-term use.

- Acetaminophen. Acetaminophen provides adequate relief for arthritis pain in many patients. At a dose of less than 4 grams a day, it is safer than aspirin or anti-inflammatory drugs and should be the initial choice for most patients with mild to moderate arthritic pain. Its use should be avoided in those with liver disease or those who routinely consume more than two alcoholic beverages a day.

- NSAIDs. Nonsteroidal anti-inflammatory drugs, such as ibuprofen, in general offer effective pain relief for arthritis patients. Numerous classes of NSAIDs exist. For reasons not well understood, individual patients vary greatly in their response, or lack of response, to different drugs within this class. Which drug to start with often is an educated guess, influenced by side effects and price. Many patients can benefit from short-term therapy and experience few side effects.

Long-term therapy can cause problems with ulcers, gastrointestinal bleeding, and liver and kidney dysfunction. Gastrointestinal bleeding is a major concern. In a study of 5,435 patients, significant bleeding occurred in 2.6 percent of patients on NSAIDs. Of those patients with bleeding, 80 percent had no warning signs; their bleeding was not predicted by indigestion or abdominal pain. Risk factors for bleeding include age greater than 60, therapy longer than one month, higher doses of drugs, the simultaneous use of prednisone or other blood thinners, and a history of previous ulcers. The risk for bleeding was not reduced by using NSAIDs with antacids or the older drugs that reduce stomach acid (H2 blockers, such as cimetidine and ranitidine) but the use of the newer acid-reducing proton pump inhibitors such as omeprazole with NSAIDs has been shown to reduce the rate of gastrointestinal bleeding.

Cox-2 Inhibitors are anti-inflammatory medications that are more selective in their action. Traditional NSAIDs are chemically activity on both Cox-1 receptors (associated with protection of the stomach from acid effects, platelet function, regulation of blood flow, and kidney function) and Cox-2 receptors (associated with the processes of inflammation, pain, and fever). Cox-2 selective inhibitors are one-half as likely to cause gastrointestinal bleeding as traditional NSAIDs. Both classes of drugs work in about 70 percent of patients to relieve the pain of arthritis. At higher doses, the current Cox-2 inhibitors begin to lose their selectivity, and gastrointestinal side effects increase. Other side effects include changes in kidney function, salt and water retention, and interference with the effects of some cardiovascular medications. Cox-2 inhibitors are expensive, and many insurance companies limit their reimbursement of them to certain medical indications or to patients who have failed a trial of the older non-selective arthritis agents due to lack of benefit or side effects experienced.

- **Topical pain relievers.** Topical pain relievers are effective for some patients with localized pain from one or a few joints. Most of these substances contain compounds that stimulate the nerves in the skin, which serves as a distraction from the joint pain. Capsaicin creams are absorbed through the skin and deplete substance P, a chemical present in small sensory nerve fibers that are necessary for the transmission of pain. Capsaicin creams must be applied routinely four times a day, take a few days to begin to work, and often stimulate the pain pathway before they begin to block it.

- **Narcotics.** Narcotics have a role in the management of arthritis pain in selected patients who either cannot tolerate, or do not benefit from, traditional therapies. When properly supervised, these medications can improve the quality of life in arthritis sufferers without creating problem addictions.

- **Steroids.** Injecting steroids into affected joints can help settle down a hotly inflamed joint and relieve the associated joint pain. These injections must be combined with other approaches, including physical therapy, to have lasting benefit. Repeated injections may damage cartilage. The repeated use of steroids in this fashion must be closely regulated by an arthritis specialist.

- **Hyaluronic acid.** Hyaluronic acid is responsible for the lubricating properties of synovial fluid. Recently, this substance has been studied and marketed for joint injection in patients with arthritis. Injection of this substance decreases inflammation within the joint and may actually stimulate the synovial lining to manufacture more of its own hyaluronate. In preliminary studies, 50 percent of patients thought that their arthritis improved after a series of five weekly injections into their knees. (38 percent of patients who received placebo injections of salt water also thought that they improved.) Significant side effects occurred in 10 percent of patients. This expensive therapy to date looks rather unimpressive; further studies are in progress.

- **Acupuncture.** Acupuncture studies for the relief of pain in arthritis patients are inconclusive but promising. Acupuncture needles stimulate larger nerves, resulting in transmitted signals to the spinal cord that confuse those signals from smaller nerves that transmit painful stimuli. This confusion apparently leads to a decreased perception of pain.

- **Magnet therapy.** Magnet therapy is a 200 million-dollar-plus industry in the United States. Promoters of magnet therapy claim that the magnets relieve pain, promote healing, and improve blood flow. The theory is that since nerves communicate sensation via electrical impulses, and magnets generate magnetic fields that can alter electrical impulse conduction, magnets may influence the pain signals transmitted in sensory nerves.

The science backing up these claims is poor. Earlier studies looked at the effects of strong magnetic fields generated by electricity pulsating through large magnetic coils and did show some influence on physical processes in the body. This data is currently being used to support the use of small magnets placed on the skin, but the application of this earlier research data to current superficial magnets is suspect. Physicists point out that the strongest magnets sold for pain relief generate only weak magnetic fields, capable of penetrating the body only 3 to 5 millimeters. This essentially limits any possible effect to the skin. Recent studies of MRI scanners, which create extremely powerful magnetic fields, show no effects on the human body. The best scientifically designed studies of magnets also do not support their benefit.

Why not try? There is probably little harm. Magnets should not be worn near pacemakers, insulin pumps, or other medical devices. They also should not be worn near drug patches, as magnetic fields can influence drug delivery from the patch. As magnetic bandages and shoe insoles age, they can wear down and chafe the skin, causing skin wounds and ulcers. Proceed with caution, and don't spend too much money.

- **Physical therapy and exercise.** Physical therapy and exercise are essential in the management of arthritis. Low-impact exercise of osteoarthritic joints does not speed the progression of the arthritis; rather, it maintains and enhances range of motion, muscle strength, and general health. Stronger muscles and supporting structures help take the load off of a joint and reduce the progression of arthritis.

- **Adaptive devices.** Adaptive devices, such as special shoes, canes, walkers, or wheelchairs, can help relieve pain. Shoes with good shock absorbing properties help. A properly used cane can reduce the amount of weight born by the opposite hip by 20 to 30 percent. (Most patients make the mistake of using the cane in the hand on the side of their problem leg. To provide the greatest assistance in walking, the cane should be placed in the opposite hand and used to bear weight simultaneously with weight bearing of the problem leg, so that the body's weight is distributed between the two.) Walkers provide stability and weight-bearing relief. The use of a wheelchair for extended distances may improve a patient's ability to negotiate shorter trips. Special training from a physical or occupational therapist can be most beneficial in maximizing current abilities.

- **Surgery.** Surgery for arthritis is indicated for moderate to severe pain and dysfunction when symptoms cannot be adequately controlled by medical therapy. Surgical options include procedures to change the alignment of a joint, arthroscopic approaches to repair cartilage tears or other mechanical symptoms, joint fusions (used for some problems in the foot, wrist, and hand), and joint replacement.

Rheumatoid Arthritis

Rheumatoid arthritis is a type of arthritis in which the immune system attacks and destroys the joint surface and other connective tissues. The concepts behind therapy for this disease are very different from those on osteoarthritis. Historically, half of the patients diagnosed with rheumatoid arthritis experience difficulty in maintaining a desired level of physical activity within five years. Half become disabled for work within 10 years and, at 15 years, two-thirds have difficulty with the activities of everyday living. Unlike in osteoarthritis, where efforts are directed toward relieving pain because current drug therapies don't affect overall disease progression, in rheumatoid arthritis it is important to institute aggressive therapy early in the course of disease to modify the progression of the disease itself. Waiting until rheumatoid arthritis causes significant disability is too late—irreparable damage to the joints has already been done.

Early symptoms that sometimes suggest the diagnosis of rheumatoid arthritis include fatigue, loss of appetite, weakness, and generalized discomfort and stiffness in addition to the joint symptoms. Involved joints—most commonly the wrist, hand, and knuckles closest to the palm—can become swollen, warm, red, and tender; patients may have difficulty making a fist and experience significant joint stiffness lasting more than 30 minutes after periods of inactivity such as sleep. Fifteen to twenty percent of patients develop nodules underneath the skin, particularly at sites subjected to pressure such as the forearms and the Achilles tendon. Other manifestations of the disease outside of joints can occur. While specific laboratory and radiographic abnormalities occur in patients with rheumatoid arthritis, the diagnosis is primarily a clinical one based on symptoms and physical exam findings; diagnosis early in the course of the disease can be difficult.

Gout

Gout is an extremely painful type of acute arthritis that usually involves one joint, typically the big toe and occasionally the ankles, knees, wrists, or elbows. The joint suddenly becomes swollen, red, and hot to the touch. The pain is of bee sting intensity, and often the joint is so sensitive that the patient can't tolerate clothing or bed sheets touching the area. Gout most commonly affects middle-aged and older men and its symptoms usually begin and peak over the first 12 to 24 hours.

CAUSE

Gout is caused by the precipitation of sodium urate crystals in the joint fluid, which are intensely irritating to the synovial lining of the joint. These crystals precipitate when their concentration becomes too high for them to remain in solution, similar to sugar precipitating at the bottom of a glass of lemonade. Uric acid levels rise in the bloodstream either from overproduction of uric acid (which can be the first signal of other serious medical problems) or lack of adequate elimination of uric acid through the kidneys. A variety of medical problems, drugs, inherited factors, and dietary indiscretions can contribute to a gout attack. For example, aspirin decreases uric acid excretion through the kidneys, and those patients who mistakenly take aspirin for their pain may prolong their gout attacks.

Gout is usually diagnosed based on clinical signs and symptoms. Although the uric acid level in the bloodstream is typically higher in those who have gout, during the acute attack itself the blood level of uric acid can be high, low, or normal—measuring it during a gout attack is not useful in making a diagnosis. As urate crystals form in the joint, the level of uric acid in the bloodstream may drop. The only way to absolutely confirm that a suddenly inflamed joint is caused by gout is to stick a needle in it, withdraw fluid, and look for crystals under the microscope. Patients aren't wild about this idea when their joint is already too painful to be touched. In most cases, only when a joint infection is being considered is it necessary to tap the fluid.

TREATMENT

Acute attacks of gout respond to nonsteroidal anti-inflammatory drugs and colchicine. Prompt relief usually begins within in the first 24 hours. For patients with infrequent attacks, all that may be needed is a readily available prescription of one of these medications for these occasional attacks. To help minimize the number of attacks, patients should avoid excessive alcohol, aspirin therapy, and other drugs that affect uric acid metabolism, such as niacin and diuretics.

For patients with frequent or severe gout attacks, tests of uric acid metabolism can be performed. To reduce the number of attacks, medicine is available to increase the elimination of uric acid by the kidneys or to decrease the production of uric acid. When one of these drugs is first started, the resultant shift in uric acid levels can actually precipitate a gout attack. For this reason, many doctors recommend that patients take colchicines or an NSAID regularly for the first month of their use until the uric acid levels stabilize.

Fibromyalgia

Fibromyalgia is a syndrome characterized by pain in muscles and tendons. Because its symptoms are nonspecific and common to many other diseases—and no single test exists to confirm or refute its diagnosis—fibromyalgia is a difficult disease to diagnose and is a frustrating condition for patient, family, and physician alike. Diagnosis is typically made solely as a result of knowing the patient's history, performing a physical examination, and excluding other possibilities. Most patients undergo a complex evaluation and see multiple physicians before the diagnosis is established.

In the United States, about 10 percent of the population reports widespread pain and 15 percent complain of chronic fatigue. Two to six percent of the population meets the criteria for fibromyalgia. It is more common in women between ages 20 to 50.

SYMPTOMS

Unlike arthritis, there is no evidence of tissue inflammation in fibromyalgia and the disease does not lead to degenerative changes in joint structure. The pain of fibromyalgia is typically described as a flu-like aching that simply doesn't go away. In the classical definition, the pain must involve both sides of the body and be present above and below the waist. It must persist for at least three months to be recognized as fibromyalgia. Soft tissue tenderness is present at points that are sensitive spots for anyone, but are tender with less force than in patients without fibromyalgia. Three-quarters of all patients with fibromyalgia experience morning stiffness lasting more than 15 minutes.

In addition to pain, patients commonly experience other symptoms such as:

- Moderate to severe fatigue, experienced by 90 percent of all patients
- Sleep disorders, including not feeling refreshed by sleep, experienced by 75 percent of all patients
- Diagnostic criteria for depression, met by 25 percent of all patients
- Complaints of difficulty concentrating and poor short-term memory
- Neurological symptoms including numbness and tingling
- Tension and migraine headaches
- Irritable bowel syndrome, with bloating, constipation, or diarrhea
- Bladder spasm and irritability
- Painful menstrual periods
- Allergy symptoms

Although no conclusive evidence exists to identify the cause of fibromyalgia's symptoms, most specialists believe that the root of the problem for fibromyalgia patients involves how their body's neurological system processes sensations. The perception of pain involves a complex interaction between sensory receptors in the skin and other tissues, the number and strength of signals they send when stimulated, and how the neurological system interprets these signals. The same touch from a loved one that is delightful on a romantic evening may be extremely annoying if you are sleep deprived or down with the flu. Likewise, for fibromyalgia patients, a sensation that others might find pleasurable or simply ignore is interpreted by the nervous system as painful. Preliminary research is focusing on chemicals responsible for the transmission of neurological messages, such as serotonin, norepinephrine, and substance P.

Fibromyalgia symptoms are generally aggravated by sleep deprivation, physical and mental fatigue, lack of physical activity, anxiety, stress, and cold or humid weather.

TREATMENT

Treatment of fibromyalgia starts with the recognition that the disease is present. The attitude and involvement of the fibromyalgia patient in his or her own disease management is the single most important determinant of success in its treatment.

Aerobic exercise is the most effective therapy for fibromyalgia. Eighty percent of fibromyalgia patients at the time of diagnosis are judged not to be physically fit. A recent 20-week study of patients with fibromyalgia divided the subjects into two groups. The first group received cardiovascular fitness training (walking, biking, water exercises, and light weights). The second group spent a similar amount of time with flexibility training (stretching, but no aerobic exercise). At the end of the 20 weeks, the exercise group significantly improved their pain threshold scores relative to the flexibility group. This makes sense. Previous studies of athletes have shown that aerobic exercise raises the levels of serotonin, norepinephrine, and the body's own steroids and opioids (narcotic-like substances).

Other therapies for fibromyalgia include:

- **Medications to reduce pain and improve sleep:**
  - Anti-inflammatory medications (NSAIDs) appear to have no major benefit in the treatment of fibromyalgia. This is consistent with the finding that inflammation does not play a major role in the pain of fibromyalgia, as it does in the pain of arthritis.
  - Tricyclic drugs (amitriptyline, doxepin, cyclobenzaprine) previously were mainstays in the treatment of depression. They have been largely replaced by more effective drugs for depression, but remain important in the treatment of chronic pain. They are given to fibromyalgia patients at lower doses, usually at bedtime, and show significant benefit in relieving sleep disturbance and modifying the pain response. Side effects are problematic and can include weight gain, dry mouth, constipation, drowsiness, urinary retention, and abnormal dreams.
- **Relaxation techniques.** Certain relaxation techniques, including controlled breathing, yoga, and other types of meditation, ease symptoms by relieving muscle tension.
- **Educational programs.** Educational programs help patients and their families understand and manage fibromyalgia. For more information about these programs, check with your local chapter of the Arthritis Foundation.
- **Alternative therapies.** As with any poorly understood chronic disease, a plethora of alternative therapies exist for the treatment of fibromyalgia. When my patients are considering these, I first ask them whether the proposed therapy could be harmful, either by keeping them from pursuing effective options for therapy or by subjecting them to procedures or chemicals ("natural supplements") with possible adverse consequences. If no harm is anticipated, I advise a scientific trial of the proposed therapy. Carefully document your symptoms at baseline in writing. Then begin therapy for an agreed upon length of time, keeping track of your symptoms. If you document significant improvement, stop the therapy to see if the original symptoms come back. If they do, resume therapy. If your symptoms again respond, you probably have a winner and should continue.

In summary, fibromyalgia is a real cause of chronic pain and fatigue. It must be dealt with like any other chronic illness. The disease is managed, not cured. Fibromyalgia does not cause deformities, is not life threatening, and rarely worsens with time. Regular aerobic exercise is the key to successful treatment, and education about the disease for both patient and family is crucial for a successful outcome.

Osteoporosis

Osteoporosis is a disease that involves bones and, as such, affects the musculoskeletal system. It is characterized by a gradual loss of bone strength and does not affect bone or joint function until the weakened bone fractures. For more information about this disease, see *Chapter 20: Glandular and Metabolic Diseases*.

Foot and Ankle Problems

On the next couple of pages, we will look at some common conditions that affect the foot and ankle.

Heel Pain (Heel Spur and Plantar Fasciitis)

Heel pain is a common problem in my practice. It can vary from a minor nuisance to a debilitating problem causing severe limitations in walking. Several problems can cause heel pain—heel spurs and plantar fasciitis are discussed below; other causes include thinning of the fat pad at the base of the heel, compression of the lateral plantar nerve in the heel, heel bone fracture (usually related to trauma or osteoporosis), tendonitis, and arthritis.

HEEL SPUR

The plantar fascia is a tough fibrous band of connective tissue that attaches to a bony prominence on the inside front portion of the heel and fans out to attach at the base of each toe. It supports the foot and helps form the arch. A *heel spur* is a bony, arthritic growth that descends down from the heel bone like a stalactite. Most patients who think that they have heel spurs actually have plantar fasciitis.

PLANTAR FASCIITIS

Plantar fasciitis is caused by the degeneration of the collagen fibers that make up the plantar fascia. This degeneration occurs when the collagen is subjected to repeated microscopic tears from activities that outpace the body's ability to repair itself. Risk factors for plantar fasciitis include age greater than 30, excessive physical activity, obesity, or a recent change from high heels to flats. When the foot is at rest (not bearing weight), the plantar fascia tightens up and shortens. This leads to exquisite pain when weight is placed on the foot and the plantar fascia stretches back out, causing the first few steps in the morning or after prolonged sitting to be the most painful. As the plantar fascia is stretched out by activity, the discomfort subsides. Excessive activity may irritate the plantar fascia further, causing pain to intensify later in the course of the day. Other activities that put tension on the plantar fascia, such as pulling the toes up or standing on tiptoe, exacerbate the pain. In contrast, the discomfort of heel spurs and most other causes of heel pain worsen with activity. The first few steps are tolerable but, as activity continues, more tissue injury and inflammation occur and pain increases.

The pain of plantar fasciitis typically lasts 6 to 18 months. Treatment requires an understanding of the cause of the condition and patience. Treatment strategies include:

- **Reduced activity level.** Reducing activities that cause excessive stress on the heel, including running and jumping, gives the plantar fascia a chance to rest, allowing time for the damaged tissue to be repaired.
- **Stretching exercises.** Stretching the heel cord and plantar fascia also reduces stress on the heel by relaxing and lengthening the involved connective tissue. Your doctor can demonstrate stretching techniques, which include placing the front part of the foot on a step and letting your weight slowly lower your heel, using a towel to form a sling around your toes and pulling them towards your body, or placing the foot behind you and leaning forward into a wall while trying to keep your heel on the ground.
- **Strengthening exercises.** Strengthen the muscles of the foot by performing exercises such as picking up marbles with your toes and placing them in a cup or placing a towel flat on the floor, anchoring it with your heel, and using your toes to scrunch it up under your foot.
- **NSAIDs.** Nonsteroidal anti-inflammatory drugs, such as ibuprofen, may speed initial relief when given as a two- to four-week course of medication.
- **Supportive devices.** Devices such as heel cups, arch supports, and splints help stabilize and protect the heel. Heel cups, inserted into your shoes for added support, are available at most sports stores and pharmacies. Arch supports should be fitted professionally. Your therapist or doctor can provide splints to keep the toes up and the heel cord extended at night.
- **Steroid injections.** Steroids injected into the base of the plantar fascia may provide limited relief but may cause the fat pad of the heel to atrophy, leading to further heel pain. Steroid injections are usually offered only after a patient has failed to respond to several weeks of the therapies described above.
- **Surgical intervention.** Surgery is usually considered only after more conservative therapy has been tried for at least 12 months and failed.

Bunions

A *bunion* is the result of arthritis at the base of the big toe, resulting in a prominence at the base of the big toe on the inside of the foot and the turning of the big toe towards the rest of the foot. In most cases, bunions are caused by shoes that have a toe box too narrow for the foot, particularly those with high heels that force the weight of the body onto the toes. This places asymmetric pressure on the cartilage of the joint at the base of the big toe, leading to its destruction and the resultant angling of the toe. Patients complain about the toe's appearance, difficulty finding comfortable shoes, and pain.

Bunions usually progress relentlessly once they develop, and efforts should be concentrated on prevention. Wear shoes that have a wider toe box. Avoid high heels. Don't sacrifice your toes, knees, and your ability to walk for fashion.

For those already developing bunions, the purchase of shoes with a wide toe box can provide some relief, as can spacers placed between the first and second toes and donut-shaped pads over the bunion itself. Arthritis medications and steroid injections typically play a very limited role. Surgery to realign or fuse the joint may be required when the ability to walk is impaired or frequent flare-ups of arthritis are occurring.

Ankle Sprain

The ankle, where the bones of the lower leg and foot meet, is a common site of injury. In addition to bearing the full weight of the body, this joint experiences many other forces which stress it front to back, side to side, and in most other conceivable directions. As with any joint, the surfaces where bones meet are lined by cartilage and are subject to damage; however, most injuries to the ankle occur to the inner (medial) and outer (lateral) ligaments that connect and hold the bones of this joint together.

An *ankle sprain* is when the ligaments are stretched or torn. This occurs most commonly when the ankle rolls in (stressing the lateral ligaments) but can occur when the ankle rolls out (stressing the medial ligaments). The risk of injury relates to several factors: previous ankle injuries and resulting instability, weak muscles, bad shoes, excessive stress (obesity or abrupt deceleration or change in direction), or inherited flaws in joint design.

Most ankle injuries will heal well if they are taken seriously. If the initial injury is ignored and not properly rehabilitated, chronic problems with ankle instability and pain may result. A *first-degree sprain* means that the ligaments are stretched but not torn. Patients are usually able to bear weight and most patients fully recover for all activities within a few weeks. A *second-degree sprain* means that the ligaments are partially torn. The ankle will swell immediately and often, within a few days, a crescent moon-shaped bruise will appear below the ankle. There is usually loss of motion and functional ability. These injuries take three to six weeks of rest, followed by rehabilitation before returning to sports. A *third-degree sprain* is a more serious tear. The patient is unable to bear weight or walk. This injury takes 8 to 12 months to heal, rehabilitation is prolonged, and occasionally surgical repair is required.

Ankle sprains are treated in three phases. The first phase is R.I.C.E.D.; this phase is begun immediately after the injury to reduce swelling and is often continued for three days.

After the proper assessment and diagnosis, the second phase of therapy begins. This phase involves bearing weight on the ankle and walking. Comfort is the best guide in how much activity is wise. Crutches, or a cane in the hand opposite the injured side, limit the force placed on the ankle until it is able to bear the full weight of the body. Stiffness often is experienced in this phase, and range of motion exercises may help relieve symptoms and speed recovery. Placing the heel on the floor and drawing imaginary numbers and letters with your big toe is a good range of motion exercise. The second phase lasts until the ankle can bear the stress of normal activity without pain.

Have You R.I.C.E.D.?

Ankle sprains are painful. To reduce the swelling and pain that accompanies an ankle sprain and help you get back on your feet, follow these steps immediately after your injury:

1. **R**est the ankle. Do not put further weight on the ankle.
2. **I**ce the ankle using crushed ice in a towel to cool the joint and minimize the initial swelling and secondary inflammation.
3. **C**ompress the ankle using an elastic bandage to further minimize the swelling.
4. **E**levate the ankle by propping it up above the level of the heart.
5. **D**ose. Drug therapy typically consists of anti-inflammatory medications to alleviate pain and reduce swelling.

The third phase involves rehabilitation exercises to gain flexibility and to strengthen muscles that support the ankle. Stretching the heel cord, working the ankle against the resistance of an elastic band, and rising up on your toes (first with both feet, then ultimately only on the injured foot) are commonly used techniques. Your physician or therapist can demonstrate safe ways to perform these maneuvers. For patients with a history of serious ankle injuries, the third phase of therapy never ends.

Knee Problems

The bone of the thigh (*femur*) and the bones of the lower leg (*tibia* and *fibula*) meet at the knee. The knee is designed as a hinge joint, with its greatest strength in movement of the lower leg forwards and backwards. It is not designed to twist. Cartilage lines the surface of the opposing bones. C-shaped pieces of cartilage (the *medial* and *lateral meniscus*) on the lower end of the joint form a cup for the rounded surface of the femur to rotate in. Strong ligaments on the sides of the knee (the *collateral ligaments*) help to stabilize the knee. Ligaments inside the knee (*anterior* and *posterior cruciate ligaments*) limit the arch of knee motion. The inner lining of the kneecap (*patella*) is covered with cartilage and slides in a groove over the front of the lower femur, providing a fulcrum in the tendon for the powerful quadriceps muscles on the front of the thigh as they attach to the lower leg. The whole apparatus is encircled by a tissue membrane (*synovial lining*) that produces a lubricating fluid for the joint. *Bursa* are additional fluid sacs that cushion key points around the joint.

Common knee problems include arthritis between the bones of the upper and lower leg, irregularities between the patella and the femur, tears of the medial or lateral meniscus cartilage, strains or tears to the supporting ligaments, inflammation of the surrounding bursal sacs or tendons, or disease of the synovial lining.

Arthritis

Arthritis of the knee occurs as the cartilage breaks down, usually from overuse and excessive wear and tear on the joint. Predisposing factors include a family history of arthritis (which may result in inherited abnormalities of the cartilage or misalignment of the joint), obesity, previous traumatic injury, or abnormal stress on the joint (excessive exercise or wearing high-heeled shoes). Often, the original knee injury may have occurred as an adolescent, leading to subtle changes in knee mechanics that then show up as arthritis 20 years later. High-heeled shoes also affect knee mechanics. This type of footwear extends the ankle, and doesn't allow it to function normally in absorbing some of the shock from walking. Thus, more force is transmitted to the front part of the knee. High heels are currently responsible for an epidemic of knee arthritis in middle-aged women. Patients with knee arthritis are typically older than 40. Pain, swelling, and a change in shape of the knee are signs of arthritis.

Abnormalities in Structure

Problems at the joint where the patella and the femur meet can occur when a patella does not tract properly in the groove on the femur. This condition often is the result of congenital abnormalities in knee structure but can be aggravated by poor muscle tone, excessive deep bending of the knee, or trauma. Patients with patellofemoral problems typically have pain in the front part of the knee, swelling, or noise with knee movement.

Tears in Cartilage

The medial and lateral meniscus in the knee are C-shaped pieces of cartilage on the lower joint surface that point toward each other, creating a cup to hold the end of the femur. Tears are usually the result of significant force on the joint or wear and tear of repetitive injuries. A meniscal tear usually appears as a loss of smooth motion in the knee, with a tendency for the knee to pop or lock up with certain movements. Smaller tears may become asymptomatic with time and proper therapy. Larger tears that interfere with joint movement often require surgery.

Ligament Injuries

Injuries to the collateral and cruciate ligaments are usually the result of direct trauma to the knee. The medial collateral ligament spans the inside of the knee joint. A direct blow to the outside of the knee joint, particularly if the foot is planted, causes the inside of the knee joint to separate, resulting in damage to the ligament. A first-degree sprain means that the ligament is stretched and irritated. A second-degree sprain implies a partial tear, and a third-degree sprain means a complete rupture of the ligament with resulting instability of the knee. Forces strong enough to damage the collateral ligaments often injure other parts of the knee, including the anterior cruciate ligament, which is frequently injured during twisting trauma to the leg. Ligament sprains are associated with acute pain and swelling. The patient may experience difficulty walking and have a sense that the knee "gives way," particularly with pivoting and twisting movements.

Bursitis

Bursitis develops from excessive friction or recurrent direct trauma to a bursa. *Prepatellar bursitis* occurs directly over the kneecap and is usually the result of direct trauma from kneeling (sometimes referred to as "milk maid's knee" to indicate occupations in which continual kneeling is common, such as flooring installers). Since this bursa is so close to the skin, it will occasionally become infected. *Anserine bursitis* occurs between the medial collateral ligament's attachment on the lower leg and tendons from thigh muscles that pass over it. This bursitis usually results from overuse such as running or walking, particularly with an improper gait.

Treatment of Knee Problems

The principles of therapy for most knee conditions are fairly similar:

- **Avoid further injury and reduce future stress on the knee.** Avoid activities such as squatting, kneeling, and pivoting maneuvers. Do not bend the knee beyond 90 degrees in exercise. Throw out those high-heeled shoes.
- **Take weight off the knee until it is ready.** Crutches are essential for serious injuries. A cane in the hand opposite the injured knee reduces weight on the injured leg. Knee braces, especially ones purchased off the shelf, usually simply serve as a knee warmer and reminder of a knee injury so that the patient doesn't attempt anything silly. Some properly designed braces can provide significant support.
- **Ice.** During the initial 48 hours of any injury, ice can reduce pain and swelling and retard the inflammatory response. For more information about icing an injury, see "Have You R.I.C.E.D.?"
- **NSAIDs.** Nonsteroidal anti-inflammatory drugs relieve pain and swelling.
- **Strengthening exercises.** Exercises to strengthen the supporting muscles, maintain range of motion, and maximize function are essential. Strong muscles splint the joint, serving as shock absorbers and minimizing the traumatic forces received by the bones, cartilage, and ligaments.
- **Surgery.** Orthopedic surgery, including an increasing number of laparoscopic techniques, plays a limited but essential role in knee health. Candidates for therapeutic surgery include patients who have a precisely identified problem that is interfering with knee health and function who can benefit from correcting it. This includes repair of significant tears in cartilage that interfere with joint function, realignment of joints to improve joint mechanics and reduce wear and tear, and partial and complete joint replacements. On the horizon are new and innovative techniques, such as cartilage transplantation.

Hip Problems

The hip is a ball-and-socket type of joint. The head of the femur is rounded like a ball and fits tightly into a cuplike cavity (*acetabulum*) in the bone of the pelvis. Cartilage covers the head of the femur, forms a horseshoe shaped ring in this cavity, and builds up the lips of the cavity to form a tight-fitting but low friction joint between the pelvis and the leg. Within a certain arch of motion, the hip moves freely. A strong, dense capsule surrounds the joint, attaching to the femur and pelvis. It is reinforced by ligaments between the two bones and is lined with a synovial membrane that secretes fluid to lubricate and nourish the joint. Further down the femur on its outside surface is a large bump of bone called the *greater trochanter*, which serves as a site of attachment for some of the strong muscles that drive hip motion. The trochanteric bursa in this region serves to allow adjacent structures to slide freely during movement.

Common hip problems include bursitis and arthritis.

Bursitis

Trochanteric bursitis is a common condition in which this bursa becomes irritated and inflamed. It is usually the result of repetitive trauma caused by excessive friction on the bursa from bending of the hip in the presence of abnormal mechanics, such as a change in gait resulting from spine or lower leg disease. Patients complain of pain over the outer portion of the thigh with walking or prolonged standing, or about sensitivity of the outside of the hip ("I can't lie on my side in bed anymore."). Treatment options include rest, anti-inflammatory medications, steroid injections, heat, stretching, and exercise. Physical therapy for trochanteric bursitis is essential to both treat the original condition and to stretch and strengthen the involved tendons to avoid recurrent bouts of bursitis.

Arthritis

Arthritis of the hip is a wear-and-tear disease characterized by loss of the cartilage lining the head of the femur and the acetabulum. Risks for arthritis include previous hip injury, obesity, a family history of hip arthritis, or an abnormal gait due to disease in the spine or leg. Patients complain of pain while bearing weight. The pain may seem to be in the hip, but commonly the pain is experienced elsewhere, such as the groin, outside of the thigh, or knee. In addition to pain, loss of range of motion in the hip and stiffness are experienced. In general, arthritis of the hip is a slowly progressive disease with intermittent flares in pain. Symptoms may respond to anti-inflammatory medications. Physical therapy is essential to maintain hip function and strengthen the muscular support of the hip to protect it and delay further deterioration. If your hip muscles are weak, all the force is transmitted to the joint. If the muscles are strong, they relieve much of the burden of day-to-day activities.

Hand and Wrist Problems

Common problems of the hand and wrist include ganglion cyst, carpal tunnel syndrome, DeQuervain's tenosynovitis, and arthritis.

Ganglion Cyst

The muscles of the forearm attach to the fingers through slender tendons. These tendons slide through sheaths, which are sleeves full of lubricating synovial fluid. If the tendon sheath develops a hole from repetitive trauma or degenerative changes, synovial fluid leaks out into the space surrounding it. The fluid is irritating to surrounding tissue and a wall develops around it, creating a *ganglion cyst*. Often the hole between the tendon sheath and the cyst remains open and fluid from the sheath continues to flow into the cyst.

Patients usually note the development of a painless lump on the back of the wrist or hand. The lump moves with the underlying tendon and rarely creates other symptoms unless it presses on an adjacent pain sensing structure.

Treatment of a ganglion cyst is optional. Occasionally, these cysts will simply resolve over time. They have been called "Bible cysts" because home remedies have included simply whacking the cyst with the heaviest book in the house, usually the Bible. This painful but effective therapy took care of the original cyst, but since the hole in the sheath was not repaired, often the cyst would recur. I don't particularly recommend this approach to my patients. Modern therapies include aspirating the fluid from the cyst with a needle and injecting steroids into it. If this fails, the cyst can be surgically removed and the defect in the tendon sheath repaired.

Carpal Tunnel Syndrome

The bones of the wrist form a tunnel through which blood vessels and nerves pass. In *carpal tunnel syndrome*, arthritis or trauma (from excessive typing, hammering, or other repetitive movements) cause the walls of this tunnel to swell and place pressure on the median nerve that passes through it. Initially, pressure on the nerve is felt as numbness or tingling in the palm and tips of the thumb and first two fingers. Pain can radiate to the wrist and up the forearm. More severe disease can lead to weakening and shrinkage of the muscles supplied by the nerve. Patients often first notice symptoms at night, awakening with numb hands. This is especially true in those who sleep with their wrists bent from tucking their hands.

Treatment involves limiting repetitive wrist motion and maintaining a wrist posture that maximizes the diameter of the carpal tunnel, thus reducing pressure on those structures within it and reducing tendencies for ongoing inflammation. Wrist splints are widely used for the purpose, particularly at night to keep the wrist open during sleep. An ergonomic review of home and office to assure proper wrist posture during keyboard and other activities is essential. Anti-inflammatory medications and steroid injections into the tunnel can be beneficial. Occasionally, surgical intervention is required if symptoms fail to respond to conservative therapy or if significant impairment of nerve function has occurred.

DeQuervain's Tenosynovitis

DeQuervain's tenosynovitis refers to inflammation of the tendons of the thumb. It is an overuse type injury that I have most frequently encountered in the mothers of new-borns, I suspect due to all the diaper changing and baby and bottle holding. "Gamer's thumb" is a similar condition seen in video game enthusiasts. With overuse, the tendons of the thumb can become inflamed from excessive friction as they pass over the wrist. This creates localized pain and swelling at the base of the thumb and wrist, and difficul-ties with gripping. Untreated, the condition can lead to scarring of the tendon and loss of motion.

Treatment centers on rest and avoiding those activities that created the problem. Splinting can be helpful in promoting rest. Ice to the tendon is quite useful to reduce pain and inflammation. Some patients respond to anti-inflammatory medications. For others, steroid injections into the tendon sheath are effective; these injections are the mainstay of orthopedic therapy for persistent cases. Occasionally, surgical intervention may be required to restore function.

Arthritis

The wrist and hand contain more than two dozen bones. Numerous synovial-lined joint surfaces among these bones allow the great dexterity and range of motion of the hands. With this many joints, and with the constant movement and stressors that they are exposed to, hand arthritis should not be surprising. Painful arthritis is particularly common at the base of the thumbs, perhaps the most common site for the development of arthritis in the body.

Symptoms of arthritis of the thumb include pain and swelling at the base of the thumb, exacerbated by movement. These symptoms tend to wax and wane over time and are treated like any other location of arthritis with rest, ice, anti-inflammatory medications, and occasionally steroid injections or surgery.

Elbow Problems

Common problems of the elbow include tennis elbow, ulnar nerve entrapment, and olecranon bursitis.

Tennis Elbow

If you feel the sides of a bent elbow, you will discover a large bump on each side. These bumps are called *epicondyles*. They are the points of attachment for the tendons of the powerful muscles of the forearm. Inflammation of these tendons is responsible for the pain of tennis elbow (*lateral epicondylitis*) and golfer's elbow (*medial epicondylitis*).

Epicondylitis is an overuse injury caused by repetitive lifting, twisting, hammering, or sports activities that require a tight grip and repeated actions. This results in microscopic tears in the tendons, which then become inflamed. Since these muscles are constantly being used in day-to-day activities, the injuries never have a chance to heal. As the degree of injury and inflammation builds, patients develop localized pain in the tendons that increases with any activity that causes the muscles attached to them to contract, such as turning a key in the door, shaking hands, or opening a door.

Treatment for epicondylitis is usually prolonged, and setbacks are common. Treatment consists of:

- **Avoiding the particular activity that aggravated the condition.** If the condition relates to a sports activity, consult a pro to see if faulty technique or improper equipment sizing is to blame.
- **Ice.** Apply ice to the epicondyle four times daily and after exercise.
- **Supportive devices.** Try a tennis elbow band, a Velcro elastic band that fits just beyond the elbow, to reduce mechanical stress on the tendons.
- **Physical therapy.** Your physician or therapist can instruct you in a series of stretching, isometric, and weight exercises to strengthen this region. This rehabilitation is important in getting relief of symptoms and is essential in avoiding recurrent difficulties.
- **Anti-inflammatory medications.** These medications are useful in the short term to treat pain and relieve inflammation.
- **Steroid injections.** Steroid injections into the elbow joint are occasionally needed for persistent cases of epicondylitis. However, they provide only temporary relief of symptoms unless combined with rehabilitation and they weaken the structure of the tendons, particularly with repeated use.

Ulnar Nerve Entrapment

The ulnar nerve passes in a groove behind the elbow and provides sensation to the outside of the forearm and the last two fingers. This nerve is easily trapped between the bone and skin, and pressure on it can lead to tingling and numbness along its course (the "funny bone"). Muscle weakness is not usually seen. This nerve injury most commonly is the result of pressure on the nerve from resting the elbow on a table, armrest, or car door ledge or console. I have seen many patients concerned that they had experienced a stroke because of numb fingers. (The brain considers the hand in regions, not as individual fingers, and strokes don't duplicate the symptoms of this nerve entrapment.) Diagnosis requires knowledge of the anatomy and recognition of symptoms. Treatment usually means avoiding reinjury of the nerve by avoiding direct pressure on the nerve or prolonged bending of the elbow. A towel splint to keep the elbow extended at night may be required. To apply a towel splint, extend the arm and wrap a bath towel centered on the elbow around it to limit bending at the elbow. Rarely, surgery may be needed to enlarge the passageway in the elbow for the nerve.

Olecranon Bursitis

The olecranon bursa is located under the tip of the elbow. When injured by excessive pressure (resting on the elbows while reading or drawing), the bursa can become inflamed. This is characterized by redness, warmth, swelling, and pain. Patients can experience the rapid development of a golf ball-sized swelling under their elbow. Treatment includes avoiding further trauma, draining the bursa, and applying pressure dressings. Because of its closeness to the skin, occasionally the olecranon bursa will become infected. This is suspected by history and confirmed by analysis of the fluid in the bursa sac.

Shoulder Problems

The shoulder joint is an amazingly versatile joint, capable of a wide range of motion while maintaining power. This versatility comes at a price. The bone surfaces of the joint, in order to allow for this great movement, are unable to provide much stability. The shoulder relies on the four rotator cuff muscles and a variety of tendons and ligaments to keep it together. These structures create a very tight joint, with little room for mishap. Because of this lack of intrinsic bony stability, the shoulder is prone to injury. It is the most frequently dislocated joint in the body.

Patients with shoulder problems usually experience pain, instability, or stiffness and loss of motion. *Fractures* are usually the result of obvious trauma. The bones of the shoulder prone to fracture include the clavicle (collarbone), scapula (shoulder blade), and humerus (bone of the upper arm). *Dislocations* occur when the bones are pulled out of their usual position; dislocations often involve tears to ligaments (connecting bone to bone) or tendons (connecting muscle to bone). A shoulder dislocation usually means that the head of the humerus has been ripped out of its sling in the shoulder, often the result of extreme force pulling the arm (a water skiing accident in which the patient lets go of the rope too late). This is most common before age 40, as the natural stiffening of tissue in the shoulder with aging results in fewer dislocations and more fractures from trauma in older patients. A direct blow to the top or side of the shoulder can separate the joint between the clavicle and the scapula (the acromioclavicular, or AC, joint). *Impingement syndrome* refers to pinching of the bursa or tendons in the shoulder between the bony structures of the shoulder blade and humerus when the arm is raised. Patients experience shoulder pain during overhead motions (can't get dishes off the top shelf or have trouble serving a tennis ball) or an inability to sleep with the arm raised above the head. *Subacromial bursitis* refers to inflammation of the bursa, or fluid sac, located over the top of the humerus. When the bursa is inflamed, it causes pain when structures move over it. This occurs when the arm is lifted to the side and rotated. The pain of bursitis can lead to decreased use of the shoulder, scarring, and loss of range of motion in the shoulder. Severe losses of motion are referred to as a *frozen shoulder*. Patients with *rotator cuff tendonitis* experience pain with reaching and evidence of impingement. Unlike the pain of bursitis, rotator cuff tendonitis pain is experienced with isometric exercise of the involved muscles (force exerted against a fixed object so that the shoulder muscles contract but no movement of the joint occurs). Tendons slide through a lubricated sleeve (the tendon sheath) as they attach muscles to bone; in tendonitis, the tendon sheath is swollen and tender, and tension on the sheath results in pain. *Rotator cuff tendon tears* occur as the result of direct trauma (a fall on an outstretched arm or vigorous pulling or pushing) or as a result of chronic impingement and inflammation. Symptoms include pain, weakness, and a sensation of popping within the shoulder during movement. *Arthritis* can occur in the shoulder and, as in any joint, is characterized by a destruction of cartilage between opposing surfaces of bone. Pain, stiffness, and progressive loss of motion are common complaints.

Many factors can contribute to the risk of shoulder injury. Overuse with repetitive overhead motions, such as in sports, assembly line work, or work around the home, seems to be the most common contributing cause. Muscle weakness leads to a less stable shoulder joint, with the brunt of force being transmitted to tendons and other joint structures rather than absorbed by the muscles. Improper technique may place excessive strain on the shoulder. Previous injuries or inherited factors may lead to a looser, less stable joint.

Courses of treatment are specific to the type of problem experienced. An examination by your physician is usually required to establish the precise diagnosis; therefore I will limit my comments to general principles of therapy:

- **Rest.** Rest is essential in the initial phases of treatment. Avoid activities that aggravate the condition by causing pain at the time of exercise, or an increase in pain later in the day, unless you are specifically instructed otherwise. However, complete immobility usually aggravates stiffness and may lead to loss of the range of motion in the shoulder. For this reason, avoid the use of slings unless medically advised and supervised.

- **Ice.** Ice relieves inflammation and swelling and is quite helpful for most painful shoulder conditions. An ice bag, a bag of frozen peas, or a commercial product such as a frozen gel pack will suffice. Place a towel next to the skin to avoid frostbite. Apply ice 30 minutes twice daily and for 15 minutes after exercise or therapy.

- **Medication.** Anti-inflammatory medications for the first few weeks after injury are helpful in reducing pain and assisting rehabilitation, and are of low risk for most patients. Short courses of steroids are also effective at minimizing inflammation. An injection of steroids into the subacromial bursa or along inflamed tendon sheaths can provide dramatic relief in selected patients.

- **Strengthening exercises.** Exercises to maintain range of motion and strengthen supporting muscles are essential to help recovery and prevent recurrence of injury. These may be provided by your doctor's office by referral to a physical therapist. In most patients, following through with an appropriate exercise program is the single most important marker for long-term recovery.

- **Surgery.** Depending on the extent of the injury, health of the patient, and desired level of physical activity, surgery may be advised for selected patients.

Spine Problems

The spine basically is a stack of bones (*vertebra*). The vertebral bones have a body and an arch, like a lopsided number eight. The bodies provide structural support and are separated by discs, which serve to cushion them and absorb shock. The arches arise from the backside of the bodies and connect to each other at facet joints. The spinal cord passes through the arches, snuggled up alongside the stack of bodies and discs. From the arches, several processes stick out, providing attachment points for ligaments and tendons and adding strength and mobility to the spine. In between each level are holes in the arches (*foramina*) through which nerves pass from the spinal cord. The greatest motion is present in the neck (*cervical spine*) and the lower back (*lumbar spine*). The mid-back (*thoracic spine*) is relatively fixed into position by the ribs and structures of the chest. As seen in the shoulder, the areas with the greatest potential for motion are also predisposed to the most injuries—the neck and the lower back.

Neck Pain

The neck is mostly muscle. Strip away the muscle and you find the equivalent of a bowling ball perched on a precarious stack of seven cervical vertebra. To keep this mass balanced, muscles are constantly at work. Quietly looking straight ahead doesn't mean that the neck is relaxed; it means that the muscles pulling it forward are balanced by an equal effort by the muscles pulling it back, and those that want to turn it to the left are balanced by their counterparts pulling to the right. This constant tension and balancing act means that most of us will experience neck pain from time to time.

NECK STRAIN

Neck strain implies a muscular injury. This is most commonly seen in a whiplash type injury. In the sudden deceleration of an automobile accident, the head is thrown forward and back, which can result in the muscles of the neck and upper back being stretched beyond their usual limits. This creates small tears within the muscle. Subsequently, swelling and some inflammation occur, triggering muscle spasm, stiffness, and pain. Whereas an arm or leg can be rested in a sling or on crutches, it is virtually impossible to fully rest the neck and upper back muscles. Injuries tend to linger and are frustrating to patient and physician alike. Patients who experience constant psychological stress have heightened muscle tone, which can both predispose to and prolong injury.

Treatment options for neck strain include:

- **Avoidance of further injury.** Help avoid further stress and injury to the neck by improving your posture.
- **Ice.** Apply ice to the neck and upper back to minimize swelling and pain initially, followed by heat and massage after the first 48 hours.
- **Stretching exercises.** Stretch the neck gently to maintain mobility. Ask your physician or therapist to provide a guide for doing these exercises.

- **Stress reduction and avoidance of sleep deprivation.** Psychological stress and sleep deprivation tense the muscles of the neck and back unnecessarily. Be aware of the contribution of these problems to your neck pain, and take measures to correct them.
- **Drug therapy.** Medications play a minor role in the treatment of neck strain. Muscle relaxants at night may improve sleep and promote healing. Anti-inflammatory medications (NSAIDs) and acetaminophen assist with pain relief. Cervical strain is not felt to have a large inflammatory component to the pain, and NSAIDs don't offer much net advantage over other types of pain medication.

Patients with persistent pain (greater than three or four weeks) should seek an appropriate medical evaluation to be certain that the cervical strain remains the most likely process causing pain. Work with a physical therapist, ultrasound, deep muscle massage, and gentle traction can also provide relief. Patients with symptoms lasting longer than six to eight weeks may benefit from referral to a pain management or rehabilitation specialist.

ARTHRITIS

Arthritis can develop in the facet joints of the cervical spine. Pain can be produced by arthritic changes in the joints themselves or from arthritic spurs of bones that poke or crush surrounding pain-sensitive structures, such as nerve roots. Arthritis in the neck accounts for 90 percent of "pinched nerves." In this condition, the nerve is unable to pass freely through its opening in the vertebra and is pinched as it exits from the spinal canal by the abnormal bone growth (spurs) or shifting alignment of the vertebrae. This pressure on the nerve root causes symptoms to develop along the course of the nerve, such as tingling, numbness, or weakness. The distribution of these symptoms helps your doctor locate the cause of the problem. For instance, irritation of the sixth cervical nerve root creates numbness on the thumb side of the forearm, weakness in bending the arm or pulling the wrist back, and the loss of a reflex in the forearm.

Initial treatment of arthritis-related pain is very similar to that employed for the treatment of acute cervical strain. In general, since nerve root irritation often involves inflammation, the use of NSAIDs or short courses of steroids proves more beneficial. Non-surgical therapy is usually successful in relieving pain and restoring function in 90 percent of patients with a pinched nerve in the neck. If the loss of nerve function is severe or progressing, a more rapid course of investigation and aggressive management may be required to preserve nerve function.

Lower Back Pain

Lower back pain is extremely common. Studies show that two-thirds of adults experience at least one episode of lower back pain, resulting in the fifth most common reason for an office visit to physicians. The cause for most lower back pain is a stretched or strained muscle (70 percent). Other causes include arthritis of the joints between spinal vertebrae, disc problems, osteoporosis-related compression fractures, and arthritic changes that encroach upon the spinal canal. Much less frequent causes of back pain include infections, cancers, and pain that the mind senses to be in the back but is actually produced from other organs in the abdomen and pelvis (prostate or kidney infection, ulcer, or aneurysm of the aorta).

Unfortunately, many types of back problems result in the same type of back pain. Thus, the initial history and examination by your doctor may be unable to pinpoint the precise cause of your pain. In addition, the use of x-rays and other imaging tests are seldom helpful in further identifying the exact cause of the pain. X-rays and MRI scans in healthy people without back symptoms commonly find abnormalities. In studies reviewed in the February 1, 2001 issue of the *New England Journal of Medicine* (Devo and Weinstein), herniated or bulging discs were found in 46 to 92 percent of healthy patients without any back complaints. Thus, it is extremely difficult to relate with certainty findings on x-ray or MRI with the patient's current pain. A ruptured disc on the MRI scan may have been there for years, having no relation to the patient's current low back strain. Plain x-rays of the spine are even less useful than MRIs and expose the patient to a significant amount of radiation, aimed directly at the ovaries and testicles. Without a clear rationale for obtaining them, x-rays, CT scans, and MRIs are at least an inconvenience and an unnecessary expense. Possible harm may arise from the radiation exposure of x-rays and CT scans and from the frequent "abnormalities" seen on those tests and MRIs, which in turn prompt additional testing and procedures to investigate often misleading test results.

Because of these and other issues, most physicians do not advise imaging tests in the initial evaluation of low back pain. Exceptions include pain associated with recent trauma, a history of osteoporosis, unexplained significant weight loss or a history of cancer, new onset incontinence (which suggests spinal cord impairment), fevers or other signs of infection, evidence of significant loss of neurological function (loss of leg strength or reflexes), severe pain radiating to the legs, or advanced age.

Fortunately, amid all this uncertainty about diagnosis and testing, there are a few reassuring facts. The overwhelming majority of cases of back pain get better on their own. Within the first week, 60 percent of back pain cases improve; within the first month, 90 percent improve. Initial therapy doesn't appear to matter much. In another study reported in 1998 in the *New England Journal of Medicine*, 321 adults with acute onset low back pain were randomly assigned to either physical therapy (40 percent), chiropractic care (40 percent), or simply given an educational book (20 percent). No difference was found in outcome at 12 weeks. Fifty percent of the patients had another episode of back pain within one year and 70 percent had another episode within two years, regardless of the initial course of treatment.

This lack of certainty in diagnosis and treatment created a fertile ground for alternative treatments of low back pain. Back adjustments, massage therapy, acupuncture, magnets, herbal treatments, and other approaches are a multi-billion dollar industry in the United States. People like hands-on care and attention, and they often report that they feel better with these therapies. However, the best scientific studies of these techniques show no or little improvements in pain, mobility, or the speed of recovery when comparing approaches to no treatment. If no risk is involved, I have no problem with my patients pursuing alternative strategies for care, but I encourage them to keep their eyes open and their hands on their wallets.

Most physicians agree upon the following points in the treatment of lower back pain:

- **Bed rest is not good.** Contrary to what I was taught in medical school, bed rest for acute lower back pain is generally a bad idea. Studies suggest that prolonged bed rest promotes stiffness and delays recovery. If bed rest helps the initial symptoms, a day or two may be a reasonable compromise. As soon as pain permits, increase activity to include gentle stretching and low-impact aerobic exercise such as walking, swimming, or biking.

- **Temperature treatments are effective.** Cold packs for the first few days can minimize pain and reduce swelling. A hot tub or heating pad set on low can help relax the powerful lower back muscles later in the course of recovery. (Warning: heating pads can cause serious burns, especially if you fall asleep while using higher settings.)

- **Anti-inflammatory medications—prescription and off the shelf—are effective for symptom relief.** Most patients tolerate these medications well and experience few side effects for the first few weeks. Muscle relaxants show variable benefit in studies of back pain. They are quite sedating, and I use them for back patients primarily at night to help promote sleep.

- **Patients should focus on proper spine positioning.** The spine is under the least amount of stress when the body is either lying down with the knees bent, standing upright with good posture, or sitting in a straight back chair. These positions either take stress off the spine or use the bony structure of the spine for support. Slouching in an easy chair maximizes strain on the muscles and ligaments that support the spine and promotes further pain and injury.

- **Formal back exercise programs are helpful to strengthen lower back muscles, improve posture, and reduce the risk of recurrent pain.** Although these programs are helpful in the long term, they are not helpful in the initial stages of back injury and should be avoided until symptoms are essentially resolved unless performed under the guidance of a physical therapist. Exercise programs for back maintenance are simple, and can be done in less than ten minutes a day. Unfortunately, most of my patients with back injuries stop paying any attention to their backs a few weeks after the pain resolves and forget all about the exercises until their next episode of pain. Bad idea!

- **Unnecessary testing or therapy risk should be avoided.** Since most back pain resolves quickly without specific therapy, you and your doctor should use caution not to pursue testing or try therapies that expose you to unnecessary risk or expense unless there are clear reasons to do so.

Healthy Habits for the Lower Back

- **Lose excess weight.** Extra fat in the abdomen creates excessive strain on the lumbar spine, often leading to poor posture and increased tension on the supporting muscles and ligaments of the lower back. Weight loss is crucial to relieve pain and prevent future injuries.
- **Maintain good posture while sitting and standing.** Your mother was right—sit up straight! The proper chair should place your knees slightly higher than your thighs. When standing, elevate one foot on a step or block; this flexes the hip, keeps the lower back from sagging forward, and allows the spinal elements to line up and function properly—reducing back strain.
- **Avoid high heels.** High-heeled shoes prevent the ankles from bending properly with standing or walking. This puts extra strain on the front of the knee—leading to premature loss of cartilage and early arthritis—and an increased forward sway in the lower back. This extra curvature transitions force in the spine from the structures designed to handle it to the supporting spinal ligaments, and wears them out.
- **Stop smoking.** Research data proves that smokers have more spinal problems and recover more slowly than nonsmokers. Most likely, this is due to the damage tobacco smoke does to the tiny arteries that supply blood to the spinal structures and to tobacco's promotion of the chemical process of oxidation within the spinal elements.
- **Sleep on a comfortable bed that doesn't lead to a stiff, painful back in the morning.** For most of us, this means a firm mattress. How firm is up to your back to decide. Lying on your side with the knees bent, or on your back with an eight-inch support under your knees, promotes a healthy resting spinal posture.
- **Be careful lifting.** Hold heavier objects close to your body, don't bend forward at the waist without bending your knees, and use the strength of your legs—not your back—when lifting. Just because you could lift it ten years ago doesn't mean you can safely lift it now; your muscles are probably weaker and your discs are drying out.
- **When performing sustained exertion, rest when you need to.** Listen to those early signals that your body provides when it is fatiguing. Use common sense.

Disc Problems

The *intervertebral discs* are the structures between the vertebral bodies in the spine. They are designed in a fashion similar to jelly-filled donuts—softest in the center (*nucleus pulposus*) and surrounded by a tougher outer shell (*annulus*). The discs act as shock absorbers and allow for the flexibility of the spine. The nucleus of the disc is liquid at birth. As a person ages, the disc begins to dry out, causing the spine to lose some of its shock-absorbing properties and flexibility. The discs degenerate and flatten out, and some height in the spinal column is lost. From a person's mid-30s to mid-50s, the weakening discs are more prone to injury and rupture. By the 60s, the discs have become worn down and tough and the risk of injury lessens. The finding of degenerating discs from an MRI in a 45-year-old person is normal.

A *ruptured disc* means that a portion of the nucleus has been pushed out from the center of the disc through the annulus, similarly to that jelly-filled donut being sat upon. If this disc portion pushes against a nerve or other pain-sensitive structure, pain is experienced. Maneuvers that increase the pressure in the spinal canal (coughing, straining, or sneezing) may aggravate the pain. Most disc ruptures will heal over time. The disc material extruded loses its water content, dries up, and shrinks—no longer putting pressure on the nerve, therefore making the pain goes away. Most patients who heal on their own will note at least some improvement within three weeks. Surgical intervention for a ruptured disc is usually delayed to see if spontaneous improvement will occur, but surgical procedures delayed more than 12 weeks after the onset of pain may be ineffective in relieving the nerve damage. Exceptions to cautious observation include large disc ruptures with signs of compromise of the nervous system, such as leg weakness, persistent numbness, or loss of bladder control or bowel function.

Sciatica

Sciatica refers to irritation of the nerve roots that exit from the base of the lumbar spine (the L5 or S1 nerve roots). Pain can be experienced along the entire distribution of this nerve, including the buttocks, outside and back of the thigh and lower leg, and outside of the foot to the toes. My patients have described the pain as a severe toothache, or as "bolts of lightning" that travel down the leg. Numbness and tingling are often experienced in the same distribution. The function of muscles supplied by these nerves can be interrupted, resulting in weakness in lifting the big toe or rising up on the toes. Maneuvers that stretch the sciatic nerve, such as sitting with the legs extended straight in front, aggravate the pain.

Causes of sciatica include any process that compresses or irritates the nerve roots at this level. A herniated disc can cause direct pressure on the nerve, or the chemical contents of the nucleus pulposus may irritate the nerve roots. Arthritic spurs, a narrowing spinal canal (*spinal stenosis*), a vertebral compression fracture, or factors outside of the spine (sitting on a too-thick wallet positioned over the nerve) are other causes of sciatica.

The proper evaluation of significant sciatica usually requires a CT scan or MRI to determine the cause. The speed with which these tests are obtained depends on the severity of the deficits in neurological function, not the degree of pain experienced by the patient.

Treatment of significant sciatica usually begins with a few days of bed rest to relieve the initial symptoms. Sitting is strictly limited; you should eat standing or lying down. Anti-inflammatory medications or a short course of oral steroids can help relieve initial symptoms related to chemical nerve irritation and swelling; muscle relaxants and pain medications may also be needed. Ice to the lower back may provide some relief. Crutches are useful while walking to limit the pressure placed on the lower spine. As you improve, more time out of bed is allowed and gentle stretching and strengthening exercises begin. Recovery requires close supervision by your doctor and therapist. Epidural steroid injections (x-ray guided injection of steroids around the nerve roots) appear to be about 50 percent effective in temporarily relieving pain. Surgical procedures are needed in only a small number of patients, typically those with progressive neurological deficits (loss of strength in the leg, or bowel or bladder control problems), large disc herniations associated with loss of muscle function or incontinence, or in patients with persistent symptoms that correlate with precise abnormalities seen on imaging procedures.

Costochondritis

Costochondritis is a common cause of chest pain, particularly in women. The first ten ribs on each side attach to the breastbone, or sternum. The section of the rib closest to the sternum is made out of cartilage, not bone. Costochondritis means inflammation of that cartilage, usually at the transition point from bone to cartilage (about a hand's width from the center of your chest). The junction between the sternum and the cartilage can also become inflamed.

Patients with costochondritis usually experience sharp pain that is increased by activities that put stress on that portion of the rib: direct pressure (tenderness to touch), twisting the chest, or a deep breath, cough or sneeze that jostles ribs in the chest wall. Most patients with this moderate to severe pain become quite concerned that something is wrong with their heart or lung. The diagnosis is suggested by the patient's history and a physical examination. It can be confirmed by making the pain transiently go away with the injection of a local anesthetic, though I have never had to do this. Since the problem involves cartilage and not bone, it does not show up on x-rays. Specialized testing, including blood work, bone scans, and other imaging procedures, is rarely helpful.

Most cases of costochondritis will resolve themselves within four to six weeks. Anti-inflammatory medications may help take the edge off the pain. Avoiding activities that stress the ribs can minimize discomfort. Occasionally, an injection of steroids at the site of pain will help relieve prolonged cases.

CHAPTER 26

Women's Health

T his chapter discusses some common health issues of interest to women: the menstrual cycle, fibroids, birth control pills, the biochemistry of estrogen, menopause, issues regarding hormone replacement therapy, premenstrual syndrome (PMS), and breast cancer screening. The issues involved in women's health topics, particularly menopause and hormone replacement therapy, are quite complex. A "one size fits all" approach to women's health issues, although the norm for many years in the United States, is no longer prudent or appropriate.

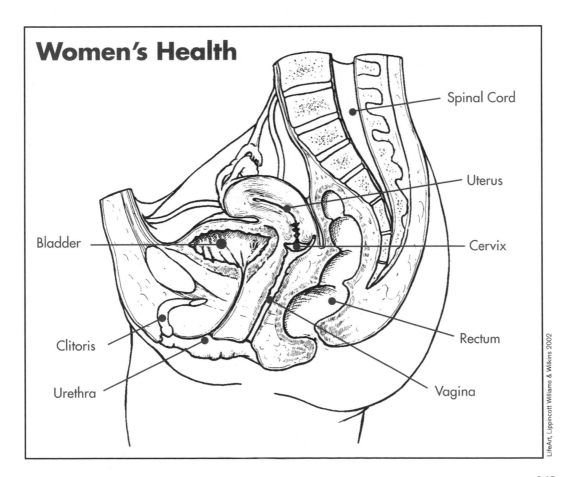

Women's Health

Spinal Cord

Uterus

Bladder

Cervix

Rectum

Clitoris

Vagina

Urethra

LifeArt, Lippincott Williams & Wilkins 2002

The Menstrual Cycle

The human menstrual cycle lasts, on average, 28 days. The cycle may shorten some-what as a woman approaches menopause. Hormones produced by the brain and ovaries, and their effects on each other, regulate the menstrual cycle. A basic understanding of how this works is useful to understand what can go wrong and how to manipulate the system to readjust it.

The hypothalamus in the brain produces Gonadotropin-Releasing Hormone (GnRH), which stimulates the pituitary gland in the brain to produce Follicle Stimulating Hor-mone (FSH) and Luteinizing Hormone (LH). Under the stimulation of FSH, several immature follicles in the ovary are stimulated to grow. These follicles are groups of cells clustering around an egg that stimulate and nurture it. For reasons not entirely clear, of the average 6 to 12 follicles stimulated during each menstrual cycle, only one or two usually make it to maturity and result in a fully developed egg.

As the follicles grow, they produce increasing amounts of estrogen. This rising amount of estrogen causes less FSH to be produced. It also stimulates the lining of the uterus to grow and become ready to accept a fertilized egg. As the follicles mature, there is a surge in estrogen production from them and levels in the bloodstream greatly increase. This is associated with a sudden surge in FSH and LH release from the pituitary gland, which leads to ovulation and preparation of the lining of the uterus to receive the egg. During ovulation, the egg ruptures from the follicle and leaves the ovary. It travels a short dis-tance through the abdominal cavity and is swept into the fallopian tube where it is transported to the uterus.

After ovulation, the levels of estrogen, FSH, and LH abruptly decline. The leftover follicle in the ovary (minus its egg) transforms into a structure called the *corpus luteum*. The corpus luteum produces progesterone and estrogen, causing the levels of these hor-mones to rise in the bloodstream again for about a week. If conception occurs, the fertilized egg leads to production of Human Chorionic Hormone (HCG), which prolongs the life of the corpus luteum and its hormone production. Otherwise, the corpus luteum begins to fail, hormone production is lost, and the lining of the uterus loses its hormonal sup-port. This lining sloughs off and menstruation occurs. As hormone levels fall, FSH begins to rise, and the cycle begins again.

I thought it was hard to describe how all those hormones interact in an understand-able fashion and looked to my wife for sympathy. Without missing a beat, she promptly replied, "You should try living it." Point taken.

Irregularities in Menstrual Cycles

Irregularities in the menstrual cycle are common and have many causes. As outlined above, the menstrual cycle involves a series of interconnected hormonal events. Irregu-larities in any of the steps, or abnormalities in the structures upon which the hormones act, can lead to changes in the menstrual cycle. Most women do not have clockwork-like menstrual cycles every 28 days. Menstrual cycle length can vary slightly from to month to month, as can the amount of menstrual flow with each cycle. If a period is skipped or significantly delayed, more time elapses for estrogen to stimulate growth in the lining of the uterus, and the next period will be heavier as this extra growth is sloughed off.

Causes of irregular menstrual bleeding:

- **Pregnancy.** The most common cause of irregular menstrual bleeding (or lack of bleeding) in women of reproductive age is pregnancy. If there is any chance of pregnancy (that is, if you have had sex in the last 9 months regardless of whatever protection was used), get a pregnancy test.
- **Hormone cycles are not yet established**. Younger girls may have irregular bleeding because their hormone cycles aren't set yet. Regular periods usually begin by a woman's 20s.
- **Physical or emotional stress.** Physical or emotional stress can affect the timing of menstrual cycles.
- **Too much exercise.** Excessive physical exercise can interfere with the hormonal cycles underlying menstruation, or a lack of sufficient body fat may interfere with adequate estrogen levels. Menstrual periods may become irregular or cease entirely.
- **Eating disorders and malnutrition.** Eating disorders, including anorexia and bulimia, can lead to a lack of menstruation, as can other causes of malnutrition.
- **Obesity.** Fat cells produce more estrogen, which may interfere with ovulation and the normal menstrual cycle.
- **Thyroid disorders.** Thyroid disorders, common in women, can affect the menstrual pattern.
- **Approaching menopause.** Women in their 40s and early 50s may experience irregularities in menstruation due to irregularities in the frequency with which their ovaries release eggs in the years leading up to menopause.

The evaluation and treatment of menstrual irregularities requires a trip to your doctor. The doctor will first take a menstrual history and ask you some general questions about your health. If you can produce a several-month calendar of your menstrual pattern, you will help your physician immeasurably in helping you. This calendar should include a record of all days of menstrual bleeding, labeled as spotting, light flow, normal flow, or heavy flow based on comparison with your usual menses. You will need a thorough physical exam, including a pelvic exam and laboratory testing to check for pregnancy, thyroid disease, anemia, and other disorders as indicated by your history. Additional testing could include ultrasound (to visualize the uterus and ovaries), an endometrial biopsy (obtained with a thin tube passed through the opening of the cervix), or fiber-optic examination of the reproductive organs through the cervix (hysteroscopy) or abdominal wall (laparoscopy).

Treatment of menstrual irregularity will obviously depend on the cause suspected. If no disorder is found, and the woman is not troubled by her irregular periods, then she may elect to simply observe her pattern over time. There is an increased risk for uterine cancer noted in some reports if periods don't occur at least every three months. A woman who goes that long without menstruating should see her gynecologist and discuss whether a menstrual period should be induced. Most causes of menstrual irregularity will respond to hormonal therapy. Thus commonly includes the use of birth control pills or cycles of progesterone.

Fibroids (Leiomyoma uteri)

Fibroids are a slang term for benign growths of bundles of smooth muscle in the uterus. We do not know why fibroids occur. They develop most commonly between the ages of 30 and 50, and are more common in black women (50 percent of those over age 30) than in white women (20 percent of those over age 30). Women who have had two or more live births are about half as likely to develop fibroids. Fibroids usually shrink after menopause unless the woman chooses to take hormone replacement therapy.

Most fibroids are not associated with any symptoms and are discovered during a routine pelvic examination. Some women experience symptoms attributed to their fibroids, including painful, heavy, or irregular bleeding, cramping, a sensation of pelvic fullness or heaviness, urinary frequency, discomfort with sexual intercourse, and low back pain. Reproductive abnormalities can occur, including infertility, spontaneous abortions, or premature onset of labor.

Fibroids are treated as follows:

- **Observation.** For a woman with asymptomatic fibroids regardless of their size, the best option may be to watch, wait, and observe over time. Previously, two arguments were given for treatment of asymptomatic fibroids: "They will grow with time anyway, and it would be easier to remove them while they are small." and "They interfere with the ability to detect uterine or ovarian cancer during your annual exams." Both of these arguments have been disproved. A study at UCLA showed no more surgical complications in women treated for large fibroids than in those treated for small ones. Besides, not all large fibroids cause symptoms, and the problem ones don't need to be addressed until they declare themselves. Second, unfortunately the routine pelvic exam has never been shown to be useful for the early detection of ovarian cancer in asymptomatic women. Screening pelvic exams looking for ovarian cancer just doesn't work, and the widespread use of ultrasounds has supplanted the clinic pelvic exam in women being checked for ovarian and uterine tumors. Remember, most fibroids decrease in size after menopause. If you are close to menopause, waiting may bring beneficial changes.
- **Symptomatic therapy.** Women with occasional pelvic pain or discomfort generally can be successfully treated with anti-inflammatory medications and other efforts for pain control. Irregular bleeding may respond to hormonal therapy.
- **Hormonal therapy.** Your gynecologist may be able to offer hormonal therapy to shrink the fibroid tumors. Estrogen blocking drugs, both in oral and injectable forms, have been used to treat problematic fibroids. Side effects, including menopausal symptoms, can be significant with these medications.

- **D&C or hysteroscopy.** D&C (dilation and curettage) and hysteroscopy are surgical procedures to evaluate for and remove fibroids. A D&C can be accomplished under local anesthesia. The cervix is dilated and a surgical instrument is passed into the uterus to scrape the lining. In a hysteroscopy, the doctor places a fiber-optic scope in the uterus to find and remove smaller fibroids. A therapeutic hysteroscopy is considered to be more sensitive and accurate than a D&C, but often requires general anesthesia.

- **Endometrial ablation.** Endometrial ablation involves the use of thermal energy or laser to remove fibroids under the lining of the uterus and destroy the remaining endometrial lining of the uterus. This procedure causes scarring of the lining of the uterus, and usually—but not always—prevents or greatly reduces further menstruation. Some of the lining of the uterus may regrow, so if the woman is of reproductive age a tubal ligation is performed at the time of an ablation to prevent the possibility of a future pregnancy in a uterus that can no longer safely support it.

- **Uterine fibroid embolization.** This procedure is performed by an Interventional Radiologist working in cooperation with your gynecologist. In this procedure, a narrow tube (catheter) is guided through the blood vessels to the arteries that supply blood to the fibroid. Those arteries are then injected with tiny plastic or sponge particles to block the flow of blood to the uterus, and thus the fibroid. Deprived of its blood flow, the fibroid shrinks. The average reduction in volume of the fibroids is about 50 percent after three months, with 78 percent to 94 percent of women reporting relief of their symptoms in the studies that are available for review. Results have only been reported in the United States since 1997; therefore, long-term follow-up data simply isn't available. The procedure seems to be safe. Patients can experience cramping, nausea, and fever related to the procedure. These symptoms can usually be controlled with medications. The recovery period is usually one to two weeks, but can take longer. In 1 percent of patients who have undergone uterine fibroid embolization, a hysterectomy has been necessary to manage complications related to the reduced blood supply to the uterus or infection.

- **Myomectomy.** This is a surgical procedure in which an incision is made through the abdominal wall to remove a fibroid and leave the pelvic organs otherwise intact. It is occasionally used to treat fibroids in younger women who still desire the ability to become pregnant. The evaluation for and performance of this surgery requires a surgeon who is experienced and skilled in this technique.

- **Hysterectomy.** This surgical procedure involves the surgical removal of the uterus and may or may not include removal of the ovaries. Historically, the treatment of fibroids accounted for about a third of the 600,000 hysterectomies performed in the United States each year, most commonly in women between the ages of 35 to 45. (Other common reasons for hysterectomy include endometriosis, uterine cancer, complications of pregnancy and delivery, and uncontrollable uterine bleeding.) In recent years, the use of hysterectomy for the treatment of fibroids has come under close scrutiny. Some studies suggested that the selection of a hysterectomy as the therapeutic response had more to do with factors other than what was most appropriate for the woman, such as physician training and abilities, physician gender, geographic location and local medical practice trends in the patient's community, and the socioeconomic status of the patient. With the development of other options for fibroid treatment and an increasing amount of education available to each woman about her options, the role of hysterectomy in the management of uterine fibroids is declining. Hysterectomy is a major surgical procedure, and is associated with a death rate of 1 to 2 per 1,000 operations in the United States. Even if a woman feels absolutely certain in her choice of a hysterectomy as her best option for treatment, she should strongly consider obtaining a second opinion before having this procedure.

Birth Control Pills

Birth control pills contain synthetic estrogens and/or progesterones at concentrations high enough to prevent the cyclic release of FSH and LH from the pituitary gland required for ovulation. They have been in use since the 1960s and are one of the most effective forms of birth control available. When used correctly, the failure rate of modern birth control pills is less than 1 in 1,000 users per year of use. The menstrual cycles of women on birth control pills are also less heavy. The pills provide less stimulation to the lining of the uterus than the normal hormonal cycle, and this lining does not grow to be as thick. Thus, there is less lining to shed during menstruation. The average menstrual flow on birth control pills is about one-eighth of the woman's previous menstrual flow.

Birth control pills were originally designed to replicate the "normal" menstrual cycle of Western societies by providing 21 days of hormones, followed by a week off of therapy during which menstruation occurs. This 12-cycle-a-year approach stuck. Actually, there is no physiological reason why a woman must menstruate each month. Worldwide, women average closer to 3 or 4 menstrual cycles a year, not 12. This includes the effects of pregnancy, prolonged breast-feeding, malnutrition, and other diseases. For many women with menstrual-related conditions (significant PMS, heavy or painful periods, and migraines associated with the menstrual cycle), doctors have long prescribed birth control pills in such a way to reduce the frequency and intensity of menstruation. The most common technique provides 12 weeks of continuous birth control pills, then 1 week off—promoting 4 menstrual periods a year instead of 12.

In general, birth control pills are safe and effective. Recent trends in birth control pills have led to the development and widespread use of pills with the lowest effective dose of hormones. This has reduced side effects, but for some women has led to breakthrough bleeding between periods, spotting, or the lack of cyclic bleeding.

The risks of birth control pills begin to rise after the age of 30, particularly in women who smoke. The bloodstream contains two chemical systems that affect blood clotting. One enables us to form a blood clot so that we don't bleed to death from a simple cut. The other system attempts to keep clots from forming in places we don't want them, such as in the blood vessels that feed the brain and the heart. Estrogens affect these systems in such a way to favor blood clotting. This leads to an increase in the relative risk for blood clots in women on birth control pills, such as blood clots in the legs (thrombophlebitis), lung (pulmonary embolism), blood vessels of the heart (myocardial infarction), or those in the brain (stroke). These occur particularly in women with inherited disorders of the blood clotting system (often unknown to them), women older than 35, and women who smoke.

Other side effects of birth control pills include elevations in blood pressure; an increased risk of gallbladder disease (but so does pregnancy); changes in how the body regulates the thyroid gland, blood sugar levels, and cholesterol metabolism; and a tenfold increase in the incidence of migraine headaches.

For a woman not on any method of birth control, the odds of pregnancy from a single act of intercourse are about 8 percent. If no birth control at all is practiced, 85 percent of sexually active women will become pregnant within one year. For most women, the risks associated with birth control pills are outweighed by the risks of pregnancy and its complications.

Benefits of birth control pills—in addition to the prevention of pregnancy—include relief of heavy, painful periods, a reduction in the rate of ovarian cancer in women who use birth control pills longer than five years, and an increase in bone density in some users.

Birth control pills are also commonly used in the perimenopausal portion of a woman's life—the five-year period around the time that menstruation ceases. Surprises do happen; 80 percent of those pregnancies that occur in a woman's 40s are unintended. In addition to effective birth control, birth control pills in the perimenopausal years offer other advantages. They help regulate the menstrual cycle, reestablishing predictability to the menstrual pattern and reducing the heavy flow that commonly occurs as menopause approaches. They also provide relief from hot flashes as the body's estrogen levels fall. Women who use birth control pills are less likely to develop ovarian and endometrial cancer and, possibly, osteoporosis. In contrast to estrogen use after menopause, no study has linked the use of birth control pills to breast cancer. Birth control pills can be used right up to the time of menopause and then transitioned over to post-menopausal estrogen replacement regimens in women who desire this therapy.

The Chemistry of Estrogens

What is estrogen? There is no single answer. Estrogen must exert its effects on a cell by binding with a receptor on the cell surface, forming a complex that is then engulfed into the cell. This complex then binds with other chemicals within the cell, which activate it as it attaches to a specific portion of the cell's DNA, turning on or off genes that regulate other cell functions.

There is no single "estrogen." Different estrogens bind to different surface receptors, creating unique complexes that may have very different effects within the cell.

Therefore, we can't look at estrogen as a single chemical. Some drugs used for estrogen replacement are composed of 10 different estrogens. Others are composed of *phytoestrogens*—chemical compounds that mimic the behavior of estrogen—derived from plants such as soy, flax, red clover, and black cohosh. Phytoestrogens are hormonally active, meaning that they, like estrogens, bind with estrogen receptors on the cells and have been shown to chemically affect cells. Also like estrogens, phytoestrogens contain the positive attributes of estrogen therapy (such as relief of the menopausal symptoms of hot flashes, mood changes, and vaginal dryness) as well as possible adverse effects (an increase in the risk of breast cancer, vascular disease, and blood clots). However, most studies of the biological effects of phytoestrogens have been limited to short-term evaluations (90 days or so), far too short to speculate the long-term effects, good or bad, from their use. Long-term trials are currently being conducted for two phytoestrogen preparations, black cohosh and red clover. Because of the lack of adequate studies evaluating the safety of phytoestrogens, I cannot medically recommend their use in the long-term management of menopausal symptoms.

Scientists have taken advantage of the fact that different tissues have different estrogen receptors to develop "selective estrogen receptor modulators" (SERMs). These chemicals bind to estrogen receptors on cells, stimulating the activity of some while blocking others so that they cannot be stimulated by the small amounts of natural estrogen that remain after menopause. Drugs in this category are currently available, and many more are being developed. The ideal SERM would stimulate those estrogen receptors responsible for estrogen's beneficial effects in the bone, brain, heart, and vaginal tissues, while blocking those estrogen receptors related to breast cancer, uterine bleeding, and blood clotting. The currently available drug raloxifene is a big step in this direction, but unfortunately still shares the risk of blood clots with traditional estrogen compounds.

Estrogen affects the body differently depending on how it enters the body. The gastrointestinal tract absorbs estrogen pills taken by mouth, and therefore the estrogen must first pass through the chemical factory of the liver before it reaches target organs. The liver can both affect, and be affected by, the estrogen. Women who smoke typically have more active enzymes in the liver that break estrogen down faster, leading to lower estrogen levels in smokers. Oral estrogen raises HDL cholesterol, a desired effect, but also raises triglycerides, which is not desired. Transdermal forms of estrogen, such as estrogen patches, deliver regulated amounts of estrogen through the skin directly into the bloodstream, bypassing the liver's activity. Transdermal forms of estrogen don't raise triglycerides as much as oral forms, but don't have the beneficial effect on HDL cholesterol either.

The effects of estrogen on a tissue depend on the estrogen receptors in that tissue. Men have few estrogen receptors and, therefore, don't benefit from estrogen therapy because their tissues can't process it. In women, the concentration of estrogen receptors in different tissues varies greatly. In the brain, estrogen receptors are concentrated in areas of the brain responsible for pain perception. In studies using rats, estrogen levels seem to modulate pain thresholds. Estrogen and serotonin levels in the brain correlate, and estrogen also affects dopamine-related neurological activity. Both serotonin and dopamine are involved in depression and other mood disorders. We are just beginning to develop an understanding of how these interactive systems work.

In summary, estrogen is a complex, multi-faceted hormone that depends upon many other factors and body processes for its activity. Just because one type of estrogen has a particular effect, it cannot be assumed that other types of estrogens will do the same thing. Published studies document significant differences in estrogen preparations in regards to breast stimulation and tenderness, as well as in the volume of menstrual bleeding. Therapeutically, this also means that women who don't tolerate one type of estrogen therapy have more options—the type of estrogen or route of administration can be changed, the dose can be regulated up or down, other hormones or medications can be added, or the therapy can simply be stopped.

Menopause and the Effects of Estrogens

My view: Menopause is a state of estrogen deficiency. There is no doubt that many women benefit from estrogen replacement therapy. The problem is that we don't know for sure how to do it safely.

Menopause refers to the end of the menstrual cycle. A woman has all of the eggs she will ever have in her ovaries at the time of her birth. When they are "used up" and the ovaries have no more remaining eggs, the possibility for pregnancy ends and estrogen production falls dramatically. Almost 5,000 women enter into menopause in the United States each day. The average age of menopause in the United States is around 51. Most women experience five to seven years of perimenopausal symptoms including irregular menstrual periods, affecting 70 percent of women, and heavy menstrual flow, affecting 20 percent.

In addition to menstrual irregularity, other common signs of menopause include hot flashes, skin changes, urogenital atrophy, and a variety of mood, sleep, cognitive, and psychological changes.

In a hot flash, the tiny blood vessels in the surface of skin suddenly dilate, and the increased blood content of the skin causes flushing (redness and warmth) and sweating. This usually occurs on the face, scalp, and front of the chest. It lasts a few minutes and is more common at night. In general, these uncomfortable events will resolve in one to two years without therapy and are fairly easily controlled with almost any type of estrogen replacement therapy.

Within the first five years of menopause, women lose about a third of the collagen content of their skin. This is due to the loss of estrogen, with a resulting relative increase in the concentration of androgens (testosterone). Collagen provides much of the support and thickness to the skin, and the loss of this amount of collagen causes the appearance of rapid skin aging—thin wrinkly skin with more visible variation in its pigmentation.

Urogenital atrophy has been labeled the most inevitable and least publicized consequence of estrogen deficiency. The vagina, surrounding tissues, and the base of the bladder have a high concentration of estrogen receptors. As estrogen levels fall, the lining of the vagina receives less hormonal support and thins. This thin tissue produces less moisture and lubrication. This can lead to pain with intercourse and more frequent infections. Eventually, the thin walls of the vagina and the shrinking of surrounding tissues don't properly support the bladder. Forty percent of postmenopausal women develop incontinence. As the lining of the vagina becomes thinner and dryer, the pH of vaginal secretions drops. This leads to a change in the type of bacteria that live in the vagina, and further increases the risk for bladder infections. By age seventy, 10 percent of women experience recurrent urinary tract infections.

Other symptoms and signs of the estrogen deficiency in menopause include dental difficulties with tooth loss due to the lack of estrogen support to the gums and teeth, insomnia, memory loss, and behavioral changes, including emotional swings and irritability. Many of my patients express unaccustomed and unwelcome variation in their emotional responses to everyday life at the time of menopause. Menopause also signals the end of childbearing years, and some women who had hoped to have children must accept the final reality that they will not.

Hormone Replacement Therapy

The use of estrogen replacement therapy began in the 1950s, primarily to reduce the discomforts of menopause discussed above. In the year 2000, between 25 and 30 percent of postmenopausal women in the United States took hormones. Many more were advised to. Studies show that after that initial trip to their doctor, 20 to 30 percent of women never filled their first prescription for estrogen, and another 50 percent stopped therapy within the first year. With the recent negative press reports about estrogen (Fall 2002), a dramatic decrease in the frequency of estrogen replacement therapy is expected.

The National Institutes of Health (NIH) established the Women's Health Initiative to address the most common causes of death, disability, and impaired quality of life in postmenopausal women. The Women's Health Initiative has been conducting an ongoing study of the effects of combining estrogen and progesterone as a hormone therapy. As I write this chapter, this study was halted based on evidence that this combination caused more harm than good. This particular study involved 161,809 postmenopausal women who were randomly given Prempro (0.625 milligrams of Premarin and 2.5 milligrams of medroxyprogesterone) or placebo (containing no hormones) and followed for an average of 5.2 years. Researchers found that this combination of estrogen and progesterone led to an increased rate of invasive breast cancer, no evidence of any prevention of heart disease, and an overall suggestion that the treatment was causing more harm than good. The chance that any single woman in the study would experience a negative effect from estrogen therapy was low, but for the group as a whole:

If 1,000 women took this hormone replacement regimen for 10 years, compared with the placebo group:

> 7 more would experience a heart attack,
> 8 more would experience a stroke,

7 more would experience a blood clot that traveled to the lungs, and

8 more would develop breast cancer.

However, some benefits were noted:

6 fewer developed colon cancer, and

5 fewer experienced hip fractures.

The study was not designed to monitor quality of life measures related to hormone replacement therapy, such as relief of hot flashes, skin changes, urogenital atrophy, and cognitive and psychological changes.

In response to this study data, the editorial in the issue of the *Journal of the American Medical Association* in which it was reported (JAMA, July 17, 2002 Vol 288, No.3) contained an uncharacteristically strongly worded statement: "Given these results, we recommend that clinicians stop prescribing this combination for long-term use" and "...do not use estrogen/progestin to prevent chronic disease."

Some physicians are cautious in interpreting the results of this study, for the following reasons:

- This arm of the study only evaluated one drug regimen. The results may or may not apply to lower doses or other forms of hormone replacement therapy.
- It is uncertain whether the estrogen or the progesterone contributed more to the effects seen. Another arm of the study, using estrogen without progesterone in women who have had a hysterectomy, was not halted and will continue until March of 2005.
- The number of events reported was quite small, and a few additional patients one way or another would have changed the findings. Data from the most recent years of the study is still incomplete. Forty percent of patients dropped out of the study before it was halted. (Researchers did look at these issues, and statistically it did not appear that they would affect study findings.)
- Most importantly, the patients enrolled in the study may have been too old to experience some of the benefits of postmenopausal estrogen replacement therapy. The average age of menopause is 51. At enrollment, patients ages 60 to 69 made up 45.3 percent of the study participants, and those ages 70 to 79 made up an additional 21.3 percent. Thomas B Clarkson, DVM, a Professor of Comparative Medicine at Wake Forest University School of Medicine in Winston Salem, North Carolina has published data from primate studies regarding hormone replacement. Hormone replacement therapy, when initiated early in the course of menopause in the primates being studied, seemed to markedly inhibit the development of heart disease. The rate of the progression of coronary artery disease in postmenopausal primates dropped 70 percent. If hormone replacement therapy was delayed until the animals were without estrogen for two years, the benefit in regards to coronary artery disease from subsequent hormone use dropped to zero. I am not aware of any human study that has looked at this question. Unfortunately, in the most scientific trial data to date (the recently reported Women's Health Initiative), the average woman in the trial appeared to be several years into menopause before estrogens

were started. If estrogens aren't started right at the time of menopause, when does it become too late to expect to see their benefits?

Most women can expect to spend at least one-third of their life after menopause. The average female life expectancy in the U.S. is 80. If a woman makes it to 65, she can reasonably expect to live another 20 years. If a woman makes it to 75, her future life expectancy approaches 90. In surveys, most women feel that they have a high likelihood of dying from breast cancer; in a Gallup poll from 1995, women estimated this risk as 40 percent when, in fact, breast cancer is the cause of death for only 4 percent of women. Cardiovascular disease (heart attack and stroke) accounts for 45 percent, more than the next 16 causes of death combined. Osteoporosis in women contributes to over 300,000 hip fractures a year in the U.S. Most of these women never regain the full ability to walk independently, and 30 percent of women with hip fractures die within 12 months, related to complications of bed rest, loss of strength and increased risk of future falls and trauma, depression and its complications, or the possibility that the hip fracture itself represented unseen deterioration in health not picked up in the comparison studies.

Previous studies show that women who take estrogen replacement therapy live longer than those who don't. Period. (Ettinger et al. *Obstetrics and Gynecology* 1996; 87:6, and others.) The how's and why's of this statement are complex and not completely understood. Let's look at some of the more controversial areas a little more closely.

Estrogen and Breast Cancer

Hormone replacement therapy and breast cancer is a confusing topic that is rife with misinformation, often supplied from well-meaning but prejudiced sources on both sides of the argument. An editorial from The North American Menopause Society (www.menopause.org) summarized that of all the published reports, 75 percent showed no estrogen-related increase in breast cancer risk, while 25 percent found an increased risk. Studies of young women on birth control pills, which contain a much higher amount of hormones than those currently used for estrogen replacement therapy, show no increase in the incidence of breast cancer after 15 or greater years of use. Several studies—including the Iowa Women's Health Study and eight other studies reported between 1976 and 1997—show that women who do develop breast cancer while on estrogen replacement therapy are less likely to die as a result of this cancer than women diagnosed with breast cancer who have not been taking hormones. This may be attributed to the earlier detection of cancers found during the more frequent mammographies and physician visits that women who take hormones are encouraged to have. Cancers detected earlier often have remained more localized, with a better outcome from cancer therapies. There are also different types of breast cancers. Breast cancers can be categorized based on their microscopic characteristics into many different types. The most common cancers are *tubular carcinomas* and *ductal carcinomas*. Women on postmenopausal estrogens appear to be diagnosed more frequently with tubular breast cancers, which are not as lethal as ductal cancers. It has been hypothesized that the extra estrogen doesn't cause these tubular cancers but does promote the growth rate of tubular cancers that do occur so that they are discovered and treated years earlier than they would otherwise have been detected.

In general, I believe that since so many smart people can so vehemently disagree about the relationship between breast cancer and estrogen replacement therapy that the influence of this therapy, if it exists, must be very small and subject to influence by many other variables unique to each woman who considers it.

A study reported in the February 2000 issue of the *Journal of the American Medical Association* shed a little light and much more heat on this issue. This study observed 46,355 women and reported the development of 2,082 incidences of cancers in these women between 1980 and 1995. Those who took estrogen had an increased risk of breast cancer, and those who took estrogen and progesterone in cycles had the greatest increase in risk. Analysis of the data showed that this risk was confined to slender women (those with a body mass index of less than 24.4). Other hormones produced in the body are converted in fatty tissue to estrogens, and those patients with a body mass index of greater than 24.4 may produce enough of their own estrogens to negate the effects of supplemental estrogens. Other facts about the study are important. Over the 15-year period of observation, the risk of cancer was only increased in those women who had taken estrogen within the four years prior to their cancer diagnosis. After four years, the rates of breast cancer diagnosis dropped to be equal to similar women who never took estrogen. This doesn't make biological sense. Like other carcinogens, if estrogen caused breast cancer the effect should remain long after the estrogen is stopped, and it doesn't.

Estrogen and Heart Disease

Over 20 studies show an average reduction in cardiac events (heart attacks and deaths from heart disease) of greater than 40 percent in postmenopausal women who take estrogens. Included in this data is the Nurses Health Study, involving 32,046 women from 1982 through 1992, which showed a 50 percent lower risk of heart disease in women who chose to take estrogens. These older studies simply observed what happened to subjects relative to the choices they made. The argument about the conclusion that estrogen reduces the incidence of heart disease centers on whether the noted benefit was due to actually taking the estrogen, or whether there were original differences in women who chose to take estrogen, that affected the outcome. To answer this question, two prospective trials of estrogen replacement therapy in postmenopausal women were launched. In a prospective trial, subjects are divided into two groups that are as similar as possible. The subjects in one group are given a therapy and followed over time to see how this intervention changes, or doesn't change, their health outcome. One of these two trials, the Heart and Estrogen/Progestin Replacement Study (HERS), looked at whether hormone replacement therapy will prevent new cardiac events in women who already have coronary artery disease. The other trial, one of the studies conducted as part of the Women's Health Initiative, looked at the same question in women who have never had heart problems.

The HERS study assigned women with known coronary disease to either take or not take hormone replacement therapy. This study, stopped after four and a half years, reported no benefit for these women from the use of estrogens. However, a year-by-year analysis of the data suggests a different story. In the first year of the study, the women who received estrogen did worse than those who did not—that is, they had more cardiac events. In the second and third years of the study, the groups were about equal. In the fourth year and beyond, the women who received estrogens did better, with fewer cardiac events. The interpretation of this study that I favor is that women fared worse in the first year because of the effects of estrogen on increasing the formation of blood clots that, in diseased coronary arteries, leads to angina and heart attacks. For these women, the protective benefits of estrogen therapy began to show up after this first year and the outcome of women taking hormones steadily improved with time. This theoretically makes sense, based on the known effects of estrogen:

- Estrogens increase the level of healthy HDL cholesterol (7.3 percent in the Women's Health Initiative data).
- Estrogens decrease the level of LDL cholesterol (12.7 percent) and Lipoprotein A, which correlate to the risk of heart disease.
- Estrogen compounds act as strong antioxidants, which are felt to reduce the risk for cardiovascular disease.
- In experimental animals, estrogens have been shown to reduce the rate of development of atherosclerosis, decrease the amount of cholesterol deposited in the walls of arteries, increase blood flow through the coronary arteries, and prevent spasm of arteries at sites of cholesterol build-up. All of these effects make sense as a mechanism in which estrogen is good for the heart.

Showing that an effect is biologically plausible does not guarantee that benefits will be seen. We need experimental proof that medical theories are correct when actually applied to people The Women's Health Initiative data provided the second set of evidence to question the belief that estrogens provide a beneficial effect in regards to heart disease. The early data from the Women's Health Initiative showed that the elevated risk for cardiovascular disease was largely limited to the first year of therapy, a similar finding to the HERS data. However, unlike the HERS study, the Women's Health Initiative found no trend toward cardiovascular benefit in later years. This may have been due to the age of the participants in the Women's Health Initiative as discussed previously. Before we draw final conclusions from this study, I would caution that not all of the data from the later years of the Women's Health Initiative study is currently available to evaluate. In addition, although the portion of the study that tests a combination of estrogen and progestin has been discontinued, the study will continue to test the effects of estrogen only until 2005 and therefore will continue to collect data that may or may not reveal estrogen's benefits on cardiovascular health.

Based on available data, it would not be wise to take long-term postmenopausal hormone replacement therapy solely to prevent heart disease. Any woman with a history of heart disease should definitely not initiate postmenopausal hormone replacement therapy for the purpose of preventing future heart problems.

Who Shouldn't Take Estrogen Replacement Therapy...

If you have any of the following conditions, you should not seek estrogen replacement therapy:

- Undiagnosed vaginal bleeding
- Current cancer of the breast or uterus
- Current disease of the liver
- Uncontrolled hypertension
- A recent history of blood clots in the legs (deep venous thrombosis) or lungs (pulmonary emboli)
- A history of cardiovascular disease (heart attack or stroke)
- Pregnancy

Irregular vaginal bleeding is a common feature of menopause and must be evaluated before hormone replacement therapy is begun. The cause can range from fluctuations in hormone levels to cancer of the lining of the uterus (endometrium). In addition to taking a history and performing an examination, evaluation can include an ultrasound evaluation of the thickness of the lining of the endometrium and an endometrial biopsy (performed in a similar fashion to a Pap smear but with a longer sampling device).

Some cancers of the breast, and most cancers of the uterus, are stimulated by estrogen. Whether a woman with a remote history of breast cancer can ever take estrogens is a subject for debate. Estrogen alone given to a woman with a uterus increases the risk of endometrial cancer by a factor of 5, though usually it is associated with a type of endometrial cancer that has a high cure rate. Because of this stimulation of the endometrium, women who have not had a hysterectomy must take estrogens in combination with a progesterone hormone to protect their uterus. The addition of progesterone actually drops the risk of endometrial cancer to less than that of a postmenopausal woman taking no hormones. The synthetic estrogen receptor modulators, or SERMs, don't stimulate the lining of the uterus at all and may make these issues irrelevant.

Estrogen, particularly taken by mouth, affects the metabolic functions of liver cells in a variety of ways, stimulating some activities and suppressing others. This form of estrogen must be used with judgment and caution in those with chronic liver disease and should not be used in women with active, unstable liver disease.

Estrogens at higher doses in birth control pills are associated with an increase in blood pressure. Several studies have been conducted to look for the same effect from post-menopausal estrogen replacement therapies. Well-designed trials have shown no significant increase in blood pressure from standard doses of estrogens in post-menopausal hormone replacement regimens. The Women's Health Initiative noted only a one-point rise in blood pressure in women who took the combination estrogen/progestin supplement. Once hypertension is controlled, replacement therapy is felt safe and possibly beneficial.

Estrogens do affect the blood clotting mechanisms, creating changes in blood vessels, blood flow, and the chemical systems that the body uses to both create and dissolve blood clots. The use of estrogens in birth control pills and hormone replacement therapy does increase the risk of blood clot formation, especially in women who have common inherited disorders of their blood clotting systems and in women who smoke.

Finally, pregnancies do occur in women in the perimenopausal years. The absence of menstruation does not prove menopause. Pregnancy must be considered before hormone replacement therapy is begun.

Other conditions that warrant caution in the use of estrogens include gallbladder disease, fibrocystic disease of the breasts, endometriosis, and migraine headaches.

...And Who Might Benefit from Estrogen Replacement Therapy

The FDA has approved estrogen replacement therapy to treat the following three conditions:

- Hot flashes (see *Menopause and the Effects of Estrogens* on page 273)
- Genitourinary changes (see *Menopause and the Effects of Estrogens* on page 273)
- The treatment and prevention of osteoporosis (see *Chapter 20: Glandular and Metabolic Diseases*)

Although not yet approved by the FDA, studies have also shown estrogen replacement therapy to be related to decreased risk of colon cancer, dementia, macular degeneration, and collagen loss. Estrogen has also been found helpful in relieving symptoms of nervousness, irritability, anxiety, and depression.

COLON CANCER

Multiple studies, including the recently published Women's Health Initiative, suggest that estrogen use reduces the risk of colon cancer by a third. In support of these findings, the rate of colon cancer deaths in women has dropped by 30 percent in the last 30 years, while the rate in men has only fallen by 7 percent. This coincides with the widespread use of postmenopausal estrogen therapy. Estrogens do affect bile acid production, which is felt to play a role in the development of colon cancer.

DEMENTIA

Studies suggest that women who take estrogens have a reduced rate of dementia, including Alzheimer's disease. However, a recent study published in the February 2000 issue of the *Journal of the American Medical Association* found no benefit to administering estrogens to women who already have Alzheimer's disease. It appears that, if there is a benefit, long-term therapy begun at the onset of menopause may be required.

MACULAR DEGENERATION

One study has shown a decrease in the incidence of age-related macular degeneration in women on estrogen replacement therapy.

SKIN ELASTICITY

After menopause, the skin experiences a generalized thinning and a loss of elasticity, with studies showing a measurable decrease in skin thickness and collagen content.

Studies demonstrate that women who use supplemental estrogens after menopause don't lose this degree of collagen and those postmenopausal women who initially did not take estrogens and experienced skin deterioration will experience an increase in the collagen content and thickness of their skin once they start them. In addition to the cosmetic benefits of thicker, healthier looking skin, it provides better protection from infections and trauma and faster healing of wounds that do occur.

UROGENITAL ATROPHY

Women have reported feeling relief from urogenital atrophy when estrogen therapy is administered systemically (using a pill or patch) or applied topically in the vagina. However, treatment may take months before a benefit is seen.

PSYCHOLOGICAL SYMPTOMS

Menopause is associated with an increase in the reporting of psychological symptoms by women, including nervousness, irritability, anxiety, and depression. Menopause usually occurs at a time of transition in many facets of a woman's family, social, and professional life. Times of transition are usually times of stress, and all psychological symptoms are not hormone related. However, several good studies have shown a benefit from estrogen therapy for mood and cognitive complaints in postmenopausal women.

The Estrogen Controversy: What's a Woman to do Now?

Women have legitimate questions about the relative risks and benefits of using estrogen during menopause. I use the following guidelines in my discussions with my patients wrestling with this issue:

- If obvious personal risks for the use of estrogens are present, I point them out. Women at higher risk include those with a personal or significant family history of blood clots or estrogen-dependent cancers of the breast or uterus, those with an established history of heart disease or multiple risk factors for heart disease, those with liver disease, and those with poorly controlled hypertension.
- I dentify women who are more likely to benefit from estrogen replacement: women who have—or are at high risk of developing—osteoporosis, women who are already having trouble with hot flashes or vaginal atrophy, women at the beginning of menopause who are concerned with a family history of heart disease or Alzheimer's disease later in life, or women experiencing significant psychological symptoms from declining estrogen levels.
- I communicate my three educated biases:
  — Except for the risk of medical problems related to blood clotting, estrogens seem pretty safe for the first five years of menopause. Breast cancer risks seem to take a longer exposure to estrogen to become significant.
  — Urogenital atrophy can be prevented or adequately treated with low-dose topical estrogens. This issue should be part of every woman's discussion with her physician at the time of menopause.

— Most women who have been taking estrogens longer than five to ten years, and who no longer experience hot flashes, are probably better off on a synthetic estrogen receptor modulator such as raloxifene coupled with topical vaginal estrogen therapy.

- I support my patient in her decision.
- If she chooses not to take estrogens, I arrange for a baseline bone density and plan a follow-up study in two years to screen for this condition. I also ask her to make sure she includes adequate calcium in her diet and coach her on the use of calcium supplements if she needs them. Lastly, I aggressively treat other risk factors she may have for atherosclerosis, such as hypertension and cholestcrol.
- All women are advised about the importance of regular physical activity in maintaining health. The ideal regimen would include at least 30 minutes of aerobically based exercise on most days, flexibility training, and weight training two days a week. Physical activity helps manage the physical and psychological symptoms of menopause. Exercise reduces the risk of heart disease and osteoporosis and combats the tendency for abdominal fat gain after menopause, and weight training has been shown to reduce the risk of injury from falls.

In summary, the use of estrogen replacement therapy after menopause is a personal decision to be made by each woman after consultation with her physician and other sources of health information. The decision must take into account each woman's individual risks and chances of benefit from postmenopausal hormones, as well as her personal fears and desires.

Premenstrual Syndrome

Premenstrual syndrome (PMS) was originally defined in 1983 as a cluster of mood, behavioral, and physical symptoms that have a regular, cyclical relationship to the time preceding menses. To meet the definition of PMS, the symptoms must be present in most if not all cycles, end by the end of menstruation, and be separated by a period of at least one symptom-free week.

PMS is most common in women between the ages of 30 and 40. It tends to worsen with age and ends at the time of menopause. Of all women, 75 percent report some menstrual-related symptoms, but only 3 to 5 percent have symptoms severe enough to interfere with daily functioning.

Bodily symptoms may include breast tenderness, bloating, weight gain, fluid retention with swelling of the extremities, headaches, fatigue, and pain in muscles and joints. Brain-related symptoms include irritability (anger, a short fuse, outbursts), depression, anxiety, crying spells, difficulty in concentrating, indecision and impulsivity, and changes in sleep patterns, appetite, or libido. These symptoms obviously can have a significant impact on the quality of life.

Many theories exist for the cause of PMS. Recent studies have concentrated on the interactions of estrogen and serotonin, a neurotransmitter in the brain involved in other mood disorders such as depression and anxiety. The evaluation of PMS primarily involves listening to the patient. It is important to rule out other medical or psychological diseases that can exist simultaneously with, or masquerade as, PMS. The most common of these are depression and thyroid disease.

Treatment options abound. Non-chemical treatments include:

- **Education.** Understanding the symptoms and patterns of PMS allows for women to plan accordingly to address them.
- **Aerobic exercise.** Studies show that regular exercise improves mood and reduces fluid retention.
- **Dietary modifications.** Increasing complex carbohydrates improves mood, reduces food cravings, and raises serotonin levels. Diets that eliminate refined sugar, salt, all sources of caffeine, and alcohol have been noted to help.

Chemical treatments are also available:

- **Calcium.** A study from Columbia showed that women who consumed 1,200 milligrams of calcium a day reported a 50 percent reduction in PMS symptoms, usually noticed within two to three menstrual cycles of beginning therapy.
- **Magnesium supplements.** Magnesium supplements are reported to reduce headaches, fluid retention, and improve mood.
- **Natural progesterone.** Natural progesterone is widely used for PMS, but controlled scientific studies do not support claims of its benefit.
- **Vitamin E.** Vitamin E has a role in reducing breast tenderness.
- **Aspirin and NSAIDs.** Prostaglandin inhibitors, including aspirin and NSAIDs (nonsteroidal anti-inflammatory drugs) such as ibuprofen or naproxen, reduce cramps, menstrual flow, breast tenderness, headaches, and generalized discomfort.
- **Diuretics.** Spironolactone, a diuretic, given regularly two weeks before each menses, can reduce water retention, breast tenderness, and weight gain.
- **Antidepressants.** The SSRI class of antidepressants helps relieve the associated mood changes of anxiety and depression.
- **Benzodiazepines.** Benzodiazepines can help relieve anxiety and irritability, but can become addictive and have other side effects including excessive sedation.
- **Nutritional Supplements.** Some nutritional supplements have been touted to help with the mood changes of PMS; however, these supplements have undergone little scientific testing.
- **Birth control pills.** Birth control pills and other hormonal manipulations can help with the physical symptoms of PMS, but have less effect on the mood changes.

Breast Cancer Screening

Breast cancer is a frightening topic. Statistics from the National Cancer Institute tell us that one in eight women in the United States will develop breast cancer at some point in her lifetime. However, breast cancer is the cause of death for only 4 percent of women in the United States. This tells us that most women who develop breast cancer do not die of the disease—in fact, 70 percent of women diagnosed with breast cancer will survive it.

An increased rate of breast cancer is associated with the following characteristics:

- A personal history of a previous breast cancer
- Age greater than 50 (two-thirds of all cancers)
- A mother, sister, or daughter with breast cancer
- Early age at onset of menstrual periods
- No children, or first child after the age of 30
- Late menopause
- The use of estrogen replacement therapy after menopause
- Alcohol use
- Smoking
- Obesity

Despite these identified "risk factors", most women diagnosed with breast cancer do not have any identifiable risks for breast cancer. Thus, routine screening to detect breast cancer is important for all women. The two major screening tools are the self-breast examination and the mammogram.

The Breast Self-Exam

Breast cancer is an abnormal tissue growth within the breast. Since the cancer is structurally different from the surrounding breast tissue, it has different physical properties that can be seen, felt, or detected by specialized testing. The breast self-exam is an important part of any screening program.

Women should perform breast self-exams every month, beginning at age 20. Ideally, the exam should be performed about one week after the menstrual period when hormone related swelling and tenderness is at its least. However, any system that fosters regular exams is acceptable. I have some women use the monthly power bill as a reminder to do the exams; others use their pet's monthly heartworm medicine as a reminder—whatever works for you.

The exam begins with an inspection. Look in the mirror for changes in breast symmetry, dimpling or puckering of the breast, or changes in the nipple such as inflammation on the surface or changes in its shape or prominence. Place your hands on your hips and push in while inspecting, then repeat the process with the arms raised above your head.

The most sensitive way to examine the breast tissue is to begin at the edge of the breast, and slowly move your hand in a spiral covering all the breast tissue to the nipple. To detect lumps in the breast tissue, it is best to use the flat part of the ends of the fingers, not the fingertips. It is also important to perform the exam in two positions to bring out or emphasize different parts of the breast. Standing up in the shower followed by lying down on the bed are two complementary techniques. Moist breasts with a little liquid soap or oil on the fingers helps to increase the sensitivity of the exam. Squeezing the nipple to look for discharge or blood finishes the exam.

Not comfortable with your technique? Most women aren't. They complain that their breasts are lumpy and bumpy anyway, and don't think that they can find anything. Just keep trying. After a few months you will at least be familiar with the normal variation in your breasts and more likely to pick up a change if one occurs. In addition to your self-exams, schedule an examination with your physician annually.

Mammograms

I frequently hear from my patients that they have read an opinion that mammograms aren't any good. This is nonsense. While mammography isn't a perfect test, it's the best we have right now for large-scale screening. The sensitivity of mammography for detecting a breast cancer is 80 to 90 percent. It is capable of detecting breast cancer-related distortions in the architecture of the breasts long before they are big enough to feel. The best proof of the benefit of mammograms comes from a study published in the August 1, 2002 issue of the journal *Cancer*. One-third of the women in Sweden were followed in a scientific study that lasted for decades. Those women who had an annual mammogram throughout the study period had a 45 percent reduction in the death rate from breast cancer compared to those women who did not obtain regular mammograms.

PREPARING FOR A MAMMOGRAM

Following are some guidelines for preparing for your mammogram:

- Schedule your visit seven to ten days after the start of your menstrual period when the breasts are least tender.
- Don't apply any body powder, cream, deodorant, or lotion to the chest—these may contain substances that show up on the mammogram as abnormal findings.
- Wear comfortable clothes; a two-piece outfit where you can remove the top works nicely.
- Research your mammography center. Seek a breast center that has been certified by the FDA (check www.fda.gov/cdrh/mammography/certified/html for a local list). Centers where radiologists who specialize in mammograms and read large numbers of them are the best. The centers I recommend have two radiologists who specialize in mammography read each film independently and then compare notes.

MAMMOGRAM RESULTS

Mammograms aren't perfect. They can suggest a problem when one doesn't exist (a "false positive"), or miss a problem when one was present (a "false negative"). A screening mammogram is done when no problem is expected. A diagnostic mammogram is done to investigate abnormal findings in the breast, such as a lump or pain. Diagnostic studies take longer, involve more views of the breast tissue, and often are combined with ultrasounds to better image the area of concern. To get the clearest views of the breast tissue with the least amount of radiation, the mammography technician must compress it between two plastic plates prior to taking the film. This is commonly done from two angles: side-to-side and top-to-bottom.

About 10 percent of screening mammograms lead to call backs for additional views. Ninety percent of these additional views look fine, and no further testing is needed. In 8 to 10 percent of patients who require additional views, an abnormality remains that requires further investigation with a biopsy. Eighty percent of these biopsies are benign; they do not show cancer. This works out to 1 or 2 cancers discovered per 1,000 mammograms.

Other Breast Evaluation Techniques

Other techniques used for evaluating and detecting abnormalities of the breasts include:

- **Breast ultrasound** uses high-frequency sound waves that penetrate the skin and bounce off internal structures, resulting in acoustic shadows of the architecture of these internal structures. No breast compression is usually needed. Jelly is placed on the skin to improve the transmission of the sound waves from the ultrasound probe. This technique is utilized primarily to determine if breast lumps felt or seen on mammogram are fluid filled cysts or solid.
- **Digital mammography** is a technique similar to traditional mammograms except that instead of x-ray film, a digital image of the breast is stored by computer. This developing technique allows the radiologist to fine-tune the image on the computer, adjusting the contrast to bring out any suspicious areas. Hopefully, this technique will increase the accuracy of mammography and reduce the need to take additional views of the breast, thus reducing the total exposure of the breast to radiation and eliminating the panic that usually occurs when the phone call requesting that a woman return for additional pictures is received.
- **Magnetic Resonant Imaging (MRI)** uses magnetic fields and their interactions with body tissues to create images of the breasts. The patient is placed in a magnetic field. The protons in the water and fat of their tissues become magnetized and align themselves with the magnetic field. A radio wave is then pulsed through the tissue, which tips the protons out of alignment, causing them to give off a radio wave that is measured as a signal. Contrast agents, such as the slightly magnetic atom gadolinium, are used to highlight blood vessels. MRIs are very sensitive in the detection of breast cancer, picking up tumors not detectable by other techniques. However, they are prohibitively expensive to use as a large-scale screening technique. MRIs currently are used in some patients with known breast cancer to clarify the extent of disease involvement in making plans for breast cancer therapy. Most patients do not need and would not benefit from an MRI test if the information being sought is available from other common assessment tools.
- **PET scanning** looks at the metabolic rate of tissues in the body. A small amount of a radioactive tracer is attached to a sugar molecule. This sugar is then injected into the patient's vein, and the body is scanned to see where the chemical accumulates. Cancerous tissues are generally more metabolically active than other tissues in the body, and the cancer and its metastases "light up" on the scan. This test can be used

in patients with known breast cancer to monitor the response to therapy and look for metastases. It is primarily useful in patients who are otherwise difficult to assess due to previous surgery, scarring, radiation therapy, or breast implants.

- **Genetic testing** is being developed as a tool in the detection of many cancers. Two genes, BRCA-1 and BRCA-2, have been identified where a mutation in the normal gene has been linked to an increased risk for breast cancer. Each person has two copies of each of these genes, one received from the mother and one from the father. If testing shows evidence of a mutation in a BRCA gene, that patient has a 50 percent to 87 percent chance of developing breast cancer. However, if the patient has a strong family history of breast cancer (multiple women in the family were diagnosed with breast cancer before the age of 50) and the BRCA gene test is negative, the negative test is really not regarded as reassuring. There are probably other genetic mutations that we don't yet know to look for.

Who should undergo genetic testing for breast cancer? This is a very controversial area. First, let me again emphasize that the overwhelming majority of breast cancers do not have known genetic causes and cannot be predicted by current genetic testing. If a woman with a strong family history for breast cancer is interested in testing, she should be referred for genetic counseling in order to make an informed decision about her options.

The bottom line: If you are a healthy woman age 20 or over, perform a breast self-exam monthly. If you are 40 or over, add an annual mammogram to your screening regimen. If you are at high risk for breast cancer, discuss an appropriate screening program with your doctor and stick to it.

CHAPTER 27

Men's Health Issues

The prostate gland is a walnut-sized organ that sits at the base of the bladder and surrounds the urethra, the tube through which urine passes from the bladder through the penis. The prostate is layered like an onion and contains glands, a series of ducts, and smooth muscle. The prostate serves to provide additional fluid volume and nourishment for sperm. Otherwise, it is a troublemaker.

This chapter discusses some common health issues of interest to men, including pros-

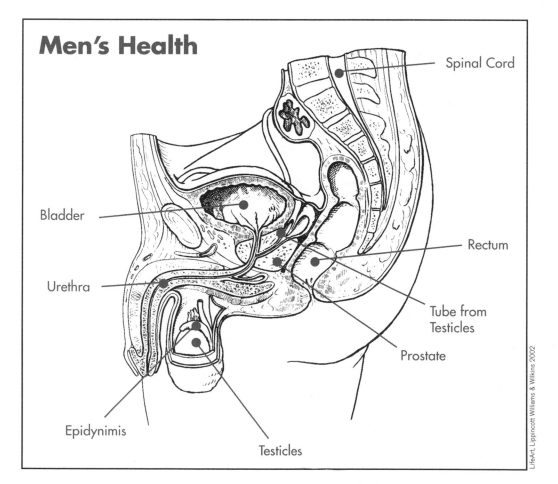

Men's Health

Spinal Cord

Bladder

Rectum

Urethra

Tube from Testicles

Prostate

Epidynimis

Testicles

LifeArt, Lippincott Williams & Wilkins 2002

tate conditions (benign prostatic hypertrophy, prostatitis, and prostate cancer), erectile dysfunction, and testosterone deficiency.

Benign Prostatic Hypertrophy

Benign prostatic hypertrophy (BPH) is an enlargement of the central zone of the prostate that lies most directly around the urethra. This enlargement appears to be due to aging and the stimulating effect of testosterone on prostate tissue. The enlarged prostate creates an obstruction to urine flow through the urethra and produces the characteristic symptoms of a decrease in the force of the urinary stream, hesitancy in initiating urination, dribbling after urination, increased urinary frequency, and nighttime urination. BPH usually affects white men after age 55 and typically begins to occur in black men about a decade earlier.

As a result of this obstruction to flow, the bladder must generate a greater force to pass urine and the muscle of the bladder wall thickens. This can initially create a smaller bladder with less storage capacity, thus contributing to the increase in urinary frequency. Bladder emptying becomes incomplete, and the leftover pooling of urine increases the risk for bladder infections. As the obstruction progresses, the bladder muscle fails and the bladder begins to balloon out and may begin to develop hernias (diverticula). Severe cases of BPH can lead to dilation of the kidneys and problems with kidney function.

The first step in treating the symptoms suggesting BPH is to eliminate other chemicals that may be worsening the obstruction. These include common off-the-shelf products such as decongestants and antihistamines, anticholinergic drugs such as those used for gastrointestinal diseases or Parkinson's disease, antidepressant medications, and some substances found in the diet such as caffeine and alcohol. Your physician will also look for prostate infections and malignancies and may also test bladder and kidney function.

Treatment options include herbal products, prescription medications, and surgical approaches. Saw palmetto is the most well studied herbal product for benign prostatic hypertrophy. It is a fruit extract that is usually taken twice a day. The chemicals in saw palmetto reduce swelling and contain a substance that blocks the stimulating effect of testosterone on the prostate gland. In one published trial of 300 patients, 88 percent of patients with BPH noted some benefit from its use.

Certain blood pressure medications (the alpha-1 blockers terazosin and doxazosin) lower blood pressure by relaxing smooth muscle in blood vessels. They also relax the smooth muscle found in the bladder neck and prostate, helping to relieve the flow obstruction. They are reasonable choices for patients who need treatment of both hypertension and benign prostatic hypertrophy. Side effects can include dizziness, a fall in blood pressure with standing, nasal congestion, and changes in ejaculation. One drug in this family in particular, tamsulosin, is selective for prostate tissue and does not affect the blood pressure.

Finasteride is a chemical that inhibits the function of an enzyme that converts testosterone to its active form. At low doses (1 milligram), this drug is marketed as a treatment for hair loss. At higher doses (5 milligrams), finasteride reduces the volume of the prostate gland and increases urinary flow. It may take from 6 to 12 months for patients to notice a benefit from this medication. A four-year study of 3,040 men with moderate to severe BPH showed that the use of finasteride reduced the incidence of acute urinary retention (being unable to pass urine at all) or the need for prostate surgery from 13.2 percent to 6.6 percent, a reduction of 50 percent.

Prostatitis

Prostatitis means inflammation of the prostate gland. It can either be acute, usually associated with signs of a bladder infection, or chronic, usually localized to the prostate and harder to diagnose.

Men with *acute prostatitis* usually experience fever, chills, discomfort in the groin and lower back, and changes in urination (pain, urgency, increased frequency, hesitancy and dribbling, nighttime urination, and urinary retention). This condition is caused by bacteria that migrate up the urethra or travel from the rectum via the lymphatic system. On examination, the prostate may feel soft and mushy. The gland is tender and examination of it can produce the sensation of an intense need to void. The treatment of acute prostatitis usually requires two to four weeks of antibiotic therapy. Because it is hard to obtain a reliable culture of the prostate secretions, physicians often choose the drugs to treat prostatitis based on the organisms they feel are most likely causing the infection.

Chronic prostatitis has more subtle symptoms and is more difficult to diagnose and treat. It can be suggested by recurrent bladder infections with the same organisms (seeded from the prostate) or an elevated prostate-specific antigen (PSA). The treatment of chronic prostatitis may require three months of continuous antibiotic therapy, and recurrences are common. Some patients required long-term daily suppressive antibiotics to keep the infection in check.

What is a Prostate-Specific Antigen?

The prostate-specific antigen (PSA) is a protein that is specific to the prostate gland. It is detectable in the bloodstream and rises in the presence of prostate gland enlargement, cancer, or infection. A normal PSA level is less than 4.0.

In addition to the absolute number value, monitoring the change in a person's annual PSA readings is a useful tool in cancer prevention. Once a trend is established over time with annual testing, a change in the rate that PSA is rising can signal a problem.

In addition to total PSA, physicians also look at the amount of PSA not bound to protein in the blood (this is referred to as "percentage-free" PSA). Lower percentage-free PSA readings correlate with an increased risk for prostate cancer.

Prostate Cancer

One in every six men will develop prostate cancer at some point in their life. The risk of death from prostate cancer is 3.2 percent in white men and about 4 percent in black men. In general, the younger the patient's age at the time of diagnosis of prostate cancer, the more aggressive the prostate cancer acts. It is impossible to predict for any individual man how soon, if ever, his prostate cancer will become problematic. Since there is a tendency for individual prostate cancers to become more aggressive with the passage of time, the patient's overall health and life expectancy is of utmost importance in deciding which treatment course to pursue for prostate cancer.

Physicians use the following techniques to test for prostate cancer:

- **The digital rectal examination.** The prostate is at the base of the bladder, snuggling up to the front side of the rectum. Although this location is somewhat awkward, it does place the majority of the gland within reach of the examining physician's finger. This exam works for cancer protection because most prostate cancers arise from the outermost "peripheral zone" of the prostate. A prostate cancer feels like a rock or nodule near the surface of the otherwise smooth and muscular prostate gland. This exam should be performed annually in all men over the age of 40. Its importance has not been replaced by the prostate-specific antigen (PSA) test (see below); I have detected a significant portion of the prostate cancers found in my patients by the rectal examination and remember two younger men who still had normal PSA readings at the time of diagnosis.

- **The prostate-specific antigen (PSA) test.** Initially, the use of PSA testing was controversial. Autopsy studies showed that greater than 80 percent of men had evidence of prostate cancer on pathological evaluation of the prostate, regardless of their cause of death. A large percentage of men will eventually develop detectable prostate cancer while they are alive. For most of these men, the prostate cancer grows slowly and harmlessly over decades, while some other cause, such as heart disease or stroke, is eventually responsible for the patient's death. A concern was raised that PSA testing would subject many of these men to unnecessary testing, surgeries, and other procedures for a disease that might never cause them problems. These concerns have been essentially laid to rest by two findings:

  — Since PSA testing became widely available, prostate cancer deaths have dropped 16 percent despite the expected sharp increase in prostate cancer diagnoses.

  — In Austria from 1993 to 1998, PSA testing was offered free to residents of the state of Tyrol, but not in other areas of the country. The prostate cancer death rate dropped 42 percent in Tyrol during this study period, whereas the rest of the country experienced no change. No other factors were identified to account for this difference other than the use of the PSA test.

  Annual PSA testing, obtained through a blood test, is thus advised for all men age 50 or older who can reasonably expect to live 10 years or longer. Higher risk men, such as black men or those with a family history of prostate cancer, should begin at age 40. The patient should not ejaculate for two days before the blood is drawn (this raises PSA); in addition, since some compounds can interfere with test results, the patient should also report the use of all drugs and supplements to the physician at the time of testing.

- **Prostate biopsy.** Prostate biopsy is performed on men with suspicious findings on physical examination and/or abnormal PSA readings. Under the setting of mild sedation, a urologist performs a series of biopsies from different areas of the prostate gland. A pathologist reviews these tissue samples. If cancer is detected, a Gleason score—a rough measure of tumor aggressiveness—is assigned. To obtain the score, the pathologist examines certain features of the tumor cells from the largest two areas of tumor in the specimen, scores each area from 1 to 5, and combines the score. A higher score suggests a more aggressive tumor and warrants consideration of more aggressive therapy.

If the patient is discovered to have prostate cancer, many factors are considered in deciding the most appropriate course of therapy. Studies have developed formulas based on the PSA level, results of the rectal examination, and Gleason score to predict the likelihood that the tumor will spread from the prostate gland. The patient's age, overall health, and personal preferences and fears are very important.

Treatment options include:

- **Radical prostatectomy.** Radical prostatectomy is the surgical removal of the prostate gland and the cancer within it. It offers the best chance for a permanent cure. This approach is suited for men without significant risk factors that would preclude surgery (such as significant heart disease, lung disease, or bleeding problems) and who are willing to undergo an operation. Patients should be expected to live long enough to experience suffering or death from the natural history of the prostate cancer despite the use of other available therapies. This usually limits this option to basically healthy men under 72 who are expected to live longer than 10 years, although exceptions obviously are made. Side effects of surgery depend on the experience of the surgeon and the clinical center where surgery is performed. On average, 10 percent of patients become incontinent with surgery and 60 percent experience impotence, though this percentage does improve with special nerve-sparing surgical techniques performed by experienced surgeons.

- **External beam radiation therapy (XRT).** Another treatment option is external beam radiation therapy. This therapy uses external beams of radiation focused to destroy the prostate gland and the tumor within it. Treatments take two to three minutes and are usually given five days a week for seven weeks. Side effects include fatigue and rectal irritation with possible fecal incontinence. The five-year survival rate from this therapy is equal to that of patients who undergo radical prostatectomy. The ten-year, disease-free survival rate is 42 percent for those who received XRT as therapy for prostate cancer, versus 69 percent for patients who have undergone prostatectomy. After age 70, the risks of general surgery and anesthesia begin to rise sharply; therefore, most men in this age group are advised to seek XRT. If the cancer recurs, options for additional therapy exist and many trials are underway for new options in the future.

- **Brachytherapy.** Brachytherapy uses the same theories as XRT, but instead of an external source of radiation, bits of radioactive material (seeds) are injected directly into the prostate gland. This material will emit radiation for a known period of time, delivering to the prostate a predetermined amount of radiation therapy. Compared to the weeks of therapy required for XRT, seeds are all implanted in one session. The long-term results of this type of therapy are not as well established.

• **Surveillance.** Watchful waiting is certainly an option for older patients with less aggressive tumors—that is, a low PSA score, a low Gleason score, and no tumor felt on rectal examination. For a patient with a decreased life expectancy (5 to 10 years or less), the risk of therapy may outweigh any foreseeable benefits.

Erectile Dysfunction

Erectile dysfunction (ED) is defined as the consistent inability to achieve or maintain an erection that is sufficient for sexual ability. Erectile dysfunction is different from libido, which describes the desire for sexual activity and doesn't depend on whether a man can follow through on that desire.

The penis is built as three parallel cylinders that contain a sponge-like tissue. Blood flows into the cylinders from arteries and flows out via veins. The sponge-like tissue is actually a network of interconnected spaces lined by the same cells that line the walls of blood vessels. The flow of blood into and out of these spaces is regulated by the tone of the blood vessels (whether they are more open or closed), which is in turn regulated by the chemicals produced in them at the direction of tiny nerves that supply each blood vessel.

To have an erection, the smooth muscles in the walls of the arteries relax. As a result, the arteries increase in size and more blood flows into the penis. This blood flow fills the spaces within the sponge-like tissue. As these spaces are filled, the pressure in them collapses the thin-walled veins connected to them, resulting in less blood flowing out. As more blood flows in and less flows out, pressure increases and the penis distends and becomes more rigid, resulting in an erection.

The stimulus to create an erection can come from the brain, as a response to sights, smells, sounds, or imagination, or from reflexes created from stimulation of sensory receptors in the penis. Regardless, the stimulus acts through the parasympathetic nervous system and its nerve connections to the tiny arteries that supply the penis. As alluded to above, the parasympathetic nervous system exerts its effects from tiny packets of chemicals released from the nerve endings and the chemical changes that these signals stimulate in the smooth muscles cells of the involved arteries.

Thus, the ability to have an erection depends on the proper and timely functioning of a network of tiny blood vessels, their neurological controls, and the complex chemistry of the interactions between the two systems. With such a delicately balanced system, lots can go wrong, and it does for an estimated 20 million American men. In 80 percent of these men with ED, a physical cause is suspected.

Erectile dysfunction can result from problems in either system—blood vessels that don't function properly or a net of nervous tissue that doesn't pass the right messages. Blood vessel problems are more likely to relate to problems increasing the blood flow into the penis, although a few problems with premature loss of erections seem to relate to "leaky veins" that allow the pressure to drain prematurely. Narrow, more rigid blood vessels (affected by atherosclerosis) may not be able to respond to the signal to dilate because they are too stiff. This can result from damage from hypertension, high cholesterol, smoking, previous groin trauma (such as bike seats), or other diseases that affect the penile blood vessels.

Some diseases affect the nerves' ability to pass messages to the blood vessels. These include strokes, spinal cord injuries, local nerve injuries (due to prostate surgery or other local trauma), diabetes, alcohol and other drug effects, and certain vitamin deficiencies.

Hormonal problems (testosterone deficiency) are fairly rare but could affect both erectile function and libido. See *Testosterone Deficiency* on page 297 for more information.

Drug side effects can interfere with erectile function. Common offenders include medications used for the treatment of depression and anxiety and certain blood pressure medications. Patients frequently face the chicken-or-the-egg dilemma when it comes to blood pressure medications. High blood pressure causes damage to the blood vessels that supply the penis, restricting blood flow through them. Early on when the disease is not too severe, further increases in blood pressure can force more blood through narrow arteries, and erectile function is maintained. Unfortunately, this is at the cost of additional blood vessel damage due to the high pressures, and eventually the system fails. If blood pressure medications are introduced after the blood vessels are damaged, they may make the damage and resultant ED more apparent by blocking the previous ability to maintain flow by jacking the pressure up. The medications don't usually cause erectile dysfunction—they just unmask it.

In order to sort out why ED has occurred, your doctor needs to know several things:

- How old were you when problems began to occur?
- Does the problem occur occasionally or all the time?
- Did problems start all at once or did they develop gradually?
- Is the problem getting an erection, maintaining it, or both?
- Do you have erections at night (while dreaming) or with a full bladder?
- Are you able to have an erection and climax with masturbation?
- Is there any history of trauma to the groin?
- Are you taking medications (prescription, herbal products, or supplements)?
- Are you a smoker? Do you drink or use narcotics?
- Are you or your sexual partner under stress?

Erectile dysfunction is a marker for disease of other blood vessels, including those that supply the heart. The onset of ED should prompt patient and physician to think about, and possibly test for, signs of heart disease.

Treatment options abound. The success of sildenafil (Viagra) has revolutionized the treatment, awareness, and willingness to discuss erectile dysfunction. The therapy is easy—take a pill—and benefits 70 percent or more of patients. It is usually well tolerated and it has removed much of the stigma and embarrassment of ED.

Viagra affects the chemical messengers responsible for dilating the blood vessels leading to arterial blood flow into the penis and restricting the venous blood flow out of the penis. The drug is best taken on an empty stomach; food or alcohol can limit its absorption. Viagra is usually ready to exert its effects one hour after ingestion, and may retain its effects up to four hours after ingestion. Contrary to what some patients may think, it doesn't cause erections spontaneously; erections occur only as a reaction to appropriate stimulation. Similarly, Viagra affects the mechanics of erections—it does not directly boost libido (sexual desire). However, a beneficial response to the drug may increase confidence and subsequent interest in sexual activity.

The same chemical system regulating blood flow in the penis exists in the heart, brain, and other organs. Viagra-induced changes in blood flow in these other locations account for its common side effects. These include headaches, flushing, gastrointestinal upset, temporary changes in blue-green color recognition, and blood pressure regulation. When combined with diseases such as diabetes or vascular disease, or medications that affect blood flow such as nitrates, Viagra can lead to dangerous drops in blood pressure. Viagra is available only by prescription, and is not a drug to borrow from a friend or obtain off the Internet or from foreign sources. Beware of imposters and herbal alternatives, which are largely ineffective. Both patient and partner should be aware when the drug is used and be familiar with its side effects in case unexpected reactions occur.

Other oral therapies exist. Yohimbine is an older medication that affects vascular tone and has been used for the treatment of ED. Studies yield conflicting evidence about its effectiveness, and the benefit above that obtained with a placebo appears low. Side effects are mild and include headache, increased blood pressure, anxiety, and gastrointestinal upset. For a few patients, Yohimbine appears to be an effective treatment, but I have not had much success with it in my patients. Other oral substances marketed for impotence, including L-arginine and a variety or herbal supplements, have not been adequately studied and results to date provide no convincing evidence of benefit. Testosterone and other hormonal supplements theoretically should help only the 5 percent of patients that have ED because of hormonal insufficiency, and must be medically supervised closely to avoid harm. It is unwise to try any supplement that claims to have hormonal effects.

Alprostadil is another chemical (Prostaglandin E1) that affects the chemistry behind the vascular mechanics of erections. It is available in a suppository that is placed into the urethra, where it dissolves and enters the penis. In general studies, this route of delivery is effective in about 40 percent of patients. About a third of patients stop using this drug due to penile pain.

Injection therapy involves training a patient to self-inject medications, such as alprostadil and other chemicals that affect blood flow, into the spongy tissue in the side of the penis. These medications directly affect blood flow in the penis and produce an erection sufficient for intercourse in about 80 percent of patients. The injection technique is easily taught and relatively painless. Fifty percent of patients using this technique report some minor discomfort. The risk of priapism (an erection that lasts longer than four hours) is about 1 percent with this technique, and requires urgent medical care in order to prevent permanent damage to the penis.

Non-medication approaches are also available to treat ED:

- **Counseling.** Of all ED cases, 20 percent are felt to relate to psychological factors and may benefit from evaluation and therapy by a trained counselor. This approach is often combined with medical therapy for the best results.
- **Partner assistance.** A rigid erection is not required for all forms of sexual activity. An innovative and willing partner may bypass the need for other therapies altogether.
- **Substance avoidance.** Habits such as smoking and excessive alcohol use, and some medications, may adversely affect erectile function. Appropriate changes can restore abilities sufficient for intercourse.
- **Mechanical devices.** Vacuum devices are mechanical pumps that produce an erection. The penis is inserted into a cylinder, and the air is pumped out of the tube to create a vacuum. This negative pressure draws additional blood into the penis; when sufficient engorgement occurs, a band is slipped off the tube around the base of the penis, holding the blood in. The response to this technique is variable. Most achieve an erection sufficient for intercourse. The advantage lies in the drug-free nature of the treatment. The cumbersome nature of the treatment requires an understanding partner.
- **Penile prostheses.** For patients who fail other techniques, penile prostheses (implants) are available. These are permanent, surgically implanted devices in the penis. They include semi-rigid rods, creating a permanent erection, and balloons with self-contained pumps. The pumps use a fluid reservoir in the scrotum that can be manually pumped to fill expandable cylinders implanted in the sides of the penis, creating an erection when full. The placement of penile prostheses destroys the natural anatomy of the penis, and once this is done, there is no going back to the above options. The failure rate of penile prostheses (that is, the incidence of infection or mechanical failure) is about 9 percent.

Testosterone Deficiency

Testosterone, testosterone deficiency, and the concept of a "male menopause" are currently hot topics in health and wellness circles. Some good science—and frankly a lot of misapplied science or outright fraud—exists behind the wealth of popular literature and numerous supplements to address these concerns.

The testicles secrete testosterone in response to the hormonal stimulation of luteinizing hormone (LH) from the pituitary gland. The amount of testosterone produced varies in a cyclical fashion during the day. Because testosterone levels are usually highest in the morning (between 8:00 a.m. and 10:00 a.m.), they should be measured then for the greatest accuracy.

Low hormone levels may result from disorders of this hormone system itself, diseases of the testicles (due to mumps and other previous infections), generalized illness (malnutrition, intestinal diseases, advanced liver, kidney, or heart disease), drug and radiation therapy side effects, emotional disorders, obesity, and from the effects of aging. Studies show that testosterone levels in men drop 1 to 2 percent per year after age 30. Testosterone levels vary considerably from day to day in healthy men and may need to be checked more than once in those with symptoms suggesting a problem.

Symptoms of testosterone deficiency are nonspecific but may include:

- Decreased libido
- Persistent fatigue and lethargy
- Erectile dysfunction
- Decreased muscle mass or strength
- Increased abdominal fat deposition
- Mood changes, including depression and irritability
- Memory impairment

Testosterone supplements come in many forms: pills, shots, topical patches, and gels. In general, I ask my patients not to take oral testosterone derivatives—prescription or otherwise acquired, including nutritional supplements. When taken by mouth, hormones must first pass through the liver. The liver can be adversely affected by testosterone and similar supplements and there are simply better, lower risk ways to administer it. Long-acting testosterone shots slowly release testosterone and can be administered every three to four weeks. The testosterone levels achieved through these injections, however, can be quite variable. Testosterone-releasing patches and topical gels are the latest means to administer the hormone. With these techniques, the testosterone is absorbed through the skin directly into the bloodstream. Hormone levels can be monitored, and the amount of supplemental hormone adjusted until the desired levels are achieved.

Studies show that most of the signs and symptoms of testosterone deficiency improve with the use of supplements, significantly improving the quality of life of those men with testosterone deficiencies. If a patient's testosterone levels are borderline, it may be worth trying a testosterone supplement for three months to simply see if he feels better. Testosterone deficiency can contribute to osteoporosis; men with hormone deficiency who cannot, or prefer not to, take supplements should be monitored for this condition.

Testosterone therapy can stimulate the bone marrow to produce more red blood cells in some individuals, increasing the blood thickness and the risk of stroke. Therapy can also raise blood pressure. The prescribing physician should monitor these issues. No evidence currently exists that testosterone supplements cause prostate cancer, but they certainly do stimulate the growth of some prostate cancers that are already present or develop during the course of therapy. Men considering testosterone therapy or those already on it should have their prostates monitored.

CHAPTER 28

The Neurological System

The nervous system is divided into the central nervous system (brain and spinal cord) and peripheral nervous system (the rest of the nerves). Some of the cells within this system are the longest cells in the body. They carry messages via electrical charges that travel through them. These charges can stimulate the nerve endings to release tiny packets of chemicals (*neurotransmitters*) that diffuse across the space between two nerve cells and stimulate specific receptors on the second cell. Depending on what a receptor is designed to do, stimulation of the receptor on the new nerve can cause it to begin its own wave of electrical activity or suppress activity in the new nerve.

The central nervous system is encased in the protective bone of the skull and vertebral column. The brain has an abundant blood supply, with two large arteries each in the front (*carotids*) and back (*vertebrals*). These blood supplies merge, theoretically allowing for the remaining vessels to fill in if the flow of blood is interrupted to one of them. The brain closely protects its own blood pressure, even to the detriment of other organ systems when necessary. The brain also constantly produces cerebrospinal fluid, which bathes and circulates through the brain and spinal cord to provide nourishment, protection, and support.

Some nerves carry messages from the body to the brain. They are stimulated by activation of special receptors in the organs in which they originate, such as temperature receptors in the skin or stretch receptors in the gut. When stimulated, they carry the message that a particular receptor has been activated to the brain, where that electrical impulse can be interpreted as a sensation, such as heat.

Once the brain has interpreted the sensation, nerves then carry instructions from the brain to the body for action. If the original signals come from a match held to the fingertip, the outgoing signals may simultaneously signal the muscles of the arm to move the hand away, direct the muscles of the neck and eyes to turn to look at the problem, dilate the blood vessels in the fingertip to speed repair, and cause the vocal cords to utter an appropriate response.

Neurological diseases occur when this system breaks down. This can occur in many ways:

- **Nerve cell death.** Common causes of nerve cell death include interruption of blood flow due to stroke or cardiac arrest, direct trauma, infection (encephalitis), or toxin exposure (drug and alcohol abuse). Unlike skin or liver cells, nerve cells cannot regenerate themselves. When they die, they are lost forever. Seriously injured cells, on the other hand, may heal partially or completely over time, but it is a slow process. An injured nerve in the leg may take 12 months or longer to repair its connections. Brain cells cannot be repaired, but sometimes the brain can be re-trained to do a task without involving the damaged portions. This retraining is the goal of rehabilitation therapies.

- **Problems with electrical conduction.** Some diseases affect the conduction of electrical impulses through the nerves. Normal nerves are wrapped in a special insulation (*myelin*) to increase the speed and efficiency with which they can transmit electrical impulses. Some diseases, like Multiple Sclerosis, destroy this insulation, slowing or blocking effective nerve transmissions. In some dementias, deposits of protein build up around the nerve cells in the brain, shutting down their communication. Seizures occur when abnormal large waves of electrical impulses travel through the brain. Some painful conditions, like migraine headaches and trigeminal neuralgia, involve abnormal electrical impulses.

- **Problems with the chemical messages between cells.** These problems can result from difficulty generating the message or difficulty receiving it. The nerve may have trouble preparing the chemical message for release, such as in Parkinson's disease with the loss of dopamine or in depression with a deficit of serotonin. The space between the nerves contains a soup of chemicals (*enzymes*) that break down the chemical message, preventing the first message from having a long-lasting effect on the receiving nerve. If these enzymes are defective, the signal may last too long, excessively stimulating the receiving nerve; if the enzymes are too active, they may break down the message before it gets across to be received. The second nerve in the series also creates its own chemical messages, which diffuse back to the first nerve and may modify its function. Problems in these "feedback loops" can occur. In other diseases, the receptors on the nerve receiving the message may fail to function. They might not work properly when stimulated, might not be present in sufficient numbers, or might be blocked or stimulated by substances other than the intended chemical message.

- **Damaged nerves transmitting false signals to the brain.** If a nerve circuit that is programmed to transmit pain is damaged, the nerve may constantly transmit a signal that is interpreted as pain. This can occur with diabetic neuropathy, in which diabetes-related damage to small nerve fibers may transmit a burning sensation from the feet, phantom limb pain after amputation, or reflex sympathetic dystrophy, where severe pain may result from a seemingly minor injury.

- **Abnormal levels of sensitivity.** The brain is responsible for interpreting the signals that it receives. The threshold for a sensation is the amount of signaling that it takes from a nerve before the brain takes notice. In some disorders, such as irritable bowel and fibromyalgia (see *Irritable Bowel Syndrome* on page 212 and *Fibromyalgia* on page 242 for more information about these conditions), there appears to be nothing wrong with the tissues that feel painful. Current research is pursuing the idea that these diseases are not caused by disorders within the tissues, but by abnormalities in the brain's interpretation of the signals that it detects from these areas—that is, the threshold for interpretation of pain may be set too low.

As we increase our understanding of how the nervous system functions in health and disease, opportunities are created to intervene as problems occur. Examples include new drugs to prevent or limit nerve cell death during stroke, enhance the amount and effect of chemical messages, improve conduction in damaged nerve cells, and help the brain reinterpret the signals that it receives.

The remaining sections of this chapter will focus on common neurological diseases, including headache, facial pain (trigeminal neuralgia and myofascial pain syndrome), dizziness, loss of consciousness (syncope), sleep disorders (insomnia and sleep apnea), attention deficit/hyperactivity disorder, dementia, Parkinson's disease, brain and spinal cord nerve disorders (peripheral neuropathies), restless leg syndrome, seizures, and Multiple Sclerosis.

Headache

Ninety percent or more of all adults have experienced one at some point in their lives—the dull, annoying throb or the sharp, incapacitating pain of a headache. Of these adults, 75 percent have recurring headache episodes, 25 percent classify their headaches as severe, over 12 percent define their headaches as migraines, and 5 percent of the U.S. population acknowledges chronic daily headaches. That adds up to a lot of headaches, and patients seeking relief of headaches consume about 4 percent of our health resources. Of all emergency room visits in the U.S., 1 to 2 percent of these visits are for the evaluation of headaches. In addition, headaches cause significant absenteeism from work and school, decreased productivity, and much pain and suffering.

Although headache complaints are common, most patients do not realize that the brain itself is not sensitive to pain. As an example, brain tumors usually do not cause headaches. They become evident as abnormalities in neurological function develop, such as confusion, loss of speech, movement disorders, or seizures. The frequency of headaches in patients with brain tumors is no greater than the frequency of headaches in the general population. Headaches arise only from pain-sensitive structures in the head—the skin and muscles of the face and scalp, the lining of the brain and skull, blood vessels, and nerve roots (cranial nerves and those of the upper spine).

Common types of headaches include migraine, tension-type and myofascial pains, cranial neuralgias, and post-traumatic headaches. Other causes include dental or sinus disease, glaucoma, diet (including excessive caffeine, alcohol, MSG, and ice cream), toxin exposure (for example, carbon monoxide or cocaine), other medical diseases (such as emphysema, sleep apnea, hypertension, certain infections), environmental causes (such as altitude or allergies), drug side effects, and sleep deprivation.

Different kinds of headaches respond to different types of therapy. Your doctor may ask you to consider the following questions to help sort out what type(s) of headaches you have:

- How many types of headaches do you have?
- Where does your head usually hurt?
- How would you describe the pain (pressure, vice-like, pounding, sharp, dull)?
- Does the time of the day or time of the month (for example, during the menstrual cycle) matter?
- How do your headaches vary from one to the other?
- How frequently do your headaches occur (per week or month)?
- How many days of work/school have you missed due to headaches?
- What are the factors that either relieve or worsen your headaches?
- Do other members of your family have patterns of headache?

Careful studies prove that the memory of headaches, and other types of pain, is unreliable. In evaluating headaches, it is most helpful to keep a dairy of your headaches for several weeks. In this diary, you should document your headaches daily as they occur, and include observations on the questions listed above. In addition to tracking the migraines, a headache diary is useful in identifying possible headache triggers.

The following warning signals associated with headaches may indicate more serious problems:

- Headaches associated with whole-body symptoms, such as fever, weight loss, stiff neck, or recent trauma to the skull
- Headaches associated with other illnesses, such as cancer, certain infections (for example, HIV), or other diseases that affect the immune system
- Headaches associated with changes in neurological function or impairment in the level of consciousness
- The sudden or abrupt onset of severe headaches
- A feeling of having "the worst headache of my life"
- The new onset of headaches after reaching age 50
- A progressive increase in the pattern of headache frequency and severity
- Headaches that are always and only on one side of the skull
- Headaches that awaken you at night
- Failure to respond to usual and appropriate treatment for headaches

Headache Management: Basic Principles

Headaches can be controlled but not cured. The objectives of headache management are to minimize the headache frequency and severity and improve quality of life. Considerations for managing headaches include:

- **Taking charge.** As with any chronic condition, the focus of responsibility for control of the condition must shift from the physician to the patient for the best results. Patients must be given the knowledge and tools to shift from an emphasis on "Cure me" to "How can I manage my headaches?" Part of this learning includes developing coping skills and the ability to function in the presence of pain.

- **Monitoring headaches and their treatment over time.** Treatment of recurrent headaches is difficult and cannot be accomplished in a single visit to the doctor. The proper diagnoses and treatment options for headaches are complex and involve good communication between the patient and physician as the headaches and their response to therapy are monitored over time.
- **Avoiding drug overuse.** Any drug therapy, whether prescribed or off the shelf, has the potential to cause "analgesic rebound headaches" if that therapy is used too frequently. The use of acetaminophen or aspirin more than five days a week, the use of combination products more than three days a week, or the use of triptans or narcotics more than two days a week has been shown to cause more frequent headaches. The headache pattern may improve once the drugs are discontinued.
- **Understanding pain thresholds.** Pain, including headache pain, is communicated, sensed, and responded to in a neurological circuit. Recurrent pain "burns a memory" in that circuit. The more frequent and prolonged the pain, the deeper that memory, and the easier the circuit is stimulated—lowering the threshold at which pain is perceived. This understanding of pain leads pain management specialists to emphasize the importance of early and adequate pain relief, in order to limit permanent changes in the brain that lead to easily stimulated pain pathways. This principle at times directly conflicts with the previous principle about avoiding drug overuse.
- **Understanding limitations of diagnostic tests.** Imaging procedures are of limited value in the evaluation of headaches. The routine use of neuroimaging techniques such as CT scans or MRIs of the brain rarely adds to the information obtained from the history and examination, and is not warranted unless atypical features are noted.

Let's take a closer look at some specific types of headaches.

Migraine Headaches

People define migraine headaches in many ways. Clinically, the most useful definition for me is to regard any established pattern of recurrent headaches as migraine until determined otherwise.

Migraine headaches usually are severe, throbbing, one-sided headaches. They typically begin between the ages of 10 and 40 and occur at least twice as frequently in women as in men. Most migraine patients average one to four attacks a month. In women, 60 percent of migraines cluster around the menstrual cycle. Family history is important—if one parent has migraines, his or her children have a 50 percent likelihood of developing them; if both parents suffer from migraines, the likelihood of their children developing them too increases to 75 percent. For women with migraines, 60 percent experience relief during pregnancy and 75 percent find that their migraines disappear when they reach natural menopause.

SYMPTOMS

Migraines usually last from 4 to 24 hours and sometimes longer. The pain can be disabling and is often associated with other symptoms, such as nausea, vomiting, sweating, cold hands, excessive sensitivity to light and sound, scalp tenderness, and extreme paleness. Migraines usually take 30 minutes to a few hours to build to full intensity and can awaken patients from sleep or develop out of other types of headaches.

Some patients with migraines may have *premonitions* 12 to 72 hours before headache begins, including feelings of well-being, talkativeness, a surge of energy, changes in appetite, drowsiness, depression, and irritability or restlessness. Premonitions are different from auras, which occur in one-fourth to one-third of patients immediately before the headache begins. Auras are neurological phenomenon that can be "positive" (for example, zigzag patterns in vision, flashing lights, or colors), "negative" (blind spots), or unusual distortions in size and shape ("Alice in Wonderland"-like). Auras gradually evolve, last 5 to 20 minutes, and may occur without the associated headache (called *optic migraines).*

Other types of migraines include *complicated migraines*, which are associated with neurological deficits that last longer than an hour, *basilar migraines*, which include symptoms such as changes in vision, vertigo, ear ringing, and difficulty with speech or swallowing, and *hemiplegic migraines*, which initially resemble strokes and can be associated with temporary paralysis and sensory deficits. Rarely, *migrainous infarction* can occur, in which the patient experiences a stroke in the region of the brain usually affected by their migraine aura. Risk factors for this awful outcome include previous migraines with auras, the use of birth control pills, smoking, and other typical risk factors for heart disease and stroke. Treatment of complicated migraines usually involves a headache specialist.

CAUSES

Although many theories exist as to how migraine headaches occur, they are best explained as an electrical neurological event with secondary vascular and inflammatory reactions. Auras are associated with electric fields that migrate across a region of the brain, stimulating the sensations felt by the patient. In a migraine, something triggers an area deep within the brain (the *dorsal raphe nucleus*) to stimulate the release of serotonin and norepinephrine within the central nervous system. This causes a variety of effects, including stimulation of the gastrointestinal tract and dilation of blood vessels in the brain. These dilated blood vessels stretch the pain sensitive nerves that surround them, activating the trigeminal nucleus and beginning a feedback loop that has an exponential effect—cascading signals to the hypothalamus (creating cravings and sensitivity to light and sound), spinal nerve roots (creating muscular tightness), and thalamus (creating headache pain). As medical scientists further characterize and explore these events, it is hoped that better migraine treatment options will be developed to both treat and prevent migraine headaches.

TREATMENT

Migraine treatment involves three components: pretreatment options, early intervention, and rescue therapy.

Pretreatment options include both drug and non-drug approaches. These options require documenting and understanding your headache patterns and triggers. Lifestyle changes, including avoiding disruptions in daily activity, help some. Sleep disturbance is frequently associated with migraine flare-ups—burning the midnight oil and creating sleep deprivation is a common trigger—but I have also seen patients who routinely trigger their migraines by extra sleep. I remember an executive who did well during the week arising daily at 5:00 a.m., but every Saturday when she finally got the chance to sleep in she experienced migraines that ruined the rest of her day. Setting her alarm clock a few hours earlier on Saturdays stopped the migraines. Dietary triggers, such as red wine and hard cheese, can be identified and avoided. Regular exercise can reduce migraine frequency. Other triggers, such as bright sunlight or altitude changes, may be identified and appropriate precautions initiated. An understanding of the potential for drug-rebound headaches can help discourage the overuse of simple analgesics.

Drug pretreatment options are useful if the migraine pattern is well established or if migraines occur frequently enough to warrant use of a daily drug to prevent them. If migraines occur mainly related to certain events, such as exercise, sex, or menstruation, patients can take medication prior to the associated event to prevent the headache. Drug therapies commonly used for this method include nonsteroidal anti-inflammatory (NSAIDs) drugs such as ibuprofen, altering how birth control pills are administered, and the drugs in the triptan family.

Prophylactic therapy for migraines involves the use of a daily medication to affect the migraine pattern. The goals of prophylactic therapy are to reduce the frequency, severity, and duration of migraines, to enhance the effectiveness of acute therapies, and to maximize a migraine patient's quality of life. Prophylactic therapy is considered when the migraines are frequent (usually three or more a month), disabling, associated with prolonged aura or severe neurological symptoms, or if the acute therapy medications affects a patient adversely. Most regimens reduce migraines by about 50 percent but may take up to three months to work. These drugs are started at a low dose to minimize side effects and increased until effective doses are achieved, intolerable side effects develop, or the maximum dose is reached without benefit. Memory is completely unreliable when it comes to pain; therefore, I recommend that my patients keep a headache diary to document their response to therapy until we can determine the effectiveness of their current migraine medication. Since most regimens work equally well, the proper prophylactic drug is chosen based on expected side effects, other patient-specific diseases and preferences, and cost. FDA-approved options include beta-blockers and the anticonvulsant drug Divalproex (Depakote). Calcium channel blockers, older tricyclic antidepressants (not the selective serotonin reuptake inhibitors, or SSRIs), Buspar, Wellbutrin, serotonin antagonists, and NSAIDs are also used. Alternative approaches have shown some success with magnesium, riboflavin, and feverfew supplements.

Early intervention refers to drug therapy initiated as soon as the headache is recognized to be a migraine. Some patients respond to plain off-the-shelf pain relievers, particularly those that include caffeine. A variety of drug therapies are available and selection is an individualized process between patient and physician. Most of the newer drugs are in the triptan class, including the brand names Imitrex, Zomig, Amerge, Axert, and Maxalt. They treat the pain and often the associated symptoms of a migraine and are available in pill, nose spray, and injectable forms. Initially, these drugs were advised for use only after the migraine headache had fully developed. However, research data showed that patients who violated the parameters of the study by taking their drug "too soon" responded better, experienced less pain, were less likely to experience rebound headaches when the drug wore off, and reported fewer side effects from this class of drugs. These observations have led to advice to use the triptan class of medications much earlier in the course of a migraine. Drug interactions and significant side effects may occur with these medications, but the chance of a serious side effect is statistically less than the chance of being hit by airplane debris.

Rescue therapy includes drugs used when the migraine has escaped early intervention and is full blown, including triptans, phenothiazines, narcotics, and other pain relievers. A plan for rescue therapy should be established between the treating physician and the migraine patient. The patient who frequently must seek emergency care for pain is not being appropriately treated.

Tension Type Headaches

Tension type headaches are the most common headaches. They tend to wax and wane during their course and—although they have no specific location—are often experienced at the temples or back of the head. They occur at some point in life in 88 percent of women and 69 percent of men. In any given year, about 40 percent of the population has tension type headaches. Like migraines, the average age for tension headaches to begin is between 10 and 40.

Tension type headaches are diagnosed as follows:

- At least 10 previous headaches
- Fewer than 15 headaches each month
- Headaches lasting from 30 minutes to a week
- At least two of the following:
  — A pressing, tightening quality—not pulsating
  — Mild to moderate severity which inhibits but does not prohibit activity
  — Involves both sides of the head
  — Not aggravated by physical activity
- No nausea or vomiting
- Excessive sensitivity to light or sound usually absent (may have one, but not both)
- No evidence of organic disease (nothing physically wrong with the patient)

Tension type headaches and migraines are felt to have a common biological root, involving a disturbance in serotonin-related nerve transmission and altered pain threshold and pain response. In patients who have both migraine and tension type headaches, the triptan class of drugs is equally effective for either type of headache. For milder headaches, simple pain relievers and a variety of other drugs work. The patient and physician must be aware of the potential of rebound headaches from frequent use of drugs. Prophylactic therapies are also available, usually with the same drugs used for migraines.

Cluster Headaches

Cluster headaches are severe, one-sided headaches that occur in waves. Patients with cluster headaches typically experience their first episode in their late 20s; men are nine times more likely to have this type of headache than women. Cluster headaches last from 15 minutes to 3 hours. Often, patients experience a headache the same time every day for weeks, and then the headaches vanish for months. Cluster headaches are characterized by severe stabbing pain, tearing, and redness around the eye. The affected side of the face is sweating, flushed, and swollen and the nose is stuffy. Cluster headaches frequently awaken the patient at night. Patients experiencing a cluster headache are usually extremely sensitive to alcohol.

Cluster headaches involve the trigeminal nerve structures on one side of the face; these atypical headaches do not respond well to usual pain relievers. They are effectively treated by administering 100 percent oxygen when the headache begins or by taking a migraine medication in the triptan family. Some patients will respond to prednisone at higher doses to break a cluster headache cycle. Prophylactic medications, similar to those used in migraine sufferers, can be tried to prevent cluster headaches.

Chronic Daily Headaches

Chronic daily headaches refer to headaches that occur more than 15 times a month. Four to five percent of the adult population in the U.S. experience chronic daily headaches. These headaches are much harder to classify and treat, and their development seems to have a lot to do with the effect of headaches themselves on increasing a person's overall sensitivity to pain and the rebound effects of the overuse of pain relievers.

Chronic headaches can take many forms, including chronic tension type headaches and chronic migraines; usually, patients with chronic headaches take multiple medications to seek relief for whichever headache type happens to be present. There is some evidence that chronic migraine and tension-type headaches occur in patients who misused their medications when previously trying to treat intermittent headaches. Studies of chronic headache sufferers also show evidence of underlying psychological problems that may have influenced the patient's pain response behavior. New daily, persistent headaches can begin suddenly in patients with no history of similar headaches; these headaches are suspected to be due to aftermaths of viral infections that involve the lining of the brain. Another type of chronic headache called *hemicrania continua* is a rare, continuous, one-sided headache that can alternate sides and responds well to the anti-inflammatory medication indomethacin.

Chronic daily headaches need evaluation and management by a headache specialist or clinic. They are extremely difficult to treat and frequently involve physical and/or psychological dependence on multiple medications.

Post-Traumatic Headaches

Three million people a year are diagnosed with post-traumatic headaches, usually related to motor vehicle accidents. No correlation exists between the development of headaches and the severity of the injury, nor with factors involved in the accident itself, such as the wearing of seatbelts, the speed of the car, and the amount of damage to the car. The risk of headache does increase, however, if the occupant of the vehicle doesn't have time to prepare for the impact, if a rear-end (whiplash) collision occurs, or if the head is rotated at the time of impact. The brain is suspended in fluid; with a sudden change in motion, the brain accelerates within the fluid and hits the inside of the skull bones. The resulting headache pain disappears in 50 percent of cases within three weeks and, in most cases, responds well to the use of simple pain relievers.

Sinus Headaches

The common cold and sinus infections are responsible for more than 35 million of-fice visits a year in the U.S., as well as countless other people who do not seek medical attention. Children typically have four to six colds a year, adults one to three. The nose is shaped around two large passageways, and the sinuses connect to these passages by much smaller openings. When the mucosal lining of the nasal passages is swollen (by infection, allergy, or other causes), the openings to the sinuses may become plugged. Air has a much higher concentration of nitrogen than blood and body tissues. When the sinuses are sealed off, the nitrogen in the air inside them diffuses according to the laws of physics from its higher concentration in the sinus to the lower concentration in the blood. This leads to a vacuum within the sinuses, pulling on the lining of the sinuses and causing pain. Thus, sinus pain does not always equal sinus infection, and therapy of this condition involves alleviating congestion in the nose, not antibiotics. Eventually, even without therapy, the pain disappears as the vacuum in the sinuses is filled with fluid weeping from surrounding tissues and equalizing the pressure.

Sinus infections can also cause pain. The major symptoms of a sinus infection include facial pressure (worsened by bending over), post nasal drainage, congestion, a change in taste or smell, eye region pain or pressure, and nasal discharge. The color of the mucus, though it gets a lot of attention, is rarely helpful. Mucus turns yellow, green, or brown because of chemicals released into the mucus by white blood cells. These cells react to inflammation, which can occur from a bacterial or viral infection, or just bad allergies. Minor symptoms of sinus infection include headache, fever, bad breath, fatigue, and tooth or ear pain.

Treatment involves relieving the obstruction with efforts to thin the mucus, reduce the swelling, and eliminate any infection that may be present. To thin the mucus, increased intake of fluids are helpful, as are room humidifiers, topical saline sprays, and medications that make the mucus more watery. Antihistamines typically thicken secretions and can make matters worse. Swelling is reduced by topical or systemic decongestants or the use of prescription nasal steroid sprays. Honestly, it is difficult for your doctor to tell if the sinuses are actually infected or if you just have a cold and sinus pain. I use antibiotics if the cold seems to be getting worse after the fifth day, if significant symptoms remain after the first 10 days, if the symptoms are unusually severe, or if the patient is at special risk due to other medical problems. If the patient doesn't respond to the first round of antibiotics, a CT scan—not plain sinus x-rays taken in the office, which are largely ineffective—may be required to visualize the sinuses. Some cases benefit from a full ear, nose, and throat evaluation and surgical intervention.

Headaches in the Elderly

Migraine headaches usually lessen in severity with aging, although migraine auras without headaches may continue. It is uncommon for people to experience migraine headaches for the first time after age 50; patients who develop this type of headache pattern need detailed evaluation and imaging of the brain to search for a cause.

Tension headaches are common with aging and may be triggered by ill-fitting dentures, arthritis in the neck, vision impairment, or many other medical diseases. A complete medical evaluation to look for underlying conditions that may respond to therapy is advised. Hypertension, low oxygen levels due to lung disease or sleep apnea, angina, thyroid and other metabolic diseases, and medication side effects are common problems.

Temporal arteritis is a disorder of the immune system, called a vasculitis, where the immune system attacks and destroys medium-sized blood vessels. It typically occurs in patients 50 years of age or older. The pain and other symptoms are fairly nonspecific and may include a headache and tenderness in the region of the temples, fatigue, and jaw pain while chewing. Other symptoms include muscular tenderness in the hips and shoulders, low-grade fever, and vision loss. Twenty to thirty percent of untreated patients with temporal arteritis will experience permanent loss of vision from it; this disease is diagnosed in time to save vision only if the patient seeks attention and the physician is alert enough to think of it. Confirmatory tests include a characteristic finding in blood work (an elevated erythrocyte sedimentation rate) and pathologic findings on biopsy of the temporal artery. Treatment requires the prompt use of high-dose steroids, usually initiated before the diagnosis is confirmed by testing in order to reduce the risk of vision loss.

Subdural hematomas are collections of blood between the inside of the skull and the brain. They occur when the veins that bridge the space between the skull and the brain rupture, and usually appear one to two weeks after trauma to the head. Advanced age and the long-term use of alcohol increase the risk for subdurals because both are associated with shrinkage in the size of the brain and more stress on the bridging veins. Patients may experience headaches, imbalance, and confusion; a CT scan can confirm the diagnosis. Subdural hematomas may require drainage by a neurosurgeon.

Trigeminal Neuralgia

Trigeminal neuralgia is characterized by bursts of intense pain in the branches of the trigeminal nerve—the side of the face from the angle of the jaw to the midline. The pain is usually described as stabbing or burning, occurs suddenly at full force, and lasts for seconds to minutes. The attacks can be triggered by certain stimuli, such as touching the face, smiling, or chewing. Each attack follows the same pattern, and patients are normal between attacks.

Most patients with trigeminal neuralgia need an MRI scan to look for any lesion that may be compressing the trigeminal nerve. Therapy involves the use of the anticonvulsant drug carbamazepine, which is taken routinely to limit the severity and frequency of attacks. Other medications and surgical procedures are available for this condition.

Myofascial Pain Syndromes ("TMJ Disorder")

Myofascial pain syndromes refer to a group of disorders involving voluntary muscle where pain is experienced in a specific region but, regardless of the region, involves the central nervous system. The theory is that the stimulation of trigger points results in the release of certain neurotransmitters within the central nervous system. These chemical messengers open previously silent pain receptors, and further signals from the region are experienced as pain.

TMJ (temperomandibular joint) disorder is a common problem that centers on the hinge-like joint of the jaw. The diagnosis of TMJ requires:

- At least two of the following:
  — Pain of the jaw precipitated by movement or clenching
  — Decreased range of motion in the jaw
  — Noise during jaw movements
  — Tenderness of the joint capsule
- Abnormal x-ray findings
- Mild to moderate pain at the TMJ site

Most patients with TMJ do quite well with a combined approach utilizing physical therapy, dental expertise, and medication.

Dizziness

The evaluation of dizziness, like headaches, is largely dependent on the history a patient provides. There are several important questions to consider and report to your doctor:

- Is the dizziness "orthostatic" in nature (that is, does it get worse when you stand up and improve when sitting or lying down)?
- Is the dizziness related to head position?
- Can you reproduce it by placing your head at a certain angle?
- Is the dizziness episodic or continuous?
- Do you have associated symptoms, such as localized numbness or weakness, difficulty with speech or vision, or palpitations?
- What other medical conditions do you have?
- Have you started any new medications or supplements?

There are many neurological and physical signals that help us detect and maintain our sense of equilibrium. Vision is important; the brain uses signals from the eyes to orient itself. *Proprioception* refers to tiny structures in the skin and joints that sense mechanical forces such as pressure, weight, and acceleration; stimulation of these structures results in signals to the brain that are used to determine position and movement. In the inner ear, the vestibular system—with its network of three semicircular canals and a sac-like utricle—also serves to maintain equilibrium. The semicircular canals are filled with fluid and are oriented as a three-dimensional structure. The inner lining is a thin membrane coated with tiny hairs, each hooked up to a nerve. When the head moves, the motion causes the fluid in the canals to swirl. This bends the hair cells, creating a pattern of signals via the nerves that the brain uses to interpret movement. The utricle, also filled with fluid and lined with tiny hairs, contains a small rock. Gravity pulls this rock downward, and the stimulated hairs send a signal to the brain to help determine which way is up. The utricle is also designed to sense linear acceleration as forceful motions pull the rock in different directions.

Dizziness can be categorized into vertigo, impending faint, disequilibrium, and ill-defined giddiness.

Vertigo

Vertigo describes an illusion of movement when the body is, in fact, still. Often, patients describe a sensation where the room seems to spin around them. There are many possible causes of this condition:

- **Motion sickness.** Motion sickness results when the brain receives conflicting signals or too many signals from its sensors, such as with the constant rocking of a boat and seasickness. Antihistamines, such as meclizine and scopolamine patches, help stabilize the vestibular system and reduce the sensitivity to motion.
- **Infection of the inner ear.** Labyrinthitis, or infection of the inner ear, is a common condition that usually follows a viral upper respiratory infection. In this condition, the lining of the inner ear becomes inflamed and swollen, causing the membrane to buckle. When the head moves, fluid swirls in the ear and the inflamed lining sends cascades of confusing signals to the brain, resulting in vertigo. When the head is still and the fluid stops swirling, the vertigo goes away. Labyrinthitis is also treated with antihistamines, such as meclizine, or with steroids.

- **Benign paroxysmal positional vertigo.** Benign paroxysmal positional vertigo causes 15 to 20 percent of dizziness in adults. With this condition, brief (30 seconds to a few minutes) periods of intense vertigo are precipitated by a certain position or change in position of the head. This type of vertigo is thought to be caused by a solid particle within a semicircular canal that makes it function like a utricle. Certain positions cause this "rock" to rest against the side of the canal, stimulating the signals for motion. Treatment of this condition involves physical maneuvers to get this material out of the semi-circular canals and back into the utricle. Experienced care providers can perform the Hallpike test and Epley maneuver to assess and treat this condition. In these maneuvers, with appropriate support the sitting patient is laid backwards suddenly so that they are flat on their back with their head hanging over the end of the bench, often inducing intense vertigo. The head is then rotated through a series of maneuvers as the patient is turned on their side. In experienced hands, these maneuvers can suddenly and permanently eliminate the vertigo.
- **Meniere's disease.** Meniere's disease is a poorly understood condition that causes hours, not minutes, of dizziness. It may be an autoimmune disease that seems to increase fluid or pressure in the inner ear and cause dizziness, tinnitus (ringing in the ears), and hearing loss. Some patients respond to antihistamines, diuretics, or steroids. Treatment usually requires the work of a team of ENT (ear, nose, and throat) and neurology specialists.
- **Central vertigo.** Central vertigo typically causes a rocking or boat-like sensation of motion when the patient is at rest. This can occur from neurological diseases such as Multiple Sclerosis, strokes to the brainstem, or masses in the back of the brain.

Orthostatic Hypotension ("Impending Faint")

Orthostatic hypotension (also called "*impending faint*") is a condition where the patient feels dizzy or lightheaded when he or she gets up too quickly after sitting or lying down. This condition usually occurs as a result of a fall in blood supply to the brain. When a person stands up, several things must happen quickly to maintain sufficient blood pressure to the brain. The heart pumps harder and more quickly; the veins in the abdomen, pelvis, and legs squeeze down, increasing the return of blood volume to the heart; and the brain allows blood to circulate more easily through it. In some patients, this system doesn't work fast enough or at all. This usually occurs in older patients and/or in those on multiple blood pressure medications that blunt the circulatory system's ability to compensate for these abrupt changes in pressure.

Treatment approaches involve carefully evaluating the circulatory system, eliminating medications that may exacerbate the condition, and increasing the effective circulating volume of blood by increasing salt intake and using compression stockings on the legs. Patients can also minimize the effects of this condition by standing up slowly, crossing the legs, and contracting muscles in the legs and abdomen to increase blood return.

Disequilibrium and Giddiness

Disequilibrium and *giddiness* refer to nonspecific complaints of dizziness or uncertainty in various bodily positions. Often these occur when neurological and cardiovascular problems—specifically, those that affect the ability to sense and maintain one's position in space—multiply. Vision may deteriorate from cataracts or macular degeneration, arthritis may interfere with joint position sense, deterioration of nerves may hamper the ability to transmit signals about joint position and movement, cardiovascular reflexes to changes in position may slow, and the patient may be on medications that worsen all of the above. In elderly patients with multiple affected systems, dizziness often cannot be eliminated entirely. Efforts are directed to improving what can be improved and promoting safety by teaching patients an awareness of their limitations and giving them tricks and tools to make up for them. The use of a physical therapist or rehabilitation specialist can be invaluable.

Sometimes, psychiatric—not physical—issues cause the dizziness experienced by patients without obvious physical problems. Studies show that the diagnosis and treatment of depression, anxiety disorders, and panic disorder benefits 20 to 50 percent of patients with unexplained dizziness.

Syncope

Syncope is a sudden, brief loss of consciousness. It is common, accounting for 1 percent of all hospital admissions and 3 percent of all emergency room visits. The loss of consciousness implies a catastrophic shutdown of the areas of brain required for conscious activity. This occurs either when the supply of blood (and therefore oxygen) is interrupted or if abnormal electrical or metabolic activity interferes with normal function in the brain.

Large studies have evaluated the frequency of identified causes of syncope. In 17 percent of the study participants, syncope was caused by cardiac problems—anatomic problems such as valves that do not open properly or disturbances in heart rhythm that interfere with the heart's ability to pump blood. Twenty-six percent had other vascular causes, such as orthostatic hypotension (see page 312) or vasovagal reflexes.

In a *vasovagal reflex*, neurological signals from the vagus nerve cause the blood vessels in the gut to dilate, shifting blood to them, while simultaneously slowing the heart rate. This suddenly reduces the blood supply to the brain and can cause loss of consciousness. Symptoms that suggest vasovagal syncope include palpitations, blurred vision, nausea, warmth, sweating, lightheadedness, or extreme fatigue just before and after the episode. In general, patients with cardiovascular causes of syncope lose consciousness only briefly and do not have impaired reasoning when they regain consciousness.

Neurological causes, including seizures and atypical migraines, accounted for less than 10 percent of syncope episodes. Patients with neurological causes of syncope generally are unconscious longer, may have seizures, and are confused for a time after the episode.

If you have been keeping track of these percentages, the math shows that the cause of many episodes of syncope remains unapparent.

The medical field has not established a standard way to evaluate a patient with syncope. As with most conditions, physicians start the evaluation by taking the patient's history and performing a physical examination, paying particular attention to any signs of underlying cardiovascular or neurological disease. The physician then reviews current medications, evaluates possible substance abuse, and looks for signs of orthostatic hypotension. The patient's family history is checked for any evidence, direct or implied, for recurrent syncope, sudden death, or cardiovascular disease. Together with the patient, the physician then gathers information about the syncopal episodes themselves, including how many episodes occurred, how much time passed between them, what triggered them, and what symptoms were experienced immediately before or after them.

Common evaluations may include the following procedures:

- **Laboratory assessment.** A complete laboratory assessment is performed, particularly looking for anemia, diabetes, thyroid disease, or other metabolic abnormalities that may affect cardiovascular or neurological function.
- **EKG.** Your doctor may order an electrocardiogram (EKG) to look for evidence of previous heart damage or abnormalities in electrical conduction in the heart.
- **Ultrasound evaluation.** Ultrasound evaluation of the carotid arteries and heart may reveal blockages to blood flow in the vascular supply of the brain, structural abnormalities in heart valves or muscle that may impede blood flow, or evidence of previous heart damage.
- **Monitors.** Holter monitors and event monitors are recording devices used to monitor the heart rhythm for longer periods. Holter monitors are usually worn for 24 to 48 hours and continuously record the heart rhythm on a tape. The patient is asked to keep a diary of symptoms, and specific attention is placed on the time periods that these symptoms were experienced during review of the tape. Event monitors can be worn for weeks. They track the heart rhythm, but must be activated by the patient in order to make a recording. When symptoms are experienced, the patient pushes a button on the monitor. The monitor the saves the last several seconds of the heart rhythm it has monitored and records subsequent heartbeats. New surgically implanted event monitors, which remain in place for up to two years, enable patients to activate the monitor when they feel an episode coming on to record the heart rhythm. In a study of 16 patients with undiagnosed syncope despite extensive conventional testing, these monitors were able to detect an abnormal heart rhythm during a syncopal episode in 9 of them, at an average of four months after the monitors were implanted.
- **EPS studies.** Electrophysiological studies (EPS) involve the placement of several catheters equipped with sensitive electronic leads into the heart. These catheters create a map of the flow of electrical activity in the heart and test for abnormal rhythms. This technique is usually used to evaluate unexplained syncope in patients with known heart disease in an attempt to identify and treat those patients at risk of sudden death from future episodes.

- **Tilt table testing.** In tilt table testing, a technician straps the patient to a table and takes an initial reading of blood pressure and heart rate and rhythm. The technician then tilts the table to 60 to 80 degrees for up to 45 minutes and measures the patient's blood pressure and heart rhythm responses. Occasionally, intravenous medications are given to enhance changes that might lead to syncope. Tilt table tests are used to evaluate recurrent syncope in patients with no evidence of heart disease and no obvious cause for syncope, or in patients with a known cardiac cause of syncope where this information would influence therapy.
- **Neurological evaluation.** Neurological evaluation, including monitoring of brain wave activity (EEG) or imaging of the central nervous system by CT scan or MRI offers limited value except in a few select patients. These tests are not necessary in most patients with syncope.

Treatment of syncope depends entirely upon what is causing—or is suspected to cause—the episodes. Treatment options include increasing the volume of fluid in the blood vessels in patients with orthostatic syncope (by ingesting extra salt and using compression stockings on the legs), eliminating drugs that decrease blood pressure, using other drugs to stabilize blood pressure and heart rhythm, inserting pacemakers, and implanting defibrillators to shock abnormal rhythms in high-risk patients.

Sleep Disorders

What is sleep? Sleep is more than simply closing the brain store for the night. The brain must continue to monitor and maintain certain vital processes during sleep, such as breathing, heart function, digestion, and other metabolic activities. While most areas of the brain decrease their level of activity during sleep, certain areas increase their

---

What Happens during Normal Sleep?

Normal sleep is divided into two basic phases:

- **REM** – In Rapid Eye Movement (REM) sleep, the brain and body are relatively active. The brain has a brain wave (EEG) pattern similar to that while awake. Heart rate and breathing increase, but as long as the pons functions normally, muscle tone and activity diminish and little movement occurs. Dreams occur in this phase.
- **Non-REM** – A time of rest, non-REM sleep is marked by the progressive slowing of brain waves in defined stages, from light sleep (Stages 1 and 2) to deep sleep (Stages 3 and 4).

During a normal night's sleep, a person will cycle through the four stages of non-REM sleep, followed by a period of REM sleep, four to five times during the night. Each cycle lasts about 90 minutes. More deep sleep occurs in early cycles, and more REM sleep tends to occur as the night progresses.

With all this activity during the night, it's a wonder anyone feels rested in the morning!

activity. At the base of the brain, the pons and the thalamus change their ability to conduct messages between the body and the brain during sleep. The thalamus becomes hyperpolarized, which means it takes more electrical activity to activate it. This decreases the brain's sensitivity to external stimuli, such as light or noise, during sleep. The pons contains cells that can turn neurological relays on or off. This area is important for suppressing motor function during sleep (thus your legs don't actually run from the monster during your nightmare).

We are certainly spending less time in bed than our ancestors. In 1910, the average adult spent 9 hours a night in bed. In 1975, this figure decreased to 7.5 hours. How much sleep is enough? A common sense definition is that you have gotten enough sleep when you feel awake and energetic throughout the next day. I see problems with this definition. Patients who chronically go without adequate sleep may not recall what it feels like to get enough sleep, and may view their daytime wakefulness and energy as "normal" when they really are not at their best. Many people mask their sleepiness with stimulants, including caffeine and nicotine. One useful measure states that the amount of sleep an individual requires is the amount of time that they sleep (without an alarm clock) towards the end of a period of vacation, once they have restored some of their "sleep deficit."

Insomnia

Insomnia refers to an inability to either fall asleep or remain asleep. By this definition, 15 to 20 percent of the U.S. population has insomnia. Of those patients with chronic insomnia, 50 percent have depression, anxiety, or other psychological problems; 10 to 15 percent have insomnia related to drug or alcohol effects; 10 percent have underlying medical conditions; 10 to 20 percent have primary sleep disorders. Stress also takes its toll on sleep, causing a condition referred to as *sleep onset insomnia*, in which it takes someone longer than 30 minutes to fall asleep. *Sleep maintenance insomnia*—where a person awakens after more than 30 minutes of sleep and cannot get back to sleep—suggests a medical problem. *Early morning awakening*—in which a person wakes up after getting less than 6.5 hours of sleep—is a common condition experienced by the elderly and by patients suffering from depression.

I firmly believe that the majority of patients that I see who complain of fatigue are suffering from chronic sleep deprivation. They live what I call late-night-to-alarm-clock lives and simply don't allow adequate time in their schedule for sleep.

Studies show that those who feel that they can function normally on less sleep in fact don't do very well on tests that evaluate physical and mental tasks. They show impaired ability to solve problems and learn and retain new information; their reaction time increases, and their stamina decreases. Motor vehicle accidents occur four to eight times more often in those with insomnia, with a higher mortality rate. Falling asleep at the wheel prohibits reacting before the crash, causing more high-speed crashes. A chronic sleep debt has physiological consequences with measurable effects on blood sugar control, balance of the sympathetic and parasympathetic nervous systems, thyroid and adrenal gland function, and function of the immune system. Those with inadequate deep sleep develop fibromyalgia-like symptoms with muscular aching and fatigue. Those with inadequate REM sleep are more agitated and aggressive.

Self-help measures for better sleep are published widely. I have summarized the best of these hints below, and take no credit for originality. Some suggestions may take weeks to improve your sleep habits; stick with it.

- **Exercise regularly.** Exercise regularly, but not too close to bedtime. Exercise raises the core body temperature, which can interfere with sleep. Exercising earlier in the day can significantly improve the quality of sleep.
- **Avoid stimulants.** Avoid foods, drinks, and medications that contain caffeine, particularly in the afternoon and evening. Caffeine stimulates the central nervous system, making it difficult to fall asleep. Caffeine in coffee, tea, and sodas is obvious; caffeine in chocolate, medication, and nutritional supplements may not be.
- **Evaluate current prescriptions.** If you take prescription drugs and can't sleep, ask your doctor to review them. Many drugs interfere with non-REM deep Stages 3 and 4 and also REM sleep. Common offenders include medications for depression and anxiety, older sleeping pills, and medications for pain.
- **Use nutritional sleep aids with caution.** Be very cautious with the use of nutritional supplements that claim to help sleep. Melatonin may have a modest benefit for sleep initiation and jet lag, but studies show that it does not lengthen overall sleep time. Some patients experience drowsiness, confusion, or headaches the following day. Kava has many drug interactions, and may impair coordination. As with any supplements, the purity and strength of these sleep preparations are not monitored.
- **Avoid alcohol.** Alcohol initially sedates, and then acts as a stimulant to the part of the brain controlling sleep, interrupting the cycles of deep sleep needed to restore you.
- **Don't go to bed on an empty stomach.** Hunger can disturb sleep; a light snack at bedtime can help. However, be careful not to eat too much—heavy meals at bedtime stimulate acid secretion and reflux, which can cause sleeplessness from physical discomfort.
- **Try bio-behavioral therapy.** Many bio-behavioral therapy suggestions can help restore a healthy sleep cycle. Patients who follow these suggestions do much better in the long term than those who take pills.
  - Avoid excessive mental stimulation in the hour before bedtime. This is the time to begin the process of relaxation, not to address problems at home or work. A pre-sleep ritual including reading, soothing music, meditation, or a warm bath may help. If problems intrude, write the subjects down in a journal to be addressed the next day, then put the journal and the thought away. This skill takes practice to develop.
  - Use the bedroom only for sleep and intimacy. Working or watching TV in the bedroom will associate it with those waking activities in your mind.
  - Keep a steady sleeping schedule, going to bed and arising at the same time each day, including weekends and holidays. This helps set and maintain your inner clock.

— Keep your sleeping environment as ideal as possible. Get a comfortable bed and wear comfortable nightclothes. Keep the room temperature as you like it. Darken the room, use shades or blinds if needed, turn the lighted clock radio away. Keep the bedroom quiet; occasional loud noises may disturb the sleep cycle even if you don't wake up completely or remember them in the morning. Heavy curtains or earplugs may help. Use white sound (a fan or vaporizer) when needed. If you typically share your bed with a snoring, kicking, cover-stealing partner, sleep somewhere else until your sleep pattern is restored—or send your partner elsewhere!

— Avoid daytime napping.

— If you don't fall asleep within 20 to 30 minutes, get up and do another relaxing activity in a different room until you feel sleepy, then go back to bed. Repeat as often as needed.

— Try progressive muscle relaxation at bedtime (for example, relax the toes, relax the feet, relax the calves, and slowly work your way up to your neck and eyes).

If these techniques do not provide adequate relief, ask yourself the following questions and write down the answers before you see your doctor:

• Describe your usual night's sleep. When do you go to bed? How long does it take to fall asleep? Do you awaken during the night? When do you wake up? When do you get up for the day? Do you take naps? Do you feel restored after a night's sleep?

• How does your sleep pattern differ on weekdays versus weekends, workdays versus vacations?

• Describe your bedroom.

• What do you do the last few hours before bed?

• Do you sleep better or worse when you are away from home?

• What troubles you about your sleep habits?

• How long have you had problems sleeping? What have you tried to improve your sleep? Include all changes in behavior, medications, and off-the-shelf products.

• List all medication and other supplements that you take. Do you consume any stimulants after noon? Consider coffee, tea, soft drinks, other caffeine-enhanced beverages, "energy bars," and any supplement marketed as an energy-booster or weight-loss aide. How many alcoholic beverages do you have in a day and when do you consume them?

• Do you have physical symptoms that interfere with sleep? Consider physical aches and pains, cough, heartburn, frequent urination, nasal congestion, loud snoring, or other difficulty breathing.

• Do you feel an irresistible urge to move your legs when you lie down? Must you get up and walk to relieve it?

• Do you get heartburn at night, or ever wake up choking or with a sour taste in your mouth?

• Do you feel anxious or depressed?

Careful consideration of the answers to these questions, and a discussion of them with your doctor, should greatly speed your diagnosis and recovery.

Treating insomnia centers on the changes in behavior suggested on previous pages. Drug therapy plays a limited role in this treatment, much to the frustration of many patients with insomnia who are tired and impatient and who want a quick, simple fix (a pill) the first night after they are seen. Most medications and supplements, prescription and off-the-shelf, have limited and short-term value at the cost of significant side effects and residual effects the next day. Most medications for insomnia (antihistamines, anti-anxiety drugs, antidepressants, and sedatives) may put you to sleep faster, but don't prolong overall sleep time and interfere with the architecture of normal sleep cycles by reducing Stages 3 and 4 deep sleep. Although some newer drugs are better at preserving the normal sleep architecture, long-term studies at sleep specialty centers repeatedly show that changes in behavior offer much better and lasting results than drug therapy.

Sleep Apnea

Sleep apnea is a condition in which there is a repeated interruption of airflow into the lungs during sleep. In most cases, this occurs because a blockage to airflow in the upper airway develops. Infrequently, the problem is located in the respiratory control center in the brain, where the signal for the lungs to breathe is not properly transmitted. This topic is covered in *Chapter 21: The Heart and Cardiovascular System*.

Sleep Disorders and Aging

Sleep disorders are common with aging. In general, older people spend more time in bed, awaken more during the night, and experience a decrease in total effective sleep time that leads to daytime sleepiness and fatigue. They are dissatisfied with their sleep, nap more, and experience a phase shift in their sleep cycle that may not be in tune with the clock everyone around them keeps. Many diseases of old age, and the medications prescribed for them, interfere with sleep. For example, it is impossible to reach Stage 3 and 4 sleep if you must awaken to urinate every 20 minutes. REM latency, the amount of deep sleep required before the first REM cycle, also shortens. Thus, sleep for elderly people simply isn't usually as restful or restorative.

In addition to the behavioral suggestions mentioned earlier in this section, it is important for elderly people to manage their medical conditions. With the help of their doctors, they should choose their medications and other supplements carefully to minimize their impact on sleep. They should also minimize the use of stimulants and alcohol after noon, exercise regularly, and seek bright light in the afternoon and early evening to keep the sleep cycle in the desired phase.

In patients with dementia, sleep disturbances are often the final straw that leads to placement in a facility. With dementia, the brain's ability to track time is impaired. EEG studies show a decreased difference in brain wave activity from the awake to sleeping state. The nervous system pathways that usually inhibit activity are impaired, and demented patients frequently experience "sundowning," agitation that is usually specific to the evening and nighttime hours.

The treatment of sleep disturbance in dementia is difficult. All of the principles we have already discussed still apply. Light is important. Most nursing homes do not provide enough bright light to drive the natural circadian rhythm. Research studies show an improvement in sleeping patterns when bright lighting is installed and used in the afternoon and early evening hours. Caregivers of patients with dementia should reduce their patient's opportunities for sleeping during the day and provide structure to the day that focuses on activity—assigning simple household tasks and engaging the patient in crafts, regular exercise sessions, and the services of adult day care. This is the opposite of what the nursing home staff or relatives may desire at the time. Grandma's afternoon nap may have been looked upon as the only opportunity to get some work done. However, if prolonged naps are allowed during the day, the nighttime sleep rhythm is disrupted. Fluid intake in the evening should be regulated to decrease nighttime urination. Finally, nighttime disruptions by caregivers (for example, to give medications or to take "vital signs" or—in a nursing home—noise at the nursing station) must be minimized.

For more information about dementia, see *Dementia* on page 321.

Attention Deficit/Hyperactivity Disorder

Attention deficit/hyperactivity disorder (ADHD) is a topic that makes most primary care physicians uncomfortable. This topic is discussed widely in the lay press, and often patients come in with this as a self-diagnosis, requesting a trial of medical therapy. In truth, most of the research and drug trials regarding ADHD have been done in children and, until recently, little information has existed about this condition in adults. The criteria for this disease are subjective and require patients to track and report their own symptoms. There is no absolute test to confirm the presence of the disease, and effective treatment requires the use of controlled substances that have a high potential for abuse. I refer most of my patients with suspected adult attention deficit/hyperactivity disorder for evaluation by a specialist.

The hallmark of this disorder in adults is disinhibition. Patients are unable to stop their immediate response to stimuli, whether these stimuli arise from their current activities, surroundings, or thoughts. Instead of reading this paragraph and making mental notes, the person with ADHD might read some of the words, think about the smear on the page, be hungry and wonder what's for dinner, be annoyed by the clock on the wall, feel the vibrations of the traffic outside, notice his shoes are scuffed, and think about morning projects undone and evening projects to follow—all at the same time, and all with equal weight as far as their importance to him at the moment.

This flurry of superficial mental activity leads to the signs of ADHD in adults. These include missed appointments and deadlines, socially inappropriate responses and comments (the first thought just blurts out), and increasing frustration with an inability to organize and prioritize.

The *Diagnostic and Statistical Manual of Mental Disorders*, 4th edition (DSM-IV) lists the formal criteria for ADHD. These are geared primarily towards children. To be diagnosed, the patient must have six or more of the symptoms of inattention listed in the manual and six or more of the listed symptoms of hyperactivity–impulsivity. Symptoms must have developed before age seven and be present in two or more settings, causing impairment in functioning in these settings.

Attempts have been made to modify these criteria for adults. For example, the research group that established the Utah criteria required a childhood history consistent with ADHD and current adult symptoms, including hyperactivity and poor concentration plus two of the following: rapidly shifting emotions, hot temper, disorganization and failure to complete tasks, stress intolerance, and problems with impulse control.

Another model of ADHD lists five central problem areas of the disorder: activation (trouble starting and organizing tasks), sustained attention (daydreaming and trouble concentrating), sustained energy and effort (drowsiness and trouble finishing projects), managing affective interference (irritability and trouble managing criticism and/or emotions), and memory difficulties.

Attention deficit/hyperactivity disorder is felt to arise from an imbalance in neurotransmitters within the brain (chemicals used to communicate between brain cells) with symptoms caused by low levels of the chemicals dopamine and norepinephrine. The medications found effective for this condition are the ones that boost the levels of these neurotransmitters. This occurs either by stimulating the release of neurotransmitters from nerve cells (the stimulant drugs), or preventing the neurotransmitters already released from being removed from the area (antidepressant medications).

In addition to medical therapy, trained therapists can help teach patients with ADHD strategies to make up for their disease's deficits. These strategies include using lists and written schedules, ensuring a proper work environment with minimal distractions, and identifying and using the time of day when each patient is naturally more effective. Patients who have developed lifelong patterns of self-doubt and poor self-worth also benefit from counseling.

In the evaluation and treatment of possible attention deficit/hyperactivity disorder, other diseases must be considered. Common problems include depression, generalized anxiety, substance abuse disorders, and thyroid disease.

Dementia

Dementia refers to a progressive disease which results in a global decline in higher cognitive function, including memory, attention and concentration, judgment and reason, speech, motor abilities, and personality. Dementia may begin subtly, with minor deficits in memory, attention, and concentration that may be hidden or dismissed by the patient and family. As cognitive function is lost, the patient loses the ability to generalize learning—to think in the abstract. Every situation or problem is new, and previous experience cannot be drawn upon to address new ones. This leads to an inability to adapt to changes in the environment. In response to difficulties handling new information, the patient's personality may become more rigid, more irritable. As dementia progresses, self-perception becomes distorted, and the patient loses awareness of his deficits. The patient may become angrier and more aggressive. In the later stages of dementia, interaction with all aspects of the environment diminishes. The patient becomes increasingly withdrawn from his or her surroundings, physical needs, and others around him or her. The pace of this decline can be slow, but is relentlessly progressive.

By age 80, one in five adults have dementia. This means that four in five do not! Old does not equal cognitively impaired. About 10 percent of cases strike before age 60, usually related to heredity or damage to the brain from toxins (alcohol) or strokes. Alzheimer's disease causes 50 to 60 percent of dementias (see *Alzheimer's Disease* on page 323 for more information). Another 15 to 20 percent relate to vascular events in the brain (see the section on strokes in *Chapter 21: The Heart and Cardiovascular System* for more information). The remaining causes are toxic or metabolic in origin, including vitamin deficiencies, thyroid disease, alcohol and other drug abuse, heavy metal (for example, lead or copper) accumulation, and infections such as syphilis or HIV. Primary neurological disorders, such as Parkinson's disease and Huntington's disease, account for a small percentage.

Common problems to all dementias include sleep disturbance (see *Sleep Disorders and Aging* on page 319), depression, delusions and hallucinations, and agitation or aggression.

Depression and Dementia

Depression occurs in 20 to 30 percent of patients with dementia. Because its clinical features can mimic worsening dementia, depression is not always apparent in dementia patients and should therefore be watched for by the patients' families and doctors. Depression is particularly common with dementia associated with Parkinson's disease, vascular dementia, and in those with strokes affecting the speech and language center of the brain. With proper therapy for depression—including an increase in physical and mental activities (such as those found in adult day care programs), bright lighting during the day, and medication—a significant improvement in cognitive function may be seen. Physicians typically prescribe antidepressant drugs in the selective serotonin reuptake inhibitors (SSRI) family according to the desired side effect—sedation or stimulation. Doses are low at first, to minimize side effects, and adjusted carefully.

Delusions and Hallucinations

Delusions refer to fixed false beliefs. *Hallucinations* are the auditory or visual false perceptions that accompany them. Frequent themes include the belief that people are stealing from or are being mean to the patient, or that dead family members or friends are present. The new onset of delusions and hallucinations should always prompt the search for a cause. Has an infection or other medical illness developed? Are side effects from a new drug becoming apparent? After investigating possible causes and before attempting to medically treat these thoughts, physicians look for a convincing argument that these delusions and hallucinations are upsetting enough to the patient (not just to the caregivers) to warrant the risk of side effects before prescribing other mood altering medications.

Agitation and Aggression

Agitation and *aggression* occur at some point in 50 percent of dementias. They may relate to delusions and hallucinations and may also signal a concurrent illness or reaction to a new medication. These behaviors are treated by providing a safe and comfortable routine for the patient, posting daily activities and simple calendars, providing a well-lit environment, and avoiding tasks that must be completed in a set amount of time or other activity with potential for frustration. Some disruptive but nonviolent behaviors simply must be tolerated. A variety of medications can help, but each provides only a fine line between improved behavior and the risk of side effects.

Normal Pressure Hydrocephalus

Normal pressure hydrocephalus is an important, reversible cause of dementia. In this process, the brain accumulates an excess of cerebrospinal fluid within the ventricles in the center of the brain. As these ventricles expand with this excess fluid volume, they press the brain tissue against the inside of the skull. This leads to dysfunction of the central nervous system, visible as what is referred to as the "classic triad"—progressive dementia, difficulty with gait, and urinary incontinence. The cause of this disease is not certain. The disease is suspected when CT scanning of the brain reveals enlarged ventricles without the usual appearance of brain shrinkage, and the diagnosis is confirmed if the patient's deficits improve after a lumbar puncture temporarily removes excess fluid. The condition is treated surgically by placement of a catheter that shunts excess fluid from the nervous system into the bloodstream.

Alzheimer's Disease

Alzheimer's disease is the most common type of dementia. Its cause is unknown. Alzheimer's disease is associated with an accumulation of the protein amyloid beta-peptide (AB42) that builds up and forms deposits that surround brain cells. This is felt to choke off the cells and interfere with their ability to communicate via chemical messages with other brain cells.

Current drug therapies for Alzheimer's disease simply boost the levels of the chemical messenger acetylcholine in the brain. These drugs can modestly improve cognitive performance in about two-thirds of those who use them, but do have side effects on gastrointestinal function and sleep. Over 50 drugs are now being tested for Alzheimer's disease. The isolation of the enzyme that forms AB42 provides a new potential target for drug therapies. In 1999, San Francisco researchers reported that healthy mice injected with tiny fragments of the protein felt to cause an Alzheimer's-like disease in mice developed antibodies that reduced the subsequent rate of the disease. This appears to lay the groundwork for the development of an Alzheimer's vaccine.

Much is written about efforts to prevent the development of Alzheimer's disease.

- **The oxidation theory.** Protein plaques may damage neurons through the chemical process of oxidation, which provokes a localized inflammatory response. Efforts to reduce oxidation and inflammation may reduce the rate of damage.

— Vitamin E and other antioxidants may be effective. Observational studies show that humans with the highest blood levels of vitamin E have the lowest incidence of Alzheimer's disease. Data does not yet exist about whether taking vitamin E supplements will lead to the same benefit.

— NSAIDs (Nonsteroidal anti-inflammatory drugs like ibuprofen) are used for the treatment of arthritis and pain. Observational studies again show a reduced rate of Alzheimer's disease in patients who have regularly taken these drugs. However, because of the costs and significant side effects of these drugs (stomach irritation and bleeding, liver or kidney damage), the possible benefits don't yet justify the risk of therapy.

• **B vitamins.** Clear deficiencies in B vitamins are known to cause dementias. Moderate deficiencies in these vitamins may contribute to cognitive decline. After age 50, the absorption of B vitamins from the gastrointestinal tract becomes less efficient. Everyone over 50 should take a B-complex multivitamin or consume B-fortified foods.

• **Estrogen replacement after menopause.** Women have a greater risk of Alzheimer's disease after menopause than men of the same age. Estrogen is known to have properties that reduce oxidation and inflammation, thus it makes sense that estrogen might affect the development of dementia. Over 15 different observational studies have shown a decrease in the frequency of Alzheimer's disease in those women who take estrogens after menopause. Studies of initiating estrogen in women who already have developed Alzheimer's disease do not show a benefit. Thus, if it is to work, it appears that estrogen replacement therapy must be begun early. Many other factors must be considered before proposing the long-term use of estrogen to prevent dementia. See *Dementia* on page 321 for more information about dementia; see *Chapter 26: Women's Health* on page 265 for more information about estrogen replacement therapy.

• **Physical exercise.** Observational studies show that those who remain physically fit remain mentally fit as well. Animal studies show an increase in the numbers of neurons and their connections in the brains of those animals regularly exercised.

• **Mental exercise.** Rats exposed to lots of toys and other mental stimulation were discovered during autopsy to have more nerve cells and more complex connections in the memory and learning centers of their brains. Mentally active people seem to retain their higher cognitive functions better than those without mental stimulation.

Improving the Lives of Patients with Dementia

Following are some helpful suggestions to improve the lives of patients with dementia and those who care for them:

• **Be educated about the disease.** Join a local support group or national organization for shared advice and updates on therapies and clinical trials.

- **Manage medications wisely.** Drug side effects emerge rapidly with declining mental abilities. Discuss with the doctor a desire to seek to eliminate all but essential medications. Don't forget about off-the-shelf drugs, supplements, and other herbal products used.
- **Watch for physical as well as mental problems.** Be alert for—and aggressively treat—concurrent physical and mental health problems such as infections, vision and hearing deficits, constipation, pain, anxiety and depression.
- **Keep the patient safe by reducing physical, visual, and noise clutter in the living environment.** Keep the room tidy and organized, eliminate throw rugs if they cause a potential for tripping, and reduce unnecessary furniture. If wandering is a problem, place big red "stop" signs at exits, or hide the doors. While a locked door may cause agitation, a door hidden behind a screen or wall hanging may not be noticed. Disable or remove the car so that it cannot be driven. Adjust the water heater so that hot water is no longer scalding. Install breakers on the stove and other electrical devices so that more than one step is needed to turn them on. Have the patient dressed in comfortable, nonbinding clothing with supportive footwear. Take control of the storage and administration of all medication and supplements. Use medical alert identification.
- **Exercise daily.** Daily exercise is important for your physical and mental well being, as well as the patient's. If possible, take walks together.
- **Be conscious of developing a calming conversation style.** Instead of asking questions that require thought, make statements—not "Do you like the weather this week?" but "I have enjoyed the warm weather this week."

The diagnosis of dementia often takes time. Many of my patients are concerned that they are showing signs of early dementia when they note trouble remembering the names of acquaintances, telephone numbers, or where the car keys are. Most patients with these "cognitive deficits" simply need reassurance. There is a difference between changes of brain function with normal aging (more repetition may be required to engrave short-term memories and the speed of recall of information from the brain's library may slow) and dementia. The hallmarks of dementia involve not only what is remembered but also how life events are interpreted. Patients with dementia can't generalize their previous knowledge and skills to new situations; they have trouble adapting to changes in their environment and thus become more rigid and at times irritable. Their perception of these events becomes distorted, and they are often unaware of their own deficits. Frequently, family members and close friends are the first to notice a persistent change. Neuro-psychological testing is available to further investigate concerns over early dementia.

Parkinson's Disease

Parkinson's disease affects 1 out of every 500 adults in the U.S. On average, the disease develops between ages 55 and 60 and its prevalence increases with age. Common symptoms include a coarse tremor at rest, slowness of movement, rigid limbs that resist smooth movement and—when bent or straightened by another person—operate in a ratcheting, cogwheel-type fashion, and changes in control of automatic reflexes such as maintaining a constant blood pressure when going from a seated position to standing.

When the disease begins, two-thirds of patients experience tremors. Tremors are typically present in the upper extremities, on one side of the body; they improve with movement and worsen at rest or while attempting to maintain a fixed position. This is in contrast to *benign essential tremor*, which is 20 times more common than Parkinson's disease. In benign essential tremor, the tremor is increased with activity, improved by rest, and usually appear on both sides of the body. Benign essential tremor follows an inherited pattern, whereas heredity doesn't play a major role in Parkinson's disease.

As Parkinson's disease progresses, other signs develop. Walking changes. There is a generalized slowness and stiffness to all movement. Less arm swing occurs with walking, the posture is bent forward, and the feet shuffle and are difficult to start—as if they are glued to the ground. Some patients develop a reflex to push backwards and tend to fall in that direction. Facial expression and blinking decrease. Speech changes, the voice is softer, and words tend to run into each other. Handwriting becomes smaller over time. Dementia develops in 20 to 25 percent of patients, and depression is common.

The cause of Parkinson's disease is unknown, but the pathological findings in the brains of Parkinson's sufferers at autopsy are constant. Patients with this disease lose an important and specific population of nerve cells in the brain—cells that are instrumental in producing the chemical dopamine, which transmits messages to the brain to help smooth body movements and coordinate posture.

In genetic studies of twins, whether one twin has the disease has little effect on the risk of disease in the other. Autoimmune disease, infections, and environmental influences are suspected to contribute to the development of Parkinson's disease. Heroin users who used heroin contaminated with MPTP developed an irreversible syndrome identical in symptoms and brain pathology on autopsy studies to Parkinson's disease, further suggesting the possible role of external factors in this disease.

Current treatment options center on efforts to increase the concentration of dopamine in the brain. Proven medications do not yet exist to protect against or slow the progression of Parkinson's disease. Most therapies are initiated when symptoms become severe enough to interfere with daily living or employment. Current drug therapies have the potential for many side effects, including gastrointestinal upset, lowering of blood pressure, vivid dreams and hallucinations, and the creation of other movement disorders. Some drugs, like levodopamine, have significant "on/off" effects, where the response to the drug may start and end suddenly. A wide variety of new treatment options are being explored, including neurosurgical procedures to block certain pathways, transplant dopamine-producing cells, and implant electrodes for long-term electrical stimulation of certain areas of the brain.

Peripheral Neuropathies

Peripheral neuropathies refer to a group of disorders that affect the health and function of nerves outside of the brain and spinal cord. Symptoms depend on what nerves are affected. Most commonly, physicians see disorders of *sensory nerves*; these disorders consist of lesions that create painful burning or numbing sensations, usually affecting the longest nerves first—thus creating symptoms in the feet. Patients notice these abnormal sensations first when they are not distracted by other activities, such as at night, and describe them as an annoying numbness or painful sensation, worsened by contact with the sheet or socks. Physicians also see disorders of *motor nerves*, which appear as weakness in the hands and feet, causing stumbling or difficulty opening lids or using keys. Muscle cramping and other movement abnormalities may occur. Lastly, physicians also see disorders of *autonomic nerves*, which cause difficulty regulating blood pressure after changes in posture, sweating and heat intolerance, impotence, or bowel and bladder dysfunction.

Causes of peripheral neuropathy are multiple:

- Entrapment of a nerve by arthritis, a prolapsed disc, or an inflamed nerve sheath
- Diabetes
- Other illness, including thyroid, kidney, liver, and connective tissue diseases
- Infections, including HIV and other viruses or leprosy
- Toxin exposure, such as alcohol, pesticides, excessive use of certain vitamins (such as B_6) and other supplements, and heavy metals (lead, mercury, and arsenic)
- Inadequate blood supply to nerves
- Vitamin deficiencies
- Side effects of certain cancers ("paraneoplastic syndromes" where the cancer produces a substance that interferes with nerve function)
- Demyelinating diseases such as Multiple Sclerosis (see *Multiple Sclerosis* on page 329)
- Inherited disorders

Evaluation includes a thorough history and physical examination and appropriate laboratory work. Doctors may also perform electrical testing of nerves and muscle tissue to see how well the nerves conduct electrical impulses or take nerve and muscle biopsies to look for certain diseases.

Treatment options center on removing the cause or optimizing management of the medical condition responsible for the neuropathy. Tricyclic antidepressant drugs, such as amitriptyline, are used at low doses. These drugs are excellent at blocking pain transmission through small nerve fibers and serve as the backbone of most therapies. Newer drugs are becoming available.

Restless Leg Syndrome

Restless leg syndrome is characterized by an irresistible urge to move the legs, associated with disagreeable leg symptoms. Symptoms are worse at rest and usually peak in the evening and early morning (midnight to 4:00 a.m.) as part of the body's circadian rhythm. They are partially relieved by movement.

Restless leg syndrome occurs in 10 percent of the population and affects men and women equally. It usually develops in the mid-thirties and is generally present lifelong thereafter. The disease frequently is inherited but some cases are caused by identifiable conditions (iron deficiency, kidney failure, pregnancy, and other neurological diseases) or medications (drugs for depression, seizures, psychosis, and asthma). It tends to occur more often in diabetics, those with rheumatoid arthritis or Parkinson's disease, smokers, the medically overweight, and people who do not exercise.

Treatment of the disease first involves identifying it and educating the patient that their symptoms are valid and due to a common disease. Some relief may come from hot baths, physical exercise, and avoiding alcohol, nicotine, and drugs known to worsen the condition. The FDA has not yet approved any drugs for this condition, but several approaches to drug therapy can offer some relief. Physicians commonly prescribe drugs used for Parkinson's disease, but some patients experience nothing more than a shift in the time of day that symptoms are experienced. Other therapies are available on a trial basis. The response and tolerance to therapy varies greatly from patient to patient.

Seizures

Seizures are sudden, abnormal electrical discharges from an area of the brain that break through the normal insulated channels of electrical communication and spread directly to other areas of the brain. Simple seizures typically last from 30 to 90 seconds. They may be preceded by an aura (a certain memory, smell, visual change, or sensation), and involve a period of impaired responsiveness to external stimuli, confusion, and amnesia afterward.

Helping Someone through a Seizure
- Place a cushion, coat, or other soft object under the person's head.
- Loosen tight clothing around the neck.
- Turn the person on his or her side to reduce the chance of aspiration into the lungs.
- Do not place anything in the person's mouth.
- Do not move the person during a seizure unless he or she is in imminent danger.
- Call for medical assistance.

A variety of movement disorders may accompany seizures. When most people think of seizures, they think of convulsions—violent contractions that involve the entire body. Other types of seizures may involve only one area of the brain. These seizures, called *complex-partial seizures*, may occur without a generalized loss of consciousness. People experiencing complex-partial seizures may be able to continue other tasks during the seizure (such as driving a car on a straight and level road), while being less attentive and responsive. They may also exhibit subconscious and repetitive behaviors, such as lip smacking, repetitive picking at clothes, fumbling with objects, or repetition of words or phrases. For some people, seizures are not accompanied by abnormal movement; these people simply lapse into a period in which they are unaware and unresponsive.

Seizures may be triggered by any irritating focus in the brain. Common causes include a previous stroke, an abnormal formation of blood vessels, a tumor, or congenital malformations in the brain such as cysts. However, a specific cause for the seizure is found in fewer than 20 percent of seizure patients. About 25 percent of people who experience seizures have a family history of seizures. Seizures can be stimulated in susceptible patients by anything that affects the conduction of electricity in brain cells. This includes sleep deprivation, alcohol use, and the use or sudden decrease in use of a variety of prescription or illicit drugs.

The treatment of seizures involves the daily use of medications that reduce the number of electrical discharges in the brain and their ability to spread to surrounding areas of brain tissue. These medications must be taken regularly to be effective, and their use monitored by drug levels and physician visits to evaluate their effectiveness and monitor for side effects. Patient and family education about the truths and myths of seizures is crucial. Legal ramifications of seizures, such as driving restrictions, can vary from state to state.

Most patients ask about whether they can come off of their seizure medications in the future. This is a difficult and involved decision, one that usually requires consultation with a neurologist. To consider withdrawal of medication, a person should have been seizure free for at least two years. His or her history should include only a single type of seizure. A current neurological exam, including EEG, must be normal. (An abnormal EEG precludes discontinuation of medication; a normal EEG provides no guarantee that seizures won't recur.) Even under these ideal circumstances, seizures are likely to recur in about 40 percent of adults who stop their medications.

Some people "fake" seizures. This usually occurs in patients with underlying psychological issues. These episodes are atypical in nature, fairly stereotypical from one event to another, and rarely occur when the patient is alone or asleep. They often last longer than two minutes and are accompanied by abnormal vocalizations. Be very careful in suspecting that someone's seizures are faked; this usually requires detailed evaluation by a seizure specialist to sort issues out. Of those patients with documented "pseudo-seizures," over 40 percent also have real seizures.

Multiple Sclerosis

Multiple Sclerosis (MS) is a disease of unknown cause that affects the myelin of the nervous system. *Myelin*, the insulating covering of certain nerve cells, functions primarily to speed transmission of electrical messages through the nerves. When the myelin is damaged, the nerves are unable to conduct electrical messages efficiently. This can affect a variety of body functions.

MS is usually diagnosed between ages 20 and 40. It occurs in women two to three times as often as in men. Racial and geographic differences exist in its incidence—it occurs most commonly in those of Northern European decent. Twenty percent of patients with MS have a family history of the disease, but the rate of an identical twin sharing the disease with an afflicted sibling is only 30 percent, indicating that there is more to it than simple inheritance. Common symptoms include numbness, loss of vision, paralysis or other muscle dysfunction, pain, and difficulties in the control of bowel and bladder function. Other diseases can mimic its symptoms, radiographic changes, and laboratory abnormalities. Although no single test exists that precisely and certainly diagnoses MS, MRI scanning of the brain is the most sensitive test to look for areas of myelin damage (called *MS plaques*). For doctors to diagnose MS, a patient must experience at least two separate symptomatic episodes of neurological dysfunction, separated in time, that involve two different areas of the brain. Physicians are cautious in establishing a diagnosis of MS—once a patient is diagnosed with MS diagnosis, significant consequences can develop regarding insurability, employment, and in how doctors view subsequent problems in MS patients. If a patient labeled with MS develops new neurological symptoms, these symptoms are usually presumed by the patient's physician to be from the MS and other possibilities are not as aggressively pursued.

The course of this disease is unpredictable and affects each individual differently. MS is characterized by sudden episodes of neurological dysfunction that resolve, partially resolve, or progress steadily onward to other episodes. These changes in neurological function can be dramatic. MS has a minimal impact on a person's expected lifespan but, for a given individual, can result in anything from no disability to severe disability. The unpredictability of the disease makes it difficult to assess a person's potential response to therapy. We can't tell for any one patient whether the therapy helped more than what the disease may have done on its own without therapy—a particular concern for MS patients who pursue alternative health strategies in addition to, or instead of, care from a specialized MS center. I caution my MS patients strongly about the use and misuse of nutritional supplements or other alternative therapies for this disease, particularly if these therapies pose any direct risk, considerable expense, or create the risk of omission of available therapies with known benefit. It is only through careful study of the responses to therapy in large groups of patients that trends can be seen and therapies evaluated. Specialty centers for MS research and treatment offer the greatest expertise in treatment, along with the use of therapies in well-controlled studies so that their potential benefits (and risks) can be more accurately assessed.

MS usually follows one of four basic patterns. Patients cannot be placed in a category until their disease experience is established.

- The most common pattern is a *relapsing-remitting* course. This is characterized by partial or total recovery after a flare in MS. Seventy percent of patients begin with this pattern.
- *Secondary-progressive* disease refers to a patient with the first pattern who then develops a steady progression in disease activity. Of those who begin with the relapsing-remitting pattern, 50 percent develop progressive disease within 10 years, 90 percent within 25 years.
- *Primary-progressive* disease characterizes those 15 percent of patients who have a progressive course in their disease from the beginning. This pattern is usually recognized in retrospect.

- *Progressive-remitting* disease involves those 6 to 10 percent of patients who have progressive disease from the outset, but also have obvious acute attacks.

In general, females who are diagnosed with MS at an early age fare better than other patients diagnosed with MS, as do patients who have fewer attacks in the first years after diagnosis, attacks separated by long periods with no new disease activity, and attacks that affect sensation rather than motor function. However, the disease is highly variable and these trends are not helpful in counseling any individual patient.

When a patient with multiple sclerosis develops worsening symptoms, the first step is to look for other disease processes that may be adversely affecting neurological function. Fevers slow the transmission of electrical impulses in nerves not insulated by myelin, and an infection with fever may make neurological function in an MS patient look worse. Urinary tract infections, constipation, and adverse reactions to medications are common causes for "pseudoflares" in MS.

Therapy for acute attacks primarily centers on the use of high-dose steroids to adjust the effects of the immune system. Current MS studies are investigating a variety of other agents that interact with the immune system's function, although we do not yet understand how this interaction changes the course of MS. Patients interested in these studies should visit the website of the National Multiple Sclerosis Society or contact their local chapter.

Other therapies are available for the symptoms that frequently accompany MS, though they have no effect on the underlying disease itself. These therapies address:

- **Fatigue.** Profound fatigue can be a prominent feature of MS at any stage. This is addressed through ensuring adequate rest (chronic sleep deprivation is a bad combination with MS), maintaining physical fitness, and avoiding subtle dehydration. Heat slows the transmission of neurological impulses through nerves, so exercise must be performed in such a way as to avoid overheating. Pool exercises, due to the heat transfer abilities of water, are ideal. Medications, such as amantadine, are helpful in some patients.

- **Pain.** Pain is a frequent component of MS due to the effects of MS on the nerve pathways of sensation. It is also an often-overlooked one; surveys of MS patients frequently detect that pain issues have been inadequately addressed. Physical therapy and hydrotherapy can help, as can many medications including the tricyclic antidepressants, some seizure medications, anti-inflammatory medications, and traditional analgesics.

- **Muscle spasm.** Movement disorders, including muscle spasticity and tremors, can interfere with purposeful movement, cause pain, and interfere with sleep. However, drug therapies that reduce muscle spasm carry a risk of decreasing muscle tone in such a way as to interfere with a patient's ability to walk or bear weight. The carefully adjusted use and monitoring of these medications can be helpful.

- **Bowel and bladder function.** MS can affect the neurological reflexes responsible for bowel and bladder control, leading to a spastic bladder that can't hold urine or a flaccid bladder that can't empty itself. Signs of trouble include urinary urgency, frequency, and incontinence. Often, evaluation by a specialist is required to assess the precise nature of the problem and design a program to compensate for it. Constipation is a common problem for MS patients due to the direct effects of MS, diet, attempts to restrict fluid to manage incontinence, medication side effects, and immobility. The treatment of constipation relies upon its prevention with fiber supplements and a regular bowel regimen.

- **Sexual dysfunction.** Sexual dysfunction is common in MS patients. In men it is treated the same way as other causes of erectile dysfunction; see *Chapter 27: Men's Health Issues* on page 289 for more information. Little research has been done in women.

- **Cognitive dysfunction.** Cognitive dysfunction may develop in two-thirds of MS patients, affecting concentration, memory for recent events, and the processing of information. No drug therapy is yet available for this problem. Awareness of it and the education of family and friends about it are important to maximize the patient's abilities and protect them from harm.

- **Depression.** Depression occurs more frequently in MS patients than in the general population. This is associated with an increased rate of suicide in those with MS, regardless of the stage of the disease. Signs of depression, such as fatigue and sleep disturbance, are common in MS and may not be recognized as being separate from the MS symptoms. Effective therapy for depression is available and can have a significant impact on the quality of life of depressed MS patients. Signs of depression should be routinely looked for as part of the ongoing comprehensive evaluation of MS patients.

CHAPTER 29

Mental Health

As an average primary care physician, most folks are surprised to learn that I spend approximately one-third of my time in the office addressing mental health issues. During my first fifteen years of practice there have been tremendous advancements in the understanding of mental health, the discovery of the biochemistry behind some mental illness, and the therapies available to assist patients with both the symptoms and biochemical aspects of their diseases. One of the most difficult parts of a primary care physician's job is to pick up the psychological issues and forces that often result in physical symptoms for which the patient has decided to seek treatment. It is a difficult and time-consuming task that, at times, can meet with significant resistance from the patient and his or her family in the recognition of the psychological basis for their physical symptoms or an acceptance of the need for therapy.

This chapter discusses some common mental health issues of interest to both men and women, including panic disorder, stage fright, generalized anxiety disorder, eating disorders, and depression.

Panic Disorder

The body has a built-in alarm system that goes off when threat is felt. This system triggers physical and emotional changes carried out through signals from the sympathetic nervous system, very similar to a shot of adrenaline. This may be useful if you hear a bump in the night, or come across a bear in the woods, in that the response heightens your awareness and primes your body for action. In patients with panic disorder, this system is triggered at inappropriate times without obvious cause. Panic disorder is understood as a chemical imbalance or instability in the brain associated with inappropriate surges in adrenaline.

Panic disorder is different from normal anxiety, such as that from taking a test or public speaking. The American Psychiatric Association defines a panic attack as an unprovoked surge of fear accompanied by at least four of the following physical or emotional symptoms:

- Racing heartbeat
- Shortness of breath or a smothering sensation

- Feeling faint or dizzy
- Hot or cold flushes
- Trembling or shaking
- Sweating
- Chest discomfort or pain
- Choking
- Tingling of the fingers, toes, or lips
- Weakness
- Nausea or abdominal discomfort
- Feelings of detachment or unreality
- Feelings of a lack of control
- Fear of dying or going crazy

Because of the number and severity of physical symptoms, most patients with panic disorder consult multiple physicians and undergo extensive testing for medical diseases before the diagnosis is made.

Panic attacks happen suddenly, last for minutes, and usually resolve quickly. The first attack usually occurs "out of the blue." The brain, usually a rational organ, tries to look for a reason for the attacks. People begin to avoid activities and circumstances that they associate with previous attacks or where they feel "escape" would be difficult if an attack occurs. They also develop secondary anxiety about when the next attack will occur. This pattern of fear and avoidance of activities and circumstances associated with attacks, and worrying about new attacks, can be paralyzing.

Four to five percent of the population has an occasional panic attack. One to two percent of the population has panic disorder, defined as four or more attacks within four weeks. Two-thirds of patients with panic disorder are women; one-third of patients with this disorder also suffer from depression. Panic disorder patients also tend to abuse drugs and alcohol. Patients who feel they might have panic disorder should visit a physician for an initial evaluation; this evaluation should include a careful review of the patient's history, a complete physical examination, and testing for medical problems that can mimic panic attacks.

The cause of panic disorder is unknown, although biologic theories exist to explain the attacks. Certain chemical substances, when administered, can duplicate panic attacks in those who are susceptible to them but have no similar effects on those without the disease. Positron emission tomography (PET) scanning, which evaluates areas of brain activity, lights up abnormal activity in a particular area of the brain in patients with panic disorder.

Treatment involves providing education and understanding for the patient and his or her family, friends, and co-workers. Involvement of family and friends in treatment and providing emotional support are essential. Cognitive and behavioral therapies from a counselor experienced in the management of panic disorder can be useful, and can provide adequate treatment without drugs in some patients.

Medical therapy for panic disorder is available in the form of both short-acting and long-acting medications. One family of drugs in particular, benzodiazepines, is often prescribed to rapidly treat the symptoms of anxiety; however, these drugs have significant side effects, tend to lose their effectiveness with continued use, and have a high addiction potential. Even after the sedative effect wears off, these drugs still slow reaction times and impair motor skills—patients taking benzodiazepines are twice as likely to have a traffic accident. Other side effects include mental confusion, risks of falls in the elderly, amnesia, disinhibition of certain behaviors, and respiratory depression (especially if mixed with alcohol).

I use benzodiazepines in carefully selected patients with anxiety and panic disorder (those whose frequency or severity of panic attacks needs rapid control but who are judged to be at low risk for addiction or medication abuse), usually in the initial course of therapy. Better long-term therapy for chronic anxiety and panic disorder is achieved through longer acting medications, such as buspirone and certain antidepressants. These drugs can work well to reduce the severity and frequency of anxiety and panic attacks but take two to six weeks to show a benefit and often heighten the symptoms before they begin to help. They are started at low doses and are carefully adjusted based on the patient's response to them. Benzodiazepines are useful in combination with these drugs to get through this initial transition period.

Stage Fright

Stage fright refers to symptoms of intense anxiety that occur in settings such as public speaking. Speaking before a group, or even the anticipation of such activity, can stimulate a whole range of symptoms of anxiety. A pounding heart, chest pain, shortness of breath, tremor, sweating, and urinary and fecal urgency are the most common physical symptoms. At times, these are so incapacitating that individuals are forced to avoid career opportunities that would force them to present to others.

Most of the symptoms of stage fright are caused by an adrenaline surge stimulated by the sympathetic nervous system. Treatment for this problem involve both cognitive—where trained counselors guide patients through a process to desensitize them to their anxieties—and medical therapies.

Medical therapies chiefly rely on drugs that block the symptoms produced by the activated sympathetic nervous system. While traditional drugs for anxiety help, their sedating side effects are most unwelcome in the public arena when you need to be at your sharpest. Beta-blockers, like propranolol, block the effects of adrenaline and therefore reduce the symptoms associated with stage fright, without the sedation of anti-anxiety drugs. They can be taken within an hour before a presentation and provide adequate relief for most patients. Longer-term therapies using the selective serotonin reuptake inhibitors (SSRI) class of antidepressants are also available. These medications must be taken daily and begin to exert their beneficial effects after two to four weeks of therapy. They work by boosting the level of serotonin in the brain, a chemical intimately involved in the regulation of emotional behaviors.

Generalized Anxiety Disorder

Generalized anxiety disorder consists of excessive worry and chronic anxiety over time, associated with physical symptoms including an increase in muscle tension, restlessness, fatigue, insomnia, impaired concentration, and irritability. Symptoms duplicate many of those in panic disorder, but instead of discrete episodes, the patient with this disorder experiences a more pervasive sense of anxiety. This disorder is also felt to be due to chemical and possibly structural changes in brain function and responds to both cognitive—where trained counselors guide patients through a process to desensitize them to their anxieties—and drug therapics.

Eating Disorders

Many varieties of eating disorders exist that share a distorted attitude toward eating that affects the patient's physical health. *Anorexia nervosa* and *bulimia nervosa* are two of the more commonly recognized eating disorders.

Anorexia Nervosa

Patients with anorexia nervosa have a distorted body image with an inordinate fear of becoming too fat, even when to the casual observer they are obviously too thin. They have a distorted attitude toward eating that overwhelms natural hunger signals. By definition, patients with anorexia are 15 percent or more below normal body weight. The disease usually begins at puberty and affects women nine times more frequently than men. The majority of patients are women under the age of 25. The cause of this disease is unknown.

Medical criteria for diagnosis include:

- Refusal to maintain body weight at or above the minimal body weight for a patient's age and height
- An intense fear of gaining weight or becoming fat
- A disturbance in body image, with an undue influence of body weight or shape on self-esteem and a denial of the seriousness of their low body weight
- In women of menstrual age, amenorrhea (the absence of at least three consecutive menstrual periods)

Other signs and symptoms of anorexia nervosa include:

- Seeming alert and active, yet unaware that there is a problem
- A desire for personal perfection—many patients are good students who are actively involved in school and community activities
- Abnormal food preoccupations—for example, may be gourmet cooks who enjoy preparing food for others but don't consume it
- Constipation
- Dry skin

- Lack of libido
- Excessive dieting and exercising
- Insomnia
- Frequent medical illness including upper respiratory infections and—as the disease progresses—anemia, palpitations, loss of bone density, tooth decay, and ultimately heart and kidney failure from nutritional deficiencies
- Increased rates of suicide and suicide attempts

Bulimia Nervosa

Patients with bulimia nervosa may have normal body weights and are more difficult for others to recognize. Whereas patients with anorexia tend to suppress all urges, patients with bulimia tend to indulge in their cravings, act on impulse, and attempt to make up for their indiscretions later. Bulimia nervosa usually begins at about age 18. The true number of women with this disease is unknown, with estimates of it occurring in up to one in five high school and college age women.

Medical criteria for diagnosis include:

- Recurrent episodes of binge eating: eating within a discrete period of time an amount of food that is definitely larger than most people would eat, coupled with a sense of lack of control over eating during the episode
- Recurrent inappropriate compensatory behavior to prevent weight gain: self-induced vomiting, abuse of laxatives, fasting, and/or excessive exercise
- Episodes occurring at least twice a week over a three-month period
- Self-evaluation and personal worth is unduly influenced by body shape and weight

Other signs and symptoms of bulimia nervosa include:

- A desire for personal perfection—many patients are good students who are actively involved in school and community activities
- An unrealistic fear of becoming fat
- Other impulsive acts, including drug abuse, risky sexual behavior, and shopping excesses
- Physical problems related to repetitive vomiting: irritation of the lining of the esophagus by stomach acid, tooth decay and gum disease, and fluid and electrolyte disturbances
- Increased rates of depression and suicide

Treatment of Anorexia Nervosa and Bulimia Nervosa

Anorexia nervosa and bulimia nervosa are serious diseases. They are tough to recognize, difficult to treat, and relapses are common. The death rate from anorexia nervosa is estimated to be between 1 and 10 to 1 in 20 patients. Family and social support is necessary to recognize the problem and get the patient to seek treatment. Patients respond better when the disease is identified and treated early—a tough job in a disease shrouded in such secrecy. As with other addictions, it is important to love and support the patient no matter what, without supporting what she is doing.

Patients with eating disorders require treatment that addresses the many facets of their disease. Medical care, psychotherapy, nutritional counseling, medication, and group therapy are all important components of the care needed. Body image improvement through Yoga, Tai Chi, or other forms of meditative exercise is helpful. It is best when these therapies can be provided in close collaboration at a center that specializes in treatment of eating disorders. Experience does matter in successfully treating these diseases.

Depression

Depression is a whole body illness, affecting the body, mood, thoughts, and behavior. It interferes with the ability to work, sleep, eat, and enjoy pleasurable activities. There are many misconceptions about depression. In reality, it is a medical illness, not a character flaw; depressed patients can't simply will themselves to get better. With therapy, recovery is the rule, not the exception. Antidepressants are not addictive, do not change personality, and do not cause suicide. Without therapy, symptoms can last for weeks, months, or years. Since the earlier depression is treated the better the symptoms respond to drug therapy, antidepressants should be used sooner rather than later in the course of depression treatment. The goal of therapy is to get well—and stay well!

Most patients with depression are seen and treated by their primary care physician. Often, patients seek treatment for the physical symptoms of depression, not for depression itself; depressed patients sometimes can't see through the cloud of their own symptoms to recognize the root of those symptoms as depression. Many things interfere with the recognition of depression. There is a historical stigma to mental illness, when it was thought of as a personal failing and not a medical, biochemical illness. Patients are fearful of the insurance ramifications and other effects of being labeled with depression; laws need to change to eliminate this as a concern.

Depression is defined as five or more of the following symptoms consistently present over a two-week period, at least one of which must be either depressed mood or loss of interest or pleasure:

- Persistent sad, anxious, or empty mood—most of the day, every day
- Markedly diminished interest and pleasure in all activity, including diminished sexual interest and disinterest in hobbies or activities that were once enjoyed
- Significant appetite changes, weight loss or gain of greater than 5 percent in a month
- Sleep disturbances, such as insomnia, early morning awakening, and oversleeping
- Psychomotor agitation or retardation nearly every day, observed by others
- Decreased energy, fatigue, feeling slowed down
- Feelings of inappropriate guilt, worthlessness, and helplessness
- Difficulty concentrating, remembering, making decisions
- Thoughts of death or suicide, perhaps resulting in suicide attempts
- Feelings of hopelessness and pessimism

- Persistent, unexplained physical symptoms that do not respond to treatment, such as headaches, digestive disorders, or chronic pain

These symptoms must cause significant distress or impairment in social, occupational, or other functions. To be attributed to depression, they cannot be the direct result of a substance (drug abuse) or other disease.

Dysthymia is the name for the condition of chronic, non-disabling symptoms of depression. Patients with many symptoms of depression but who don't reach the established criteria for a diagnosis of depression may still be experiencing a significant reduction in the quality of their lives. I have treated many patients in this category with antidepressant therapy with significant benefit. *Manic-depression* is a condition with wide and repeated swings of mood from depression to extreme elevations of mood. It is associated with irrational beliefs and actions. This condition is talked about a lot, but in 16 years of patient care I haven't seen more than a few patients with it. It is much more popular in movies than in fact.

The exact cause of depression is not understood, although contributors are thought to include defects in chemical systems in the brain involving serotonin, norepinephrine, and dopamine. Risk factors associated with an increased incidence of depression include:

- A prior history of other episodes of depression. Of those patients who fully recover from depression, 50 percent will have a second episode later in life. In those with two episodes, 75 percent will have a third. If more than three episodes have occurred, the subsequent risk of recurrence is greater than 90 percent, and ongoing medical therapy is advised.
- A family history of depression
- Previous onset of depression before age 40
- Female gender
- A recent pregnancy (postpartum depression)
- Stressful life events, such as serious loss, chronic illness, relationship difficulties, or financial hardship
- Lack of social support
- Current substance abuse
- Certain medical conditions. Fifty percent of patients with a recent heart attack become depressed; Parkinson's disease and early Alzheimer's disease are strongly associated with depression, as are thyroid disease, diabetes, and certain cancers.
- Exposure to certain medications

Treatment for depression involves several approaches, often pursued simultaneously.

Self-help efforts revolve around gaining an understanding of the disease and protecting yourself from harm until you are better. Educate yourself—know that your symptoms are part of a disease, not personal failure. Be patient with yourself; recovery takes time. Symptoms and the negative thinking associated with them fade gradually. Do not set difficult goals with deadlines or take on greater responsibilities until you are better. Write down priorities, break large tasks into small ones, do what you can. Remain involved with people and activities that you enjoy and avoid isolation. Let friends and family know what you are facing; educate them and rely upon them. Begin a regular exercise program; several studies show that regular exercise affects the levels of neurotransmitters in the brain and can be an effective tool in managing depression.

All types of depression can benefit from psychotherapy—I encourage all of my patients with depression and anxiety disorders to explore this option. It usually takes three or four visits with a therapist to decide if this is a person that you can effectively work with. Although studies show that cognitive therapy for depression can have the same long-term success rates as medical therapy in some patients, I usually favor a combination of medical and psychological therapy. I think that my patients get better faster this way.

As for antidepressant medications, many classes exist. They differ not so much in effectiveness as in side effects. Patients respond very differently to the various antidepressant medications, and physicians can merely guess as to which drug will perform best for an individual patient. This guess is improved by patient–physician collaboration to choose the most likely drug to target the main symptoms bothering the patient and to avoid the side effects the patient would find the most troubling.

Antidepressant medications act slowly. It usually takes four to six weeks before any benefit is seen and even longer to reach maximum benefit. Although the side effects of these medications often fade within a few weeks, they usually begin right away and there is a strong possibility that, overall, a patient will feel worse rather than better in the early parts of therapy. The patient and physician must work closely during this time period to adjust the dose appropriately and deal with side effects.

Most antidepressants must be taken for an initial course of 6 to 12 months. Patients often want to stop therapy prematurely once they feel better, but stopping a drug too early significantly increases the risk of a relapse of the depression. Don't do this.

Side effects of antidepressants are usually mild and most bothersome right at the beginning of therapy, fading after one or two weeks. The newer drugs, including selective serotonin reuptake inhibitors (SSRIs), are the drugs of choice for most patients. Their initial side effects may include nausea, headache, nervousness, insomnia, sexual dysfunction (decreased libido and difficulty reaching orgasm), and weight gain. There are ways to minimize most of these symptoms. Older classes of antidepressants (the tricyclics) have different side effects including urinary retention, constipation, dry mouth, blurred vision, blood pressure drops with upright posture, weight gain, and sedation. These drugs have limited use now, mostly as supplemental therapies to increase the benefit of some of the newer drugs.

Many antidepressants have withdrawal symptoms if they are stopped too abruptly, including dizziness, headache, nausea, sensory changes, and mood changes. At times, it is difficult to separate patients having a withdrawal from their medications with those experiencing an early relapse of depression.

In summary, depression is a many-faceted disorder that has a biochemical basis and is as real as hypertension or diabetes. Therapy for depression is complex but can offer tremendous benefit. A close working relationship between patient and physician is required to most successfully diagnose and treat depression.

Glossary

A

Acne – a chronic infectious and inflammatory disorder of the skin, commonly affecting the sweat and oil glands of the face, chest, and back.

Actinic keratoses – red, sandpaper-textured skin lesions that come and go, frequently peeling off and then growing back in the same spot. Actinic keratoses are related to sun exposure and are felt to be precursors to skin cancer.

Acquired immune deficiency syndrome – *See* HIV.

Acute – having a sudden, abrupt onset; not long-term.

Addiction – a compulsive disorder in which a person is preoccupied with using substances that lower the quality of their life.

Adrenal gland – a triangular-shaped gland covering the top of each kidney. Adrenal glands are composed of two layers. The outer layer, or cortex, produces hormones that influence almost all body systems. The inner layer, or medulla, produces chemicals that regulate blood flow, heart function, and several other body functions.

Aerobic exercise – sustained exercise in which energy is obtained from inhaled oxygen rather than only from energy sources already stored in the body.

AIDS – *See* HIV.

Airway remodeling – permanent adverse changes in the architecture of the lungs that occur over time due to uncontrolled inflammation.

Aldosterone – a hormone that regulates the balance of salt and water in the body.

Allergic rhinitis – the local allergy reaction that occurs when an antigen floating in the air is inhaled through the nose.

Alopecia – absence or loss of hair.

Alternative medicine – medical diagnostic and therapeutic approaches that lie outside the standard training of most United States medical graduates, often relying on theories or philosophies that have not been developed through objective scientific principals that allow for validation of their effectiveness by commonly accepted means. Examples include homeopathy, aromatherapy, and faith healing.

Amenorrhea – the absence of at least three consecutive menstrual periods.

Anabolic steroid – steroid hormone utilized to promote muscle mass development, commonly associated with side effects including acne, mood swings, liver toxicity, heart disease, premature closing of the growth plates and stunted growth in teens, and possibly an increased risk of prostate cancer.

Anaphylaxis – an immune reaction to an antigen that results in dilation of large numbers of blood vessels. Symptoms include skin flushing; hives and angioedema; excessive secretions, swelling, and spasm in the respiratory airways; chest pain and palpitations; and effects on the gastrointestinal tract including abdominal cramping, nausea, vomiting, and diarrhea; shock and death.

Androgen – a substance leading to the development of male characteristics (for example, testosterone).

Androstenedione – a testosterone precursor that can increase strength and muscle mass.

Aneurysm – a localized swelling in a blood vessel of greater than 50 percent of its usual diameter.

Angina – chest pain, pressure, numbness, or other symptoms caused by a temporary insufficiency of blood flow to the heart.

Angioedema – localized immune reactions composed of dilated blood vessels and localized tissue fluid that extend deeper into the skin and subcutaneous tissues than hives and typically involve the face, tongue, and genitals.

Angiogram – a procedure in which a contrast material is placed in a blood vessel to allow an x-ray picture of its internal shape to be taken.

Angioplasty – a procedure during which an incision is made under local anesthesia to gain access to a diseased blood vessel, a catheter is passed to the area of blockage in the vessel, and a balloon is inflated to crush the blockage open. *See also* Atherectomy.

Anorexia – a lack or loss of appetite

Antibiotics – medications that kill bacteria or stop them from growing so that your immune system can destroy them. Antibiotics work by chemically interfering with the key steps that a bacterium follows to get energy, grow, or reproduce.

Antigen – a substance that the immune system's allergy mechanisms recognize and react to.

Antihistamines – medications that block the effects of histamine. Antihistamines are used to help relieve symptoms of the allergy response, such as sneezing, itching, and drainage.

Antioxidants – chemicals that prevent or slow the process of oxidation by donating extra electrons to free radicals, in theory before they have a chance to cause much damage. *See also* Free radicals.

Aortic valve – a one-way heart valve between the left ventricle and the aorta

Aphthous ulcers (canker sores) – small, shallow, painful ulcers that occur in the lining of the mouth.

Artery – a blood vessel, typically with a thick muscular wall, that carries blood away from the heart.

Asthma – a chronic inflammatory disease of the small airways with symptoms including wheezing, shortness of breath, chest tightness, and cough.

Aspiration – 1) a diagnostic technique where fluid or tissue is obtained from the body with a needle and suction. 2) the process when solids or liquids are introduced from the oral cavity into the airway and lungs.

Atherectomy – similar to an angioplasty, except that a drill-like device is used to grind up and remove plaque. *See also* Angioplasty.

Atherosclerosis – a life-long process leading to thickening of the artery walls and subsequent narrowing of the artery by accumulations of lipids, connective tissue, and other substances.

Atopic dermatitis – a chronic, inflammatory condition of the skin that usually begins before age 5 and typically involves the neck, creases of the elbows and knees, wrists and ankles, and hands and feet. Atopic dermatitis is characterized by red, shallow erosions in the skin and tiny blisters filled with clear fluid. Intense itching leads to red, scratched, thickened areas, skin dryness, and changes in skin pigmentation.

Atrial fibrillation – a condition in which the underlying heart rhythm from the sinoatrial node completely breaks down and the heartbeat has an irregular rhythm.

Atrium – the first chamber on each side of the heart, which receives the blood and functions as a primer pump for the main pumping chamber (the ventricle).

Autonomic nervous system – the portion of the nervous system concerned with the regulation of involuntary body functions, such as gland and the cardiovascular and gastrointestinal systems.

B

Bacteremia – the presence of bacteria in the bloodstream.

Bacteria – self-contained microscopic organisms, some of which are capable of living within the human body, either with beneficial (manufacturing vitamins) or detrimental (causing disease) effects.

Barrett's esophagus – precancerous changes to the lining of the esophagus, often related to gastroesophageal reflux.

Basal cell carcinoma – a locally aggressive skin cancer that can appear as a pearl-like growth or non-healing sore.

Benign – the opposite of malignant—a growth that does not follow an aggressive course, does not produce disease or death, and is not cancerous.

Benign prostatic hypertrophy (BPH) – age-related enlargement of the prostate gland, often affecting urine flow.

Benzodiazepines – a group of drugs with sedative properties, used to treat anxiety and promote sleep. Propensity towards lack of sustained effect with time, addiction, and abuse limit their usefulness.

Bimodal intermittent positive airway pressure – *See* BiPAP.

Biopsy – obtaining a sample of tissue for analysis though an incision, needle, or other surgical technique.

BiPAP (Bimodal intermittent positive airway pressure) – a device that increases the positive pressure in the airways, worn at night by sleep apnea patients to keep their airways open.

Body mass index – a calculation of weight in comparison to height used to measure the health risks associated with an individual's weight.

Bone density – a measure of calcium content of bone, correlating to the risk of fracture.

BPH – *See* Benign prostatic hypertrophy.

Bronchia – the upper airway beyond the trachea as it divides to reach the left and right lungs.

Bronchitis – an infection of the large- and medium-sized upper airways in the lung, commonly caused by a virus.

Bronchodilators – medications that relax the smooth muscle in the airways to reverse or prevent airway narrowing.

Bronchoscopy – the use of a flexible, fiber-optic tube to examine the inside of the upper airways.

Bursa – sacs filled with fluid and positioned around joints to allow structures to smoothly slide over one another.

Bypass – surgical placement of a new blood vessel to route blood flow around an area of obstruction.

C

CA-125 – a protein associated with ovarian cancer that can be measured in blood. Current testing has proven useful to monitor the response to therapy for patients with known ovarian cancer. It has not proven effective as a screening test for the early detection of ovarian cancer.

Calcium – an element important in numerous body processes, including bone growth and development, blood clotting, acid-base balance, nerve and muscle function.

Canker sores – *See* aphthous ulcers.

Capillaries – the tiniest of blood vessels, with very thin walls so that oxygen and other nutrients can easily pass into the tissues that they supply.

Carbon dioxide – a waste gas produced by the body and eliminated via breathing.

Carbon monoxide – a poison in tobacco smoke that interferes with the blood's ability to carry oxygen.

Carcinogens – cancer-causing substances.

Cardiac catheterization – a diagnostic and therapeutic procedure performed in the hospital using thin catheters introduced in a major blood vessel and guided up to the heart for testing and treatment.

Carotid – the major blood vessels in the front of the neck that supply the brain.

Carpal tunnel – a tunnel formed from bones in the wrist through which nerves, tendons, and blood vessels pass.

Carpal tunnel syndrome – a condition in which arthritis or trauma cause the walls of the carpal tunnel to swell and place pressure on the median nerve that passes through it.

Cartilage – a specialized type of dense connective tissue forming the smooth surfaces on the ends of bones at a joint and at other sites (nose, ears, airways) for structural support.

Cataract – clouding of the lens of the eye, caused when the proteins that make up the lens clump together.

Cathartic – a chemical that stimulates bowel movements.

Cellulitis – a bacterial infection that typically appears as a red, hot, painful swelling on the surface of the skin and often spreads rapidly.

Chemoprevention – the use of chemicals to reduce the rate of cancer occurrence or prevent the development of other diseases.

Chemotherapy – the use of chemicals to treat a disease, most commonly used to describe cancer therapies.

CHF – *See* Congestive heart failure.

Chlamydia – a microscopic organism that is the most common sexually transmitted disease in the United States

Cholecystitis – inflammation of the wall of the gallbladder.

Cholera – a disease acquired from contaminated food (particularly shellfish), water, or milk causing severe diarrhea, cramps, and vomiting. It can lead to profound dehydration and death.

Cholesterol – a chemical in foods or produced in the liver. It serves as the building blocks for the production of certain hormones. High levels of cholesterol are associated with heart and other blood vessel diseases. *See also HDL cholesterol, LDL cholesterol.*

Chromosome – a structure in the cell nucleus containing genetic material that codes for the structure and function of the body.

Chronic – of long duration.

Chronic bronchitis – a lung disease defined by cough and sputum production for at least three consecutive months for more than two consecutive years.

Chronic fatigue syndrome – a disease defined by a cluster of symptoms including: 1) severe chronic fatigue of six months or longer in duration, not explained by other known medical illness, and 2) four or more of the following symptoms: reduced short-term memory or impaired ability to concentrate, sore throat, tender lymph nodes, muscle pain, joint pain without signs of inflammation, headaches, sleep that does not refresh, and excessive, prolonged (more than 24 hours) fatigue after physical exertion.

Chronic obstructive pulmonary disease (COPD) – chronic bronchitis and/or emphysema.

Cilia – tiny, microscopic hairs that line some areas of the upper respiratory tract.

Circadian rhythm – pertaining to usual variations in the body seen over a 24-hour period, particularly in reference to hormone levels.

Cirrhosis – the result of many chronic diseases of the liver, characterized by scar formation in the liver and a decrease in liver function.

Cluster headaches – severe, one-sided migraine-like headaches that occur in waves, often associated with tearing, facial flushing, and sweating on the involved side.

Collagen – a protein found in connective tissues, a key component of skin, bones, cartilage, and ligaments.

Colonoscopy – examination of the colon with a flexible fiber-optic scope. This procedure requires intravenous sedation and can be used for diagnostic and therapeutic purposes.

Co-morbid conditions – other illnesses occurring simultaneously as the primary illness. These conditions may be related or completely independent of each other.

Congestive heart failure (CHF) – a condition in which the heart cannot effectively pump blood to the body, usually because the heart is weakened or damaged by disease. Occasionally occurs when the body's demand for blood flow exceeds the abilities of a normally functioning heart.

Conjunctivitis – inflammation of the conjunctiva, the visible portion of the moist tissue surrounding the eyeball. Conjunctivitis can be caused by infection stemming from a virus or bacteria, or by allergies or other immune reactions.

Constipation – the passage of dry, hard bowel movements, usually fewer than three times a week.

COPD – *See* Chronic obstructive pulmonary disease.

Coronary arteries – blood vessels that begin off of the first part of the aorta and supply blood rich with oxygen to the heart muscle.

Coronary artery disease – atherosclerosis affecting the arteries that supply blood to the heart muscle.

Costochondritis – inflammation of the cartilage that connects the ribs and the breastbone, a common cause of chest pain.

Cox-2 inhibitors – anti-inflammatory medications that are more selective for inflammation in the joints, with fewer side effects on the gastrointestinal tract and platelets.

CPAP (Continuous positive airway pressure) – a device that increases the positive pressure in the airways, worn at night by sleep apnea patients to keep their airways open.

Crohn's disease – an inflammatory bowel disease which may involve the entire gastrointestinal tract.

CT scan – an x-ray technique that creates three-dimensional images of internal body structures.

Cystoscopy – a procedure in which a flexible fiber-optic tube is inserted through the urethra into the bladder to allow for inspection of the bladder or procedures within it.

D

Delirium tremens – a syndrome that may occur one to three days after the abrupt cessation of alcohol intake in an alcohol dependent person. Patients experiencing this syndrome are hyperactive, tremulous, combative, disoriented, and confused. Other signs include dilated pupils, sweating, increase in heart rate and breathing, fever, and repetitive seizures.

Delusions – fixed, false beliefs.

Dementia – a progressive disease which results in a global decline in higher cognitive function, including memory, attention and concentration, judgment and reason, speech, motor abilities, and personality.

Depression – a biochemical disorder of the brain, defined by depressed mood and/or a loss of interest or pleasure, as well as a series of associated symptoms.

Dermatitis – inflammationof the skin, usually characterized by itching and redness.

Dermis – the skin.

Diabetes – a disorder of carbohydrate metabolism, characterized by tissue resistance to the effects of insulin, and/or insulin deficiency.

Diagnosis – 1) The term relating the condition that a patient is believed to have. 2) The process of identifying what condition afflicts the patient, involving obtaining a history of the illness, a physical examination, testing, and deductive reasoning.

Diaphragm – a dome-shaped muscle at the base of the lungs that separates the chest and abdominal cavities, providing the force for breathing.

Diarrhea – the frequent passage of poorly formed stools.

Diastolic blood pressure – the lowest blood pressure that occurs in the arteries prior to the next contraction of the heart muscle.

Diastolic hypertension – a lower blood pressure (diastolic) measurement of greater than or equal to 90. *See also* Systolic blood pressure.

Dietary supplement – under the 1994 Dietary Supplement Health and Education Act, this term is used to describe any product marketed for and claimed to affect the structure or function of the body, as long as the labeling includes a disclaimer saying that it has not been evaluated by the FDA and the product is not intended to diagnose, treat, or prevent any disease.

Differentiation – the process of turning on and off select portions of DNA within a cell as it becomes more specialized in structure or function.

Diphtheria – a respiratory illness acquired from exposure to respiratory secretions from an infected patient, characterized by fever, sore throat, painful swallowing, blockage of airway with respiratory distress.

Discs, intravertebral – structures between the vertebral bodies in the spinal column that act as shock absorbers and allow for flexibility.

Dislocation – when bones are pulled out their usual position, often involving tears in ligaments.

Diuretics – medications that affect kidney function in such a way as to increase the elimination of salt and water.

Diverticulitis – infection of a diverticulum.

Diverticulosis – the condition when diverticulum are present.

Diverticulum – a small hernia or pouch in the muscular wall of the colon.

DNA – deoxyribonucleic acid, containing the genetic code for an organism. *See also* RNA.

Dopamine – a neurotransmitter in the brain, associated with movement disorders (Parkinson's disease), emotions, and the rewarding effects of addictive substances.

Dysphagia – difficulty swallowing.

Dysplasia – a precancerous state, where the tissue is abnormal but not cancerous.

Dysthymia – chronic symptoms of depression that are not disabling and aren't severe or numerous enough to meet the formal definition of depression.

E

Eczema – a chronic, inflammatory condition of the skin that lasts for months to years and typically involves the neck, creases of the elbows and knees, wrists and ankles, and hands and feet. Eczema is characterized by red, shallow erosions in the skin and tiny blisters filled with clear fluid. Intense itching leads to red, scratched, thickened areas, skin dryness, and changes in skin pigmentation.

Edema – a condition in which the body tissues contain excessive fluid in the loose space between cells. This fluid is pulled down between cells by gravity, often resulting in swollen ankles.

EKG – *See* Electrocardiogram.

Electrocardiogram – a surface recording of the electric impulses generated by heart muscle. Changes from normal in this recording can be clues to past or present heart disease.

Electrolytes – ionized salts in blood and body fluid, such as sodium, potassium, chloride, or magnesium.

Emphysema – defined anatomically as distention of the alveoli (air sacs of the lung) with breakdown of the fine membranes separating them.

Endometrial biopsy – an office procedure in which a thin tube is passed though the opening of the cervix into the cavity of the uterus and suction is used to obtain a sample of the uterine lining cells.

Endoscopy – the use of a flexible fiberoptic tube passed through the mouth or anus, to examine or perform procedures on portions of the upper or lower gastrointestinal tract.

Enzyme – a protein chemical produced by living cells that is capable of promoting a chemical reaction.

Epicondylitis – an overuse injury causing inflammation in the elbow where tendons from the forearm muscles attach.

Epidemic – an infectious disease or condition that strikes many people simultaneously in an identified geographic area.

Epidermis – the outermost layer of the skin.

Erectile dysfunction (ED) – the consistent or intermittent inability to obtain or sustain an erection sufficient for sexual intercourse.

Esophagitis – inflammation of the lining of the esophagus, usually caused by acid reflux or noxious chemicals or medications.

Estrogen – the female sex hormones, which control body changes related to the reproductive cycle and have a variety of effects on many other body systems.

Eustachian tube – a small tube providing ventilation between the middle ear and the back of the nasal passages.

Family history – a health history of other blood-related family members that serves to alert your physician to inherited disease trends.

Fats – a class of chemical structures, as opposed to protein or carbohydrate, present in animals and plants. Dietary fats are grouped into categories based on their chemical composition that relate to their effects on the body. Rated from healthiest to worst fats are:

Monounsaturated fats – olive, peanut, canola, and flax seed oils
Polyunsaturated fats – sunflower, safflower, corn, and soybean oils
Saturated fat – animal proteins, palm oil, and coconut oil

Fecal occult blood test (Guaiac test) – a chemical test of stool samples to detect microscopic amounts of blood.

Fibrocystic breast disease – a nonspecific condition in which there are benign lumps in the breast tissue, usually associated with pain and tenderness, that fluctuate with the menstrual cycle and generally resolve at menopause.

Fibroid – a benign tumor in the muscular wall of the uterus that may be associated with pain, regional pressure, and irregular menstrual bleeding.

Fibromyalgia – a syndrome characterized by pain in muscles and tendons without evidence of inflammation or degenerative changes in the joints.

Flexible sigmoidoscopy – an evaluation of the lower colon using a flexible fiber-optic scope.

Flu – *See* Influenza.

Folic acid – a member of the B complex vitamins, essential for health and development.

Free radicals – a chemical compound that has lost an electron in it's chemical structure, often damaging to other tissues as it attempts to steal an electron from them. *See also* Antioxidants.

Fungus (yeast) – parasitic plants that typically cause infections of body surfaces, but can also cause invasive disease when the body is not functioning properly.

G

Gallbladder – a small sac-like organ at the base of the liver that stores bile.

Gallstones – rock-like collections of cholesterol that may form in the gallbladder

Ganglion cyst – a cyst formed around synovial fluid that has leaked from a tendon sheath.

Gastroesophageal reflux (GERD) – malfunction of the protective mechanisms between the esophagus and stomach, allowing for contents of the stomach to wash up into the esophagus.

Gene – *See* Chromosome.

GERD – *See* Gastroesophageal reflux.

Gestational diabetes – diabetes that occurs during pregnancy, and resolves with the end of pregnancy.

Glaucoma – a disease of the eye related to abnormal fluid circulation within the eyeball.

Goiter – an enlarged, lumpy thyroid gland.

Gout – a type of inflammatory arthritis caused by the precipitation of sodium urate crystals in the joint fluid.

Grave's disease – the body's immune system produces an antibody that stimulates the thyroid gland in the same way that TSH does, leading to excess production and release of thyroid hormone that is not controlled by the body's usual feedback mechanisms and results in hyperthyroidism.

Guaiac test – *See* Fecal occult blood test.

H

Halitosis – continuous bad breath.

Hallucinations – false auditory or visual perceptions that accompany delusions.

HDL cholesterol – the "good" cholesterol, associated with beneficial effects on blood vessels. A protein that carries cholesterol from the arteries to be metabolized in the liver. *See also* Cholesterol.

Heart attack – *See* Myocardial infarction.

Hematoma – a collection of clotted blood inside the body but outside of a blood vessel, usually the result of a trauma.

Hemochromatosis – a metabolic disease of iron metabolism in which the intestine absorbs excessive iron leading to a gradual overloading of iron in the body. Iron overload has been associated with cancers, heart disease, arthritis, chronic fatigue, diabetes, liver damage, and impotence.

Hemoglobin – a chemical that carries oxygen in the bloodstream, the red part of a red blood cell.

Hemoglobin A1c test (HgbA1c) – a test that provides a measure of the average blood sugar readings over the past three months by measuring changes in hemoglobin caused by elevated blood sugars.

Hemorrhoids – distended veins at the end of the gastrointestinal tract

Hepatitis – inflammation of the liver, most commonly caused by a drug reaction or viral infection.

Hernia – a defect in the structure of the wall of an organ or body cavity, so that the contents of that cavity can bulge through it. Hernias are classified according to their location within the body:

Femoral hernia – located at the junction of the leg and pelvis.
Inguinal hernia – located at the groin.
Umbilical hernia – located at the belly button.
Ventral hernia – located in the midline of the abdomen.

HgbA1c – *See* Hemoglobin A1c test.

Hirsutism – excessive growth of facial and bodily hair.

Histamine – a substance released from cells responsible for many of the symptoms of an allergic reaction. The actions of this substance are blocked by medications referred to as anti-histamines.

HIV (Human Immunodeficiency Virus) – a virus that attacks the immune system, the causative agent of AIDS (acquired immune deficiency syndrome).

Hives – localized immune reactions that are itchy, red, raised spots composed of dilated blood vessels and localized tissue fluid (edema). Individual lesions come and go in less than 24 hours.

Holter monitor – a portable external monitor worn to record the heart rhythm for 24 to 48 hours.

Homocysteine – an amino acid produced in the body, high levels of which are associated with heart and other vascular diseases.

Hordeolum (stye) – a localized infection in the eyelid.

Hormone – a substance, made in one part of the body, which is carried in the bloodstream to another part of the body where it chemically affects the function of local tissues.

HPV – *See* Human papilloma virus.

Human Immunodeficiency Virus – *See* HIV.

Human papilloma virus (HPV) – a sexually transmitted virus that can infect the cervix and is responsible for changes that may lead to cervical cancer. Also causes genital warts.

Hypertension – a sustained elevation in blood pressure above the normal range. Classically defined as a blood pressure greater than 140 systolic or 90 diastolic.

Hyperthyroidism – when too much thyroid hormone is present, resulting from an irritated thyroid gland that is releasing previously stored hormone, a thyroid gland that is being excessively stimulated to manufacture and release extra hormone, or consumption of too much thyroid hormone in pill form. Symptoms of hyperthyroidism include tremor, sweating, fast heartbeat, diarrhea, anxiety, poor sleeping and concentration abilities, and weight loss. *See also* Hypothyroidism

Hypoglycemia – a syndrome that refers to a symptomatic lowering of the blood sugar.

Hypothalamus – a specialized portion of the brain that produces substances that regulate metabolic activities in the body.

Hypothyroidism – the under-production of thyroid hormone, characterized by fatigue, sluggishness, weight gain, hair loss, skin thickening, enlargement of the thyroid gland, constipation, and depression. *See also* Hyperthyroidism.

I

Immune system – the system of cells and chemicals in the body responsible for protecting the body from disease. The immune system is also involved in the allergy response, monitoring for and destroying early cancers, and diseases in which the immune system falsely identifies a component of the body's structure as foreign and attacks it, resulting in an "autoimmune disease" such as Rheumatoid Arthritis.

Immunotherapy – giving repeated injections of antigens under the skin. Over time, this decreases the allergy response through several changes in the immune system.

Impingement syndrome – the pinching of the tendons or bursa between bony structures of the shoulder.

Impotence – *See* Erectile dysfunction.

Incidence – the frequency that a disease occurs in a certain population over a set period of time.

Incontinence – an involuntary loss of urine.

Infection – the presence of another organism within the body that causes disease.

Inflammation – a tissue response to injury, often characterized by increased blood flow to the region, an increase in the amount of fluid, white blood cells, and connective tissue present between cells, and a red, warm appearance.

Inflammatory bowel disease – including ulcerative colitis and Crohn's disease, is a chronic, relapsing disorder characterized by inflammation of the wall of the intestine.

Influenza ("the flu") – a viral infection of the respiratory tract that occurs in epidemics in winter months, usually accompanied by headache, fever, chills, muscle aches, and coughing.

Insomnia – an inability to fall asleep or to remain asleep.

Insulin – a hormone produced by the pancreas that transfers glucose from the bloodstream into cells.

Intrinsic Factor – a carrier protein made in the stomach necessary for the absorption of vitamin B_{12}.

Irritable bowel syndrome – a functional bowel disorder characterized by crampy abdominal pain and associated with alternating painful episodes of diarrhea and constipation often accompanied by bloating.

Isoflavones – a group of estrogen-like chemicals, found in high concentration in some soy products.

J

Jaundice – a yellow discoloration of the skin, eyeballs, and mucus membranes produced by an increased level of bilirubin in the blood. Bilirubin is a waste product of red blood cells that is normally cleared by the liver; jaundice can be a sign of liver disease.

Joints – where two bones come together and may allow for movement.

K

Kegel exercises – exercises designed to strengthen the pelvic floor muscles to foster urine continence.

Ketoacidosis – an acid condition in the body created by disordered metabolism resulting from uncontrolled diabetes in susceptible patients or alcohol toxicity.

Ketones – a chemical product in the metabolism of fatty acids.

Ketosis – the accumulation of excessive ketones in the body, most frequently related to uncontrolled diabetes or alcohol toxicity.

L

Labyrinthitis – inflammation of the inner ear, often producing vertigo.

Lactic acid – a chemical byproduct of metabolism that can cause acidosis, which can suppress heart function, result in irregular heartbeat, and cause changes in brain or muscle function.

Laxative – a chemical substance that speeds passage of fecal contents through the bowel to treat or prevent constipation. Overuse of laxatives can lead to permanent damage the normal function of the bowel.

LDL cholesterol – the "bad" cholesterol, associated with detrimental effects on blood vessels. A protein that carries cholesterol to be deposited into the wall of arteries. *See also* cholesterol.

Leukotrienes – a potent class of chemicals in the body that are involved in the process of inflammation.

Ligaments – tough, fibrous bands that connect bones, holding them together.

Lipids – fats or fatlike substances, including cholesterol, fatty acids, and phospholipids.

Lithotripsy – a procedure using ultrasound shock waves to shatter stones in the urinary tract into smaller pieces that can be passed or removed more easily.

Lyme disease – a disease transmitted by infected ticks. It is sometimes associated with a characteristic "bulls-eye" skin lesion, flu-like symptoms, headache, and enlarged lymph nodes. Late effects of untreated disease include problems with the musculoskeletal system, brain, and heart.

M

Magnetic resonance angiography – *See* MRA.

Magnetic resonance imaging – *See* MRI.

Macula – the area of the retina capable of the most precise vision, located in the center of the visual field.

Macular degeneration – the breakdown of vision in the macula, resulting in the loss of high-definition vision such as that used for reading, driving, watching television, and recognizing faces.

Magnesium – an element important in the function of enzymes involved in energy production, regulation of body temperature, and muscular function. Magnesium is widely available from a variety of foodstuffs, deficiency is rare except in alcoholics.

Malaise – a generalized sensation of persistent fatigue.

Malaria – a parasite infection acquired in the tropics from the bite of a mosquito, characterized by chills, fever, fatigue, and anemia.

Mammogram – an x-ray technique to examine the breasts for structural abnormalities.

Managed Care – originally, a type of health insurance where access to health services are coordinated to maximize the efficient and effective use of health resources in a cost-conscious manner. In current practice, many managed care companies are turning to management paradigms of specific diseases, with emphasis on wellness, disease prevention, and standard pathways for chronic disease management.

Malignant – the opposite of benign, a growth that follows an aggressive course, tends to produce disease or death, and is cancerous.

Mast cells – specialized white blood cells that live in the tissues and participate in the allergic reaction by releasing certain chemical mediators of inflammation when they are stimulated.

Measles – a viral infection spread by respiratory secretions and characterized by initial nasal congestion, high fever, and fatigue followed by a rash on the trunk that spreads to the extremities.

Meniere's disease – a poorly understood but probably autoimmune disease characterized by dizziness, tinnitis, and hearing loss.

Meningitis – inflammation of the lining of the brain and spinal cord, often in response to an infection.

Menopause – formally defined as when ovulation has ceased and there has been a lack of menstruation for 12 months.

Metabolism – formally defined as the sum of all changes that occur in the body, including physical changes in substances and changes in energy forms. Commonly used to refer to the level of energy expenditure in the body, both at rest and with activity.

Microalbumin – a protein that can be measured in the urine. Abnormally high levels are a sensitive marker for early kidney disease in diabetics, and can be followed to monitor response to therapy.

Microvascular disease – atherosclerotic disease affecting tiny arteries and thus the structures that they supply: nerves, kidneys, eyes, heart, and brain.

Migraine headache – a recurrent headache with a repeating pattern of headache development and associated symptoms.

Mitral valve – a one-way heart valve between the left atrium and left ventricle.

Mitral valve prolapse (MVP) – a common (3 percent to 6 percent of the population) structural abnormality of the mitral valve related to how the valve closes between the two heart chambers during the normal heartbeat. Usually asymptomatic, MVP can be associated with chest pain or palpitations.

MMR – a combination measles, mumps, and rubella vaccine.

MRA (magnetic resonance angiography) – a technique that couples MRI with contrast material in the blood vessels to create three-dimensional images of the blood vessel structure.

MRI (magnetic resonance imaging) – a technique that uses magnetic fields and computer imaging to create three-dimensional reproductions of body regions. Unlike x-rays and CT scans, no radiation is involved in MRI.

Mucosa – a moist surface lining, such as the lining of the nose, which contains glands.

Mucus – the substance secreted by a mucosa to provide moisture and protection.

Multiple Sclerosis – a disease of unknown cause that affects the myelin of the central nerve system, thus reducing the speed and efficiency with which electrical signals can be conducted.

Mumps – a highly contagious viral infection characterized by fever, malaise, headache, and swollen salivary glands. Complications include inflammation and damage to the testicles in males infected after adolescence, meningitis, hearing loss, pancreatitis, and arthritis. The disease is largely prevented by childhood vaccination. .

MVP – *See* Mitral valve prolapse.

Myelin – the insulating covering of certain nerve cells.

Myocardial infarction (heart attack) – heart muscle damage due to interruption in its blood supply.

Myofascial pain syndrome – a group of disorders involving the central nervous system where pain is experienced in a specific region of skeletal muscles.

N

Narcotics – *See* Opioids.

Neurons – nerve cells.

Neuropathy – a disorder of the peripheral nerves leading to altered sensation or loss of motor control in the extremities.

Neurotransmitters – chemicals used to communicate between nerve cells.

Nonsteroidal anti-inflammatory medications – *See* NSAIDs.

Norepinephrine – a neurotransmitter in the brain associated with emotional disorders; also produced by the adrenal gland and related to muscular tone in the blood vessels.

Normal flora – bacteria that live within the body but do not cause disease. Typically present in the upper respiratory tract and gastrointestinal system, these organisms may help assist the body (vitamin production in the gut) or protect it from harmful organisms by taking up available space and nutrients.

Normal Pressure Hydrocephalus (NPH) – the accumulation of an excessive amount of cerebrospinal fluid within the ventricles within the center of the brain, accompanied by progressive dementia, giat difficultes, and incontinence.

NSAIDs – Nonsteroidal anti-inflammatory medications, like ibuprofen or naproxen, with chemical properties that relieve pain and inflammation.

O

Observational studies – experimental studies during which of group of people are observed, without active intervention, over time to understand how certain factors or attributes affect their health.

Omega-3 fatty acids – Oils that are healthier for the body, particularly in the processes of atherosclerosis and inflammation, found in high concentration in certain fish oils and olive and safflower oil.

Opioids (narcotics) – the most effective drugs for the treatment of severe acute pain and some types of cancer pain. Patients can develop a tolerance or physical addiction to these drugs over time. Side effects include sedation, nausea and vomiting, and constipation.

OPV – oral polio vaccine.

Osteoarthritis – a chronic disease of joints physically characterized by destruction of cartilage and disordered growth of new bone. Symptoms include joint pain and reduction in joint range of motion and function. Most common in weight-bearing joints (hips, knees, ankles, and feet), spine, and small bones of the hands, particularly the base of the thumbs.

Osteoblasts – bone cells that create new bone.

Osteoclasts – bone cells that chemically break down bone, developing crevices in existing bone so that it can be remodeled.

Osteopenia – low bone density, but not sufficiently low to be classified as osteoporosis (A bone density between −1.0 and −2.5 standard deviations below expected bone mass).

Osteoporosis – a bone density (the amount of bone per unit volume) that is more than 2.5 standard deviations below expected bone mass.

Otitis externa ("swimmer's ear") – an infection of the outer ear canal between the outer ear and the eardrum.

Otitis media – infection of the middle portion of the ear, frequently following a nasal, sinus infection, or other conditions that block the opening of the eustachian tube.

Oxidation – a chemical process involving the loss of electrons from an atom; creates damage to cell structures and is involved in the aging process.

P

Palpation – an examination technique where an organ or gland is felt to determine size and features, such as feeling for a lump in the breast.

Palpitation – an irregularity in the heartbeat perceived by the patient.

Pancreatitis – inflammation of the pancrease, often from blockage of the pancreatic drainage system by gallstones or the chemical effects of alcohol. Symptoms include severe upper abdominal pain, nausea, and vomiting.

Panic attack – an unprovoked surge of fear accompanied by physical or emotional symptoms.

Panic disorder – four or more panic attacks within four weeks.

Pap smear – a test obtained from a microscopic examination of cells obtained by brushing the cervix to look for cervical cancer or other precancerous abnormalities.

Parasympathetic nervous system – a part of the nervous system that is involved in the control of involuntary functions. Stimulation of parasympathetic nerves produces vasodilation (enlargement of blood vessels), decreased heart rate, an increase in gastrointestinal activity, constricted pupils, and an increase in saliva.

Parkinson's disease – a disease of the central nervous system resulting in the destruction of a certain population of neurons containing high concentrations of dopamine. Characterized by tremor, muscular weakness and stiffness, gait disturbance, and depression.

Peak flow meter – an airflow-measuring device used by asthmatics to monitor their airway function.

Pelvic inflammatory disease – a serious infection of the upper genital tract in women, involving the fallopian tubes, ovaries, and surrounding tissues.

Peptic ulcer disease – ulceration of the upper gastrointestinal tract.

Percussion – an examination technique in which the physician taps or thumps on the surface of the body, recognizing the sound qualities produced over different body structures.

Peripheral Vascular Disease (PVD) – disease that occurs in the blood vessels supplying blood to the body, typically in the legs.

Peristalsis – a series of coordinated contractions by circular muscles within the gastrointestinal tract to propel contents through it.

PET scan – positron emission tomography, a procedure that produces three-dimensional images of the body by measuring characteristics of their chemical structure.

pH – a measure of the acid content of a substance.

Photoaging – the process of affecting skin structure through chronic ultraviolet irradiation (that is, sustained sun exposure). Photoaging leads to thickened, pebbly, coarse skin with prominent wrinkles and irregular pigmentation, with eventual loss of skin thickness and other secondary changes.

Phytoestrogens – plant compounds that are converted to estrogens in the gastrointestinal tract. Common varieties include isoflavones (soybeans), lignans (flax seed), black cohosh, and red clover.

Pituitary gland – a small gland at the base of the brain that secretes hormones that regulate a variety of body processes, including growth, reproduction, and thyroid function.

Placebo – a pill or device that, usually unknown to the user, has no active ingredient or other effect on a physical process.

Placebo-controlled trials – studies where the effects of chemical substance are compared with the effects of a placebo, while all other variables remain the same. Usually the researchers and subjects do not know which subjects only receive the placebo until the end of the trial.

Plantar fasciitis – inflammation of the fibrous band that supports the arch of the foot.

Platelets – components of the blood that help form blood clots.

Pleurisy – pain produced from inflammation of the lining of the lung, often sharp in character, and worsened when the lung expands as in breathing or coughing.

PMS – *See* Premenstrual syndrome.

Pneumonia – a respiratory tract infection involving the air sacs (alveoli) of the lung, usually caused by viruses or bacteria.

Positron emission tomography – *See* PET scan.

Post-phlebitic syndrome – a collection of long-term signs and symptoms due to the damage to a vein caused by a previous blood clot. May include pain, edema, formation of varicose veins, and skin changes including discoloration and ulcer formation.

Potassium – a mineral element that is found in high concentration within cells. It is essential for the function of muscle and nerve tissues.

Premenstrual syndrome – a cluster of mood, behavioral, and physical symptoms that have a regular, cyclical relationship to the time preceding the menstrual period. Symptoms are present in most if not all cycles and end by the onset of menstruation.

Prevalence – at any one time, the frequency of a disease in a defined population.

Primary care provider – the health provider responsible for the basic or general health care of an individual, including the coordination of specialty care when required.

Progesterone – a hormone produced from the ovary after ovulation of an egg, and by the placenta, responsible for changes in the lining of the uterus during the second half of the menstrual cycle.

Prophylaxis – the use of a medication or vaccine before exposure to prevent a disease or side effect of another medication.

Prostaglandins – a large group of biologically active substances that have their effects in the local tissues in which they are produced. Prostaglandins affect blood flow, blood clot formation, and gastrointestinal and kidney function and are involved in the inflammatory process.

Prostate gland – a walnut-sized gland through which the urethra passes that sits at the base of the bladder. It provides additional fluid volume and nourishment for sperm.

Prostate-specific antigen (PSA) – a protein measurable in the bloodstream produced only by the prostate gland, used for the detection of prostate cancer and the monitoring of its therapy.

Prostatitis – inflammation of the prostate gland, usually related to infection.

PSA – *See* Prostate-specific antigen.

Psoriasis – a chronic skin disease that usually begins in young adults, characterized by inflamed, raised areas of skin with silvery scales commonly on the scalp, elbows, and knees.

Psoriatic arthritis – an inflammatory type of arthritis that occurs in 5 to 10 percent of patients with psoriasis, characterized by involvement of the spine and the joints of the hands and feet.

Pulmonary embolism – a blood clot that has traveled to the lungs.

Pulmonary function testing – a series of tests that measure air flow rates, lung volumes, and gas exchange abilities to assess lung structure and function.

Pulmonic valve – a one-way heart valve between the right ventricle and pulmonary artery (leading to the lungs).

PVD – *See* Peripheral vascular disease.

R

Radiation therapy – the therapeutic use of high doses of x-ray radiation focused on malignant tumors.

Receptors – the chemical structure in a cell or on its surface that is able to combine with a specific substance to lead to changes within the cell.

Relapse – a recurrence of a disease or symptoms after initial improvement or recovery.

Resistance – 1) A description of the body's ability to prevent invasion, growth, and damage from infectious organisms. 2) The ability of an infectious organism to acquire means to survive an antibiotic that may have been previously effective against it.

Restless leg syndrome – a neurological disorder characterized by an irresistible and disagreeable urge to move the legs, usually in the early nighttime hours.

Retina – a complex, multi-layered structure on the inside of the eyeball that collects visual images and transmits them as electrical signals along the optic nerve to the brain.

Rheumatoid arthritis – a type of arthritis in which the immune system attacks and destroys joint surfaces.

Risk factors – habits, traits, or conditions that increase the likelihood of a specific disease.

RNA – ribonucleic acid, a message copied from a portion of DNA that carries information for the production of proteins and enzymes within the cell. *See also DNA.*

Rosacea – an acne-like condition of the skin that usually begins in middle-aged adults. It is characterized by tiny bumps and pustules on the cheeks, chin, nose, and forehead, excessive flushing, and the development of tiny superficial blood vessels.

Rotator cuff – the four muscles that provide strength and flexibility to the shoulder.

Rubella – a viral infection spread by respiratory droplets, that is manifested by rash, enlarged lymph nodes, and mild flu-like symptoms. Infection of a pregnant woman can cause severe birth defects or loss of the fetus. This disease has been largely eliminated in the United States by vaccination.

S

Sciatica – irritation of the nerve roots that exit from the base of the spine, causing pain that radiates along the buttocks, outside and back of the leg, and outside of the foot.

Screening – the use of diagnostic testing to detect a disease or condition in a patient.

Sebaceous glands – larger structures in the skin that produce sebum, a lipid mixture important in maintaining hydration of the skin.

Seborrheic dermatitis – a chronic inflammatory disorder of the skin that appears as red and itchy areas with white, fine scales on a greasy base. It affects areas where sebaceous glands are most prominent—the scalp (dandruff), eyebrows and lashes, mustache and beard, forehead, ear canals, chest, and body folds.

Seizure – a sudden, abnormal electrical discharge from an area of the brain that spreads directly to other areas of the brain and may be associated with alterations in consciousness or body movement.

Sensitivity – refers to the ability of a test or procedure to detect a condition if it is present. A test with a sensitivity of 100 percent would detect all cases of a disease, while a test with a sensitivity of 50 percent would only detect half of them. *See also* Specificity.

Sepsis – a serious infection with the presence of bacteria in the bloodstream along with a series of biochemical and physical changes in the body having an adverse effect on blood pressure and organ function.

Serotonin – a neurotransmitter within the brain and a chemical present in the gastrointestinal tract and other locations. Disorders of serotonin are associated with diseases such as depression and irritable bowel syndrome.

Shingles – a common viral infection of the skin seen caused by the reactivation of the Varicella-zoster (chickenpox) virus. Shingles begins with exquisite skin sensitivity in a band-like region on one side of the body, followed by intense and tiny white blisters that appear in clusters on a reddened base.

Side effects – unintended effects of a therapeutic or diagnostic intervention. Side effects may be beneficial but are often detrimental to the patient.

Sigmoidoscopy – examination of the lower colon with a flexible fiberoptic scope. Performed in the physician's office, this examination requires minimal preparation and no sedation, but doesn't reach as far into the colon as the colonoscope.

Signs – objective evidence of a disease process in the body that can be seen, heard, measured, or felt. Examples include a fever, rash, or mass. *See also* symptoms.

Sinoatrial node – the natural pacemaker region of the heart.

Sinusitis – infection of the sinus cavities

> Acute sinusitis – less than 4 weeks in duration.

> Recurrent acute sinusitis – 4 or more episodes within 12 months, each lasting 7-10 days, with at least 8 weeks of no symptoms between infections.

> Subacute sinusitis – last between 4 and 12 weeks.

> Chronic infections – last longer than 12 weeks

Sleep apnea – a disorder in which there is repeated interruption of airflow into the lungs during sleep

Spasm – an involuntary, sustained, and often painful muscular contraction.

Specificity – refers to the ability of a test or procedure not to show evidence of a condition if it is not present. A test with a specificity of 100 percent would never show evidence of a disease if it weren't there. A test with a specificity of 50 percent would mean that half the time that the test was positive, the disease really wasn't there. *See* also Sensitivity.

Spirometry – a test involving forceful expiration into a measuring device to examine airflow through the lungs airways. Diseases that inflame or narrow the airways reduce airflow rates.

Staging – the process of determining how far a cancer has spread.

Statin drugs – cholesterol-lowering medications.

Stent – a small spring or tube placed in an artery after angioplasty to help hold it open.

Stress test – a test to exercise the heart muscle while monitoring for signs of heart disease

Treadmill stress test – the patient walks on a treadmill while the heart is monitored by EKG

Stress echocardiogram – before and after echocardiograms are added to look for changes in heart muscle motion.

Nuclear stress test (often with thallium) – x-ray images of regional blood flow are added to increase the sensitivity of the stress test

Chemical stress test – instead of a treadmill, intravenous medications are used to exercise the heart

Stroke – death of brain tissue caused by an interruption of blood flow to the brain. A hemorrhagic stroke is a particularly deadly form of stroke involving a weakened blood vessel that bursts and bleeds into the brain.

Stye – *See* Hordeolum.

Subdural hematoma – a collection of blood between the inside of the skull and brain.

Swimmer's ear – *See* Otitis externa.

Sympathetic nervous system – a part of the nervous system that is involved in the control of involuntary functions. Stimulation of sympathetic nerves produces vasoconstriction (narrowing of blood vessels), increased heart rate, slowing of gastrointestinal activity, and dilated pupils.

Symptoms – any perceptible change in the body, subjective or objective, that may indicate evidence of a disease. *See also* Signs.

Syncope – a sudden but reversible loss of consciousness related to a shutdown of the parts of the brain required for conscious activity.

Syndrome – a disease identified by a recurring collection of signs and symptoms rather than by a known cause.

Synovial capsule – the lining that surrounds a joint and encompasses the joint space, secreting synovial fluid to nourish and lubricate the joint surfaces.

Systolic blood pressure – the peak blood pressure that occurs in the arteries when the left ventricle contracts. *See also* Diastolic blood pressure.

Systolic hypertension – an upper blood pressure (systolic) measurement of greater than or equal to 140.

T

T-suppressor cells – specialized cells that help regulate the allergy immune response.

Temporal arteritis – a disorder of the immune system where the temporal artery and associated medium-sized blood vessels are attacked and destroyed. Usually causes headache and tenderness in the temples, fatigue, and pain with chewing and can progress to blindness.

Tendons – tough, fibrous bands that hold connect muscle to bone.

Testosterone – male sexual hormone that is responsible for the development of the male reproductive system, as well as secondary characteristics of men such as body hair distribution, muscle development, voice, and behavior.

Tetanus – a disease that is acquired from contaminated wounds, characterized by painful and sustained muscle spasms.

Therapeutic range – a range of concentration of a substance that is felt to offer a net benefit to the patient. Lower levels offer little measurable benefit; higher levels lead to excessive toxicity.

Therapeutic trial – the experimental use of a medication to see if a benefit is noted in regards to the disease being treated.

Thrombolytics – drugs that dissolve blood clots.

Thrombophlebitis – a blood clot in a vein accompanied by inflammation.

Thyroid gland – a butterfly-shaped gland located over the windpipe in the front of the neck that produces, stores, and releases thyroid hormone.

Thyroid releasing hormone (TRH) – a hormone from the hypothalamus that controls production of TSH.

Thyroid stimulating hormone (TSH) – a hormone from the pituitary that stimulates thyroid hormone production and release.

Tinea Versicolor – a superficial skin disease that usually affects the trunk and central portions of the extremities. It is caused by a superficial yeast infection and characterized by circular areas of altered skin pigmentation.

Tinnitus – the perception of sound in the ears or head (typically ringing or hissing), when no external sound is present, related to damage of, or irritation to, the hearing nerve.

Tolerance – a chemical adjustment in the body to a drug, often resulting in a shorter duration of action and an overall decrease in the effectiveness of the drug. Can also refer to a decreased perception to the side effects of a drug that occurs over time.

Toxicity – unwanted, harmful side effects from a drug or therapy.

Trachea – the upper airway or windpipe, before it divides into the bronchi.

TRH – *See* Thyroid releasing hormone.

Tricuspid valve – a one-way heart valve between the right atrium and right ventricle

Tricyclic antidepressants – a group of older antidepressant medications that are no longer used as first-line therapy for treatment of depression due to their side effects and the availability of more effective drugs. These medications are currently used to manage chronic pain, sleep disturbance, bladder dysfunction, and as an add-on therapy to enhance the effects of other drugs.

Trigeminal neuralgia – paroxysmal attacks of intense, one-sided facial pain along the trigeminal nerve.

Triglycerides – constitutes a large portion of the lipids in the bloodstream, ingested in food or manufactured by the liver. Associated with vascular disease.

TSH – *See* Thyroid stimulating hormone.

Tympanic membrane – the eardrum.

Typhoid fever – a bacterial infection spread by contaminated food or water, characterized by fever, often higher than 103 degrees Fahrenheit, weakness, headache, stomach pain, and loss of appetite.

U

Ulcer – a breakdown in the surface lining of the body, most commonly the skin, gastrointestinal tract, urogenital tract, or cornea.

Ulcerative colitis – an inflammatory bowel disease primarily affecting the colon.

Ultrasound – a diagnostic technique using sound waves and their reflections from different structures to examine internal components of the body.

Ureters – the tubes transporting urine from the kidneys to the bladder.

Urethra – a tube that drains urine from the bladder for elimination.

Urethritis – an infection of the urethra.

V

Vaccinations – shots or pills that prime the immune system to respond faster if exposed to certain infectious agents in the future.

Vaginitis, atrophic – thinning and drying of the vaginal lining related to a lack of estrogen support.

Valvular regurgitation – when a heart valve does not close properly, which allows blood to leak backward through it when the heart contracts.

Valvular stenosis – when a heart valve does not open completely, which makes it harder for the blood to flow through it.

Varicella virus – a virus in the Herpes family responsible for chicken pox and shingles.

Varicose veins – dilated superficial veins.

Vascular dementia – cognitive dysfunction related to a series of tiny strokes that had occurred in the brains, often seen in patients with hypertension.

Vasculitis – a process of inflammation and destruction of blood vessels, often related to attack by the immune system.

Vasoconstrictors – chemicals that cause the smooth muscle in arteries to contract, decreasing the size of arteries and restricting blood flow.

Vasodilator – chemicals that cause the smooth muscle in arteries to relax, increasing the size of arteries and improving blood flow.

Vasovagal reflex – a reflex involving the vagus nerve that dilates the blood vessels in the gut while simultaneously slowing the heart rate, leading to a drop in blood pressure and possible loss of consciousness.

Vein – a blood vessel that carries blood back to the heart, typically thin walled.

Ventricles – the second, larger and more powerful chambers on each side of the heart that pump blood throughout the lungs or body.

Vertebra – the bones of the spine.

Vertigo – an illusion of movement when the body is in fact still.

Virus – a tiny infectious agent made up of an outer protein core surrounding genetic material. Because they must use the cellular machinery of their host to reproduce, viruses can grow and multiply only within living cells.

Yeast (fungus) – a parasitic plant that typically causes infections of body surfaces, but can also cause invasive disease when the body is not functioning properly.

Resource List

Items are listed for informational purposes only; inclusion does not imply endorsement by *Health Basics* or Dr. Richardson

Chapter 1   Physical Fitness

www.aaos.org   *American Academy of Orthopedic Surgeons*
The "Prevent Injuries America" section has excellent advice on exercise safety tips and injury prevention.

www.aapmr.org   *American Academy of Physical Medicine and Rehabilitation*
Access the "Consumers/Public" tab for information on the rehabilitation of spine and brain injuries, including general overviews, diagnostic testing, and treatment options.

www.acefitness.org   *American Council of Exercise*
A nonprofit organization committed to promoting active, healthy lifestyles. Check out the "Ace Fit Facts" section for a wealth of information about fitness and exercise techniques.

www.fitness.gov   *The President's Council on Physical Fitness and Sports*
Site provides access to download multiple resources about exercise fundamentals, fitness guides, and motivational literature for designing and maintaining a fitness program for yourself or others.

www.hoptechno.com/book11.htm   *Fitness Fundamentals*
Developed by the President's Council on Physical Fitness and Sports, this is a good resource for someone just getting started in a fitness program.

Chapter 2   Common Sense Nutrition

www.eatright.org   *American Dietetic Association*
The "Healthy Lifestyle" tab provides access to nutrition tips, fact sheets, an updated reading list for in depth books about a variety of topics, including special interests such as vegetarian diets, food sensitivities, and nutrition in common medical conditions such as diabetes.

www.nal.usda.gov/fnic/etext/fnic.html **U.S. Department of Agriculture Site**
Website of the Food and Nutrition Information Center, with extensive information on food composition, dietary guidelines, and specialty topics.

www.governmentguide.com
Click on "Health and Safety", then select "Health Topics", then select "Nutrition and Dieting" for a wealth of information on nutrition, dietary supplements, and weight loss. A very thorough site with up to date information.

www.olen.com/food/index.html **Fast Food Facts – Interactive Food Finder**
Calorie and nutritional information for your favorite fast food restaurant selections.

Chapter 3   Obesity and Weight Loss
www.weightwatchers.com **Official site of Weight Watchers**
If you're serious about long-term healthy eating, check out this site for information about Weight Watchers, and general information on foods, recipes, healthy lifestyles and fitness.

www.obesity.org **American Obesity Association**
A comprehensive site on obesity as a chronic illness, addressing education, patient advocacy, research, prevention, and treatment topics. Very professional and thorough in it's approach to understanding obesity and its management.

Chapter 4   Allergies
www.aaaai.org **American Academy of Allergy, Asthma, and Immunology**
Check out the "Patients and Consumers" tab to access reliable information about allergic conditions and treatment options.

www.niaid.nih.gov **National Institute of Allergy and Infectious Disease**
National Institute of Health site with a good search engine to research specific diseases, treatment options, and up-to-date information about research results and how to participate in ongoing clinical trials.

www.aafa.org **Asthma and Allergy Foundation of America**
Asthma and allergy educational information, patient advocacy, and research links.

Chapter 5   Infections and Antibiotics
www.cdc.gov/ncidod/diseases/index.htm **Centers for Disease Control**
Site with detailed information about individual infectious diseases and other topics in infection management.

www.nfid.org **National Foundation for Infectious Diseases**
Sponsored by a non-profit organization to support education, research, and training about infectious diseases. "Factsheets" provide good informational summaries about topics in infectious disease, although some are more geared toward health care providers than the general public.

Chapter 6   Pain

www.sepaincare.com   *Southeast PainCare*
Provides general information about acute and chronic pain, pain management strategies, specific conditions and alternative medicine approaches. Portions of the site remain under construction at time of publication.

www.pain.com
General information about pain management. Includes pain assessment tools and a useful section on what to expect after common surgical procedures.

www.aapainmanage.org   *American Academy of Pain Management*
General information on pain management. Provides links to other websites for associations and other general informational resources on pain. Directory for finding a local pain management program.

Chapter 7   Smoking

www.lungusa.org/tobacco   *American Lung Association*
Smoking cessation information and resources.

www.cancer.org   *American Cancer Society*
Enter the website, type "tobacco" in the search box, and select "Tobacco and Cancer" for several resources on tobacco health issues and tobacco cessation.

www.hhs.gov   *Department of Health and Human Services*
Select "Agencies" for descriptions and links to each of the HHS agencies, including the Administration on Aging, Agency for Healthcare Research and Quality, the Food and Drug Administration, and the Centers for Disease Control and Prevention

www.surgeongeneral.gov/library/reports.htm   *Office of the Surgeon General*
A list of the reports published by the U.S. Surgeon General, including smoking and health.

Chapter 8   Alcohol

www.alcoholics-anonymous.org   *Alcoholics Anonymous*
A wealth of information about alcohol abuse, support for alcoholics and those around them, and the Alcoholics Anonymous approach to alcohol addiction treatment.

www.niaaa.nih.gov   *National Institute on Alcohol Abuse and Alcoholism*
Comprehensive site for information about alcohol abuse including clinical research trials for addiction management.

www.nmha.org/substance/factsheet.cfm   *National Mental Health Association*
General information about alcohol abuse and related disorders.

Chapter 9   Cancer

www.cancernet.nci.nih.gov   *National Cancer Institute*
Excellent site covering information on cancer types and treatment, prevention, genetics, and causes, screening and testing, support and resources available to patients and their caregivers.

<u>*www.cancer.org*</u>   ***American Cancer Society***

The website of the American Cancer Society, offering information about cancer, treatment options, and coping as well as easy access to cancer statistics and support programs.

<u>*www.peoplelivingwithcancer.org*</u>   ***American Society of Clinical Oncology***

Another excellent site providing disease specific information by cancer type, as well as a comprehensive overview of cancer prevention, detection, and treatment as well as an extensive database of cancer specialists and clinical trials.

<u>www.astro.org</u> American Society for Therapeutic Radiology and Oncology

The "Patient Information: section provides a useful guide to radiation therapy.

Chapter 10   Travel Health

<u>*www.cdc.gov*</u>   ***Centers for Disease Control***

Click on the "Travelers' Health" tab on the opening page for access to travel health information organized by destination or disease. An excellent source for vaccination information, travel safety trips, and up-to-date information about regional disease outbreaks.

<u>*www.travel.state.gov*</u>   ***US State Department***

Under "Services", click on the "Travel warnings/Consular Info Sheets" tab for up-to-date information by country about health conditions, political issues, currency and entry regulations, crime and security. Includes warnings of an particular threats to the security of American travelers .

Chapter 11   Vaccinations and Associated Diseases

<u>*www.cdc.gov/nip/*</u>   ***Centers for Disease Control***

The CDC's National Immunization Program's Website. Information on recommended vaccination schedules and individual vaccine information statements.

Chapter 12   Herbals, Vitamins, and other "Nutritional Supplements"

<u>*www.consumerlab.com*</u>

This site provides comprehensive information on herbals, vitamins and minerals, and other supplements. Provides a list of commercial products that are "approved" based on Consumer Lab's testing of quality, label accuracy (for ingredients), freedom from contaminants, and consistency. Includes the "Natural Products Encyclopedia" that provides detailed, science-based information on hundreds of nutritional supplements, and provides drug interaction information.

<u>*www.cfsan.fda.gov/~lrd/advice.html#dietary*</u>   ***Food and Drug Administration***

Site provides general information about the regulation of dietary supplements and safety issues in regards to their use.

<u>*www.nal.usda.gov/fnic/etext/000015.html*</u>   ***U.S. Department of Agriculture***

Food and Nutritional information center site providing scientific information on various herbs, vitamins, and mineral supplements as well as a database of published literature regarding their use. No nonsense information about the possible benefits and risks of nutritional supplements.

Chapter 13   Health Assessment

www.labtestsonline.org   *Lab Tests Online*
A non-commercial site providing in depth information on laboratory testing. The most useful aspect of this site is a library of tests that provides detailed information on why a test might be ordered and how to interpret its results.

www.nlm.nih.gov/medlineplus/healthtopics.html   *National Library of Medicine*
Excellent resource for in depth information on a comprehensive list of health topics, organized alphabetically or by body system, procedures, demographic group, or general health and wellness groups.

www.aafp.org   *American Society of Family Physicians*
Click on the "Periodic Health Exam" tab under the "Clinical Care and Research" section for an expert discussion on current recommendations for medical testing in health assessment.

www.ahrq.gov   *Agency for Health Care Policy and Research*
A site with an emphasis on medical services with proven validity. Topics include evidence-based medicine, technology assessment, and guidelines for clinical practice.

www.preventdisease.com
General information on wellness and a variety of health topics, including screening tools to calculate your personal risks for cancer and other diseases.National Library of Medicine

Chapter 14   How to Get What You Want From Your Doctor

www.ama-assn.org   *American Medical Association*
The "Patients" section provides access to health information, as well as a description of the training of physicians and a review of the principles of medical ethics.

Chapter 15   The Skin

www.nih.gov/niams   *National Institute of Arthritis and Musculoskeletal and Skin Diseases*
Comprehensive patient information about skin diseases. Click on "Health Information", then choose a topic from the alphabetical list.

www.aad.org   *American Academy of Dermatology*
Excellent informational sections on acne, actinic keratoses, aging skin, eczema, melanoma, and psoriasis. Physician locator available through the website.

www.psoriasis.org   *National Psoriasis Foundation*
Psoriasis specific information and support.

www.asds-net.org   *American Society for Dermatologic Surgery*
Excellent fact sheets on dermatologic surgery procedures, complete with before and after photographs, as well as articles on cosmetic skin techniques and surgeries.

Chapter 16   The Eye

www.nei.nih.gov   *National Eye Institute*

The Health Information section provides comprehensive information about common eye conditions.

www.glaucoma.org   *Glaucoma Research Foundation*

Glaucoma specific information and support.

www.ascrs.org *American Society of Cataract and Refractive Surgery*

Comprehensive information about expectations, benefits, costs, and the technology behind surgical techniques to improve vision.

Chapter 17   The Ear

www.nidcd.nih.gov   *National Institute on Deafness and other Communication Disorders*

Basic and advanced information on hearing, balance, speech, and language.

www.entnet.org   *American Academy of Otolaryngology & Head & Neck Surgery*

Click on the Health Information section for detailed information about the ear and conditions that affect it.

www.ata.org   *American Tinnitis Association*

A good source of general information about protecting healthy hearing, and a thorough reference for the understanding of tinnitis and its management.

Chapter 18   The Nose and Sinuses

www.entnet.org   *American Academy of Otolaryngology & Head & Neck Surgery*

Click on the Health Information section for detailed information about the nose and sinuses and conditions that affect them.

Chapter 19   The Throat

www.ada.org   *American Dental Association*

Click on "Oral health topics" for information on diseases and conditions of the mouth.

www.entnet.org   *American Academy of Otolaryngology & Head & Neck Surgery*

Click on the Health Information section for detailed information about the throat and conditions that affect it.

Chapter 20   Glandular and Metabolic Diseases

www.diabetes.org   *American Diabetes Association site*

General information on diabetes, connections to community groups and info

www.niddk.nih.gov   *National Institute of Diabetes & Digestive & Kidney Diseases*

Click on "Diabetes" under the "Health Information" heading for comprehensive information on diabetes topics and research.

www.irondisorders.org   *Iron Disorders Institute*

Specialized information on hemachromatosis and other diseases of iron metabolism.

www.the-thyroid-society.org   *The Thyroid Society*

Specialized information on the thyroid gland, diseases that affect it, and principles of treatment.

www.thyroid.org   *American Thyroid Association*

Click on "For Patients" for concise and informative information sheets on the thyroid gland, diseases that affect it, and principles of treatment.

www.nof.org   *National Osteoporosis Foundation*

Specialized information on osteoporosis, its prevention, diagnosis, and treatment.

www.hormone.org   *The Hormone Foundation*

Site contains information about various topics in endocrinology, including diabetes, growth, menopause, obesity, osteoporosis, pituitary hormones and thyroid as well as valuable links to other sources of information.

Chapter 21   The Heart and Cardiovascular System

www.americanheart.org   *American Heart AssociationSite contains excellent* resources on diseases and conditions affecting the cardiovascular system, articles promoting a healthy lifestyle, and a neat "Heart and Stroke Encyclopedia" with links to detailed articles for an extraordinary complete list of topics.

www.nhlbi.nih.gov   *National Heart, Lung, and Blood Institute*

Provides detailed health information of cardiovascular topics, clinical guidelines for accepted treatment protocols, and referrals to clinical studies currently seeking patients.

www.scvir.org   *Society of Cardiovascular & Interventional Radiology*

Click on the "Patients and Public" tab to access up-to-date information about procedures trained physicians perform by guiding narrow tubes (catheters) through blood vessels to various sites in the body to treat medical problems – including aneurysms, clogged vessels, uterine fibroid tumors, infertility, cancers, and stroke.

www.sts.org   *Society of Thoracic Surgeons*

The Patient Information section contains valuable information about cardiothoracic surgical procedures, including techniques and discussions on what to expect after surgery.

Chapter 22   The Respiratory System

www.nhlbi.nih.gov   *National Heart, Lung, and Blood Institute*

Click on "Health Information", then under "For Patients and the General Public – Lung Diseases" for in depth information about common and uncommon lung diseases. Disease specific brochures can be ordered or reviewed online.

www.chestnet.org   *American College of Chest Physicians*

Click on "Clinical Information" on the sidebar, then "Patient Education Guides" for simple, easy to understand articles on asthma, COPD, cough, lung transplantation, and procedures used to evaluate lung disease.

www.lungusa.org   *American Lung Association*

The most comprehensive site on lung topics, this web site is thorough and easy to navigate. An excellent resource for school and other educational projects.

Chapter 23   The Gastrointestinal System

www.niddk.nih.gov   *National Institute of Diabetes & Digestive & Kidney Diseases*

Click on "Digestive" under the "Health Information" heading for comprehensive information on gastrointestinal topics and research.

www.fascrs.org   *American Society of Colon and Rectal Surgeons*

Click on "Patient Information" for easy to understand brochures on diseases that affect the colon along with a description of diagnostic and therapeutic procedures.

www.ccfa.org   *Crohn's and Colitis Foundation of America*

Specialized information on inflammatory bowel disease, including information on clinical trials and finding a doctor.

www.gastro.org   *American Gastroenterology Association*

Click on the "Public Section" for access to detailed information about gastroenterological diseases and procedures. This site includes a series of video presentations in the multimedia library.

Chapter 24   The Urinary System

www.niddk.nih.gov   *National Institute of Diabetes & Digestive & Kidney Diseases*

Click on "Kidney" or "Urologic" tabs under the "Health Information" heading for comprehensive information on topics and research regarding the urinary system.

www.prostatehealth.com   *The Prostate Health Council*

Information on prostate conditions, symptoms, diagnosis and treatment. Through, easy to negotiate site with understandable text, useful graphics and videos, and a self-assessment area for prostate disease.

www.afud.org   *American Foundation for Urologic Disease*

The site of a nonprofit organization providing general information about urinary tract disorders, research updates, and access to clinical trials.

www.ichelp.org   *Interstitial Cystitis Association*

Disease specific information on Interstitial Cystitis, with useful information on disability issues and support groups.

www.ashastd.org   *American Social Health Association*

A comprehensive site about sexually transmitted diseases, including access to hotlines for instant assistance with questions about STDs.

www.nafc.org   *National Association for Continence*

Click on "About Incontinence" for a review of incontinence and its treatment.

Chapter 25   The Musculoskeletal System

www.rheumatology.org   *American College of Rheumatology*

Click on the "Patient Information" tab on the sidebar for access to Fact Sheets covering topics in rheumatology and common joint procedures.

www.nih.gov/niams   *National Institute of Arthritis and Musculoskeletal and Skin Diseases*

Click on "Health Information" for a complete information on a variety of topics about the musculoskeletal system and diseases that affect it.

www.aaos.org   *American Academy of Orthopedic Surgeons*

Checkout the Patient/Public information tab for access to joint specific fact sheets and brochures on common orthopedic conditions. Information is concise, well written, and very practical.

www.arthritis.org   *Arthritis Foundation*

An excellent general source for information on arthritis and related diseases. The "Surgery Center" describes surgical procedures in detail, and has on-line animations of common procedures. The "Pain Center" section is an excellent source reviewing pain management through lifestyle changes, medications, and surgery as well as alternative therapies. Online purchase of books and videos is available. Site facilitates referrals to local programs

www.apma.org   *American Podiatric Medical Association*

Provides detailed information about foot and ankle conditions and treatments.

www.aofas.org   *American Orthopedic Foot and Ankle Society*

Another excellent site on foot and ankle health, with a practical section on proper footwear.

www.lupus.org   *Lupus Foundation of America*

Well-organized site with specialized information about Lupus and patient support resources.

Chapter 26   Women's Health

www.asrm.org   *American Society for Reproductive Medicine*

Comprehensive site about infertility and treatment options.

www.menopause.org   *North American Menopause Society*

Click on the "Consumers" icon for comprehensive information about the health issues surrounding menopause. A bit technical in some sections, but informative.

www.4woman.gov   *National Women's Health Information Center*

An up-to-date site on all issues affecting women's health, with access to detailed and reader friendly information. Site includes "hot topics" and a weekly newsletter. Click on "Frequently Asked Questions" to reach the topic index.

Chapter 27   Men's Health Issues

Try Keyword "Men's Health" on your internet service for well organized sites.

www.menshealthnetwork.org Men's Health Network
Provides links to information on health and social issues important to men.

Be cautious in Internet sites about Men's Health. Most of the sites that I reviewed did not provide access to reliable, scientifically based information.

Chapter 28   The Neurological System
www.ninds.nih.gov   National Institute of Neurological Disorders and Stroke
Click on "Browse all disorders" to access the index, a very complete site with listings of clinical trials looking for patients.

www.aans.org   American Association of Neurological Surgeons
Click on "Health Resources" then "Patient Resources" to access detailed information about neurological issues, with an emphasis on the neurosurgical techniques used to address them.

www.biausa.org   Brain Injury Association
Excellent information and support resources for brain injury patients and their families.

www.epilepsyfoundation.org   The Epilepsy Foundation
Click on "Answerplace" for detailed information on seizure disorders, their treatment, and associated lifestyle issues.

www.sleepfoundation.org   National Sleep Foundation
Specialized information and links about sleep disorders. Articles are thorough and easy to read.

www.ifmss.org.uk   International Federation of Multiple Sclerosis Societies
Specialized information and support for Multiple Sclerosis patients and their families.

www.stroke.org   National Stroke Association
Specialized information and videos about stroke and related topics.

www.parkinson.org   National Parkinson's Foundation, Inc.
Specialized information and resources about Parkinson's disease.

www.alzheimers.org   Alzheimer's Disease Education and Referral Center
                      (ADEAR) 1-800-438-4380
Information about Alzheimer's disease.

www.alz.org   Alzheimer's Association   1-800-272-3900
Information about disease therapies and ongoing studies for Alzheimer's disease.

www.nmss.org   National Multiple Sclerosis Society
Information about disease therapies and ongoing studies for Multiple Sclerosis, as well as assistance in finding a local chapter.

The following sites provide useful information and resources on aging:
www.americangeriatrics.org American Geriatrics Society
www.nih.gov/nia   National Institute on Aging
www.aoa.dhhs.gov   U.S. Administration on Aging

Chapter 29   Mental Health

www.nmha.org   *National Mental Health Association*
Mental health information, including screening tools, prevention, and substance abuse.

www.nimh.nih.gov   *National Institute of Mental Health*
Comprehensive site for information on Mental Health issues, including summaries of "breaking news" and links to clinical trials.

www.anad.org *National Association of Anorexia Nervosa and Related Disorders*
Specialized information of eating disorders.

www.adaa.org *Anxiety Disorders Association of America*

General resources

www.medlineplus.gov *National Library of Medicine*
Extraordinarily comprehensive site on medical conditions, diseases, and wellness, a medical encyclopedia, drug information, physician and hospital directories, and links to other useful resources.

www.aafp.org   *American Society of Family Physicians*
Health Topics, a 506-item index on medical issues, provides access to general information on specific health topics in easy to read and understand terms. Enter the main website, click on the "Patients" tab, and then select "Health Topics".

Other reliable sites for comprehensive information:

www.clevelandclinic.org   *Cleveland Clinic*
www.cpmcnet.columbia.edu   *Columbia-Presbyterian Medical Center*
www.mayoclinic.com   *Mayo Clinic*
www.hopkinsmedicine.org/healthinformation   *John Hopkins University*
www.cdc.gov/niosh   *National Institute for Occupational Safety and Health*
www.webmd.com   *A comprehensive health resource.*
www.merck.com   *Merck Manual*

Index

E

O

P

USE THIS FORM IF THIS BOOK IS NOT AVAILABLE AT YOUR LOCAL BOOKSTORE

Order Form

SHIP TO: _____

YOUR NAME: _____

NAME OF ORGANIZATION: _____

STREET ADDRESS: _____

CITY: _____ STATE: _____ ZIP: _____

TELEPHONE: _____

Please send the following:

_____ copies of *Health Basics* at $22.95 per book

Shipping charges: $5.00 for first book, $1.00 for each additional book.

A check for $_____ is enclosed.

Credit Card payments: ☐ Visa **VISA**   ☐ MasterCard MasterCard

Credit Card # _____ Expiration Date: _____

Name on Card: _____

Signature: _____

Orders must be prepaid unless using an official purchase order.

Mail to:

Next Decade, Inc.
39 Old Farmstead Road
Chester, NJ 07930
TELEPHONE (908) 879-6625 • FAX (908) 879-2920
EMAIL: info@nextdecade.com